Richard Sharpe. August. 1996.

Serono Symposia USA
Norwell, Massachusetts

Springer

New York
Berlin
Heidelberg
Barcelona
Budapest
Hong Kong
London
Milan
Paris
Santa Clara
Singapore
Tokyo

PROCEEDINGS IN THE SERONO SYMPOSIA USA SERIES

Continued after Index

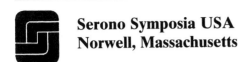

Serono Symposia USA
Norwell, Massachusetts

Claude Desjardins
Editor

Cellular and Molecular Regulation of Testicular Cells

With 107 Figures

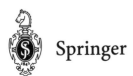

Springer

Claude Desjardins, Ph.D.
Department of Physiology
University of Virginia
School of Medicine
Charlottesville, VA 22908
USA

Proceedings of the XIIIth Testis Workshop on Cellular and Molecular Regulation of Testicular Cells sponsored by Serono Symposia USA, Inc., held March 30 to April 1, 1995, in Raleigh, North Carolina.

For information on previous volumes, please contact Serono Symposia USA, Inc.

Library of Congress Cataloging-in-Publication Data
Cellular and molecular regulation of testicular cells/Claude
    Desjardins, editor.
        p.   cm.
    "Proceedings of the XIIIth Testis Workshop on Cellular and
Molecular Regulation of Testicular Cells, sponsored by Serono
Symposia USA, Inc., held March 30–April 1, 1995, in Raleigh, North
Carolina"—T.p. verso.
    Includes bibliographical references and index.
    ISBN 0-387-94648-9 (hardcover: alk. paper)
    1. Testis—Physiology—Congresses.   2. Testis—Molecular aspects—
Congresses.   3. Spermatogenesis—Congresses.   4. Testis—Cytology—
Congresses.   I. Desjardins, Claude, 1938–   .   II. Serono
Symposia, USA.   III. Testis Workshop on Cellular and Molecular
Regulation of Testicular Cells (1995: Raleigh, N.C.)
    [DNLM: 1. Testis—cytology—congresses.   2. Spermatogenesis—
physiology—congresses.   3. Germ Cells—physiology—congresses.
4. Leydig Cells—cytology—congresses.   5. Steroids—biosynthesis—
congresses.   WJ 830 C394   1996]
QP255.C457   1996
612.6'1—dc20   95-46670

Printed on acid-free paper.

Production coordinated by Chernow Editorial Services, Inc., and managed by Francine McNeill; manufacturing supervised by Joe Quatela.
Typeset by Best-set Typesetter Ltd., Hong Kong.
Printed and bound by Braun-Brumfield, Inc., Ann Arbor, MI.

Printed in the United States of America.

9 8 7 6 5 4 3 2 1

ISBN 0-387-94648-9 Springer-Verlag New York Berlin Heidelberg   SPIN 10524836

XIIIth TESTIS WORKSHOP ON CELLULAR AND MOLECULAR REGULATION OF TESTICULAR CELLS

Scientific Committee

Claude Desjardins, Ph.D., Chairman
University of Virginia

Andrzej Bartke, Ph.D.
Southern Illinois University

William J. Bremner, M.D., Ph.D.
University of Washington

Glenn R. Cunningham, M.D.
Baylor College of Medicine

Maria L. Dufau, M.D., Ph.D.
National Institutes of Health

Michael D. Griswold, Ph.D.
Washington State University

Mary Ann Handel, Ph.D.
University of Tennessee

Diana G. Myles, Ph.D.
University of Connecticut

Deborah A. O'Brien, Ph.D.
University of North Carolina

Marie-Claire Orgebin-Crist, Ph.D.
Vanderbilt University

Barry R. Zirkin, Ph.D.
Johns Hopkins University

Organizing Secretary

Leslie Nies
Serono Symposia USA, Inc.
100 Longwater Circle
Norwell, Massachusetts

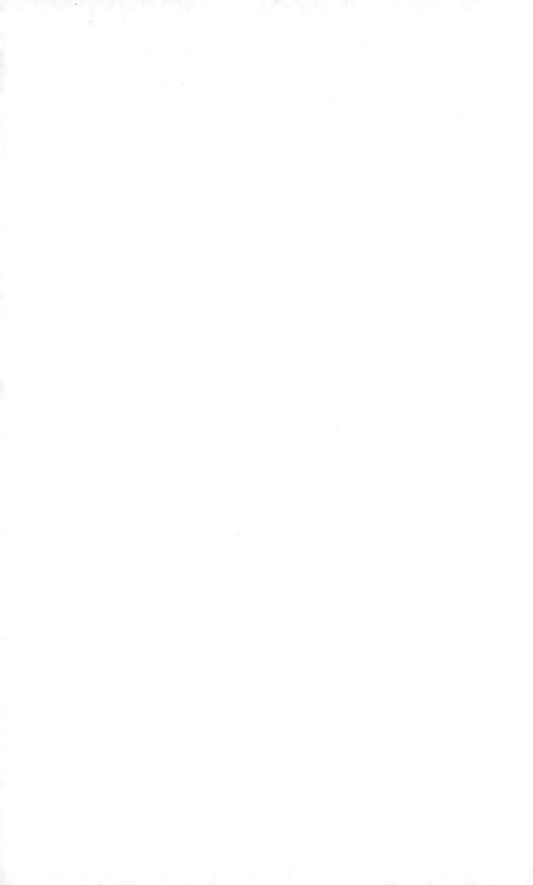

Preface

Conceptual advances in the biological sciences are marked by the application of new techniques and experimental strategies. Nowhere has this generic principle been more apparent than in the study of testicular cells, as judged by the evolution of themes presented at the Testis Workshop over the past 23 years. Like its predecessors, the 1995 Testis Workshop was structured to offer fresh insights and approaches for understanding the mechanisms of spermatogenesis and steroidogenesis. The chapters presented in this book emphasize three aspects of testicular cell function: first, the molecular analysis of the cell cycle; second, examination of the cell cycle, including the function and identification of specific macromolecules that direct the proliferation and differentiation of germ cells; and third, the development of Leydig cells and the role of specific macromolecules in the formation of testicular steroids.

Each chapter is based on a lecture presented at the XIIIth Testis Workshop held on March 30 to April 1, 1995, at the Radisson Plaza Hotel in Raleigh, North Carolina. The selection of topics reflects the recommendations of the workshop's organizing committee. Sincere thanks are due to the speakers who agreed to lecture and prepare chapters. This book also represents the summed efforts of the many individuals who supported the 1995 Testis Workshop, the participants who took part in the scientific sessions, the investigators whose work was presented in more than 150 posters, and the Council of the American Society of Andrology, which made it possible to convene the 1995 workshop prior to the society's annual meeting. The cooperation between the Local Arrangement Committees for the society and the Testis Workshop was achieved through the efforts of their representatives, Dr. Sally Perreault Darney and Dr. Deborah O'Brien, respectively.

Financial support for the 1995 workshop was provided by Serono Symposia USA, Inc., under the leadership of Leslie Nies. Symposia's support included the skillful coordination of all conference arrangements and the expertise of the publications staff in the production of the program abstract book and this volume of proceedings.

Special thanks go to colleagues Ellen Barber, Meredith Beam, and Susan Hobbs at the University of Virginia who handled correspondence with many of the participants and supplied imaginative energy throughout the planning of the workshop.

CLAUDE DESJARDINS

Contents

Part III. Macromolecules and Organelles Unique to Germ Cells

Part IV. Hormone Action and Transport Mechanisms

Contributors

DONARA ABRAMIAN, La Jolla Cancer Research Foundation, Cancer Research Center, La Jolla, California, USA.

KARIN M. AKMAL, Department of Genetics and Cell Biology, Washington State University, Pullman, Washington, USA.

CRISTINA ALBANESI, Department of Public Health and Cellular Biology, University of Rome "Tor Vergata," Rome, Italy.

HAKIMA AMRI, Department of Cell Biology, Georgetown University Medical Center, Washington, D.C., USA.

JOHN G. BARTELL, Department of Chemistry and Biochemistry, University of South Carolina, Columbia, South Carolina, USA.

ROBERT M. BELL, Department of Molecular Cancer Biology, Duke University Medical Center, Durham, North Carolina, USA.

NOUREDDINE BOUJRAD, Department of Cell Biology, Georgetown University Medical Center, Washington, D.C., USA.

WILLIAM J. BREMNER, Department of Medicine, Medical Service (III), Department of Veterans Affairs Medical Center, Seattle, Washington, USA.

A. SHANE BROWN, Department of Cell Biology, Georgetown University Medical Center, Washington, D.C., USA.

SHARON E. CLARE, Department of Chemistry and Biochemistry, University of South Carolina, Columbia, South Carolina, USA.

BARBARA J. CLARK, Department of Cell Biology and Biochemistry, Texas Tech University Health Sciences Center, Lubbock, Texas, USA.

Jacqui Clegg, Glaxo Research and Development Limited, Ware, Hertfordshire, UK.

Claude Desjardins, Department of Physiology, University of Virginia, Charlottesville, Virginia, USA.

Michael J. Dewey, Department of Biological Sciences, University of South Carolina, Columbia, South Carolina, USA.

Susanna Dolci, Department of Public Health and Cellular Biology, University of Rome "Tor Vergata," Rome, Italy.

Hui-Bao Gao, Center for Biomedical Research, The Population Council, New York, New York, USA.

Martine Garnier, Department of Cell Biology, Georgetown University Medical Center, Washington, D.C., USA.

Raffaele Geremia, Department of Public Health and Cellular Biology, University of Rome "Tor Vergata," Rome, Italy.

Marco Giorgio, Regina Elena Cancer Institute, Rome, Italy.

Erwin Goldberg, Department of Biochemistry, Molecular Biology and Cell Biology, Northwestern University, Evanston, Illinois, USA.

Kenneth M. Grigor, Department of Pathology, University of Edinburgh, Edinburgh, UK.

Paola Grimaldi, Department of Public Health and Cellular Biology, University of Rome "Tor Vergata," Rome, Italy.

Matthew P. Hardy, Center for Biomedical Research, The Population Council, New York, New York, USA.

Wendy R. Hatfield, Department of Chemistry and Biochemistry, University of South Carolina, Columbia, South Carolina, USA.

Marie-Claude Hofmann, La Jolla Cancer Research Foundation, Cancer Research Center, La Jolla, California, USA.

Yayoi Ikeda, Department of Medicine, Duke University Medical Center, Durham, North Carolina, USA.

Diane S. Keeney, Department of Biochemistry, Vanderbilt University School of Medicine, Nashville, Tennessee, USA.

KWAN HEE KIM, Department of Genetics and Cell Biology, Department of Biochemistry and Biophysics, Washington State University, Pullman, Washington, USA.

MALATHI K. KISTLER, Department of Chemistry and Biochemistry, University of South Carolina, Columbia, South Carolina, USA.

W. STEPHEN KISTLER, Department of Chemistry and Biochemistry, University of South Carolina, Columbia, South Carolina, USA.

SHINJI KOSUGI, Department of Laboratory Medicine, Kyoto University School of Medicine, Kyoto, Japan.

DONG LIN, Department of Pediatrics, University of California, San Francisco, California, USA.

XUNRONG LUO, Department of Biochemistry, Duke University Medical Center, Durham, North Carolina, USA.

SIMON MADDOCKS, Department of Animal Science, Waite Agricultural Research Institute, Glen Osmond, South Australia.

GREGOR MAJDIC, Medical Research Council (MRC) Reproductive Biology Unit, Edinburgh, UK.

KAREN H. MARTIN, Department of Molecular Cancer Biology, Duke University Medical Center, Durham, North Carolina, USA.

TANYA T. MCLAREN, Medical Research Council (MRC) Reproductive Biology Unit, Edinburgh, UK.

MICHAEL MENDENHALL, Department of Biochemistry and Markey Cancer Center, Chandler Medical Center, University of Kentucky, Lexington, Kentucky, USA.

JOSÉ LUIS MILLÁN, La Jolla Cancer Research Foundation, Cancer Research Center, La Jolla, California, USA.

MICHAEL R. MILLAR, Medical Research Council (MRC) Reproductive Biology Unit, Edinburgh, UK.

WALTER L. MILLER, Department of Pediatrics, University of California, San Francisco, California, USA.

PETER B. MOENS, Department of Biology, York University, Downsview, Ontario, Canada.

CARLOS R. MORALES, Department of Anatomy and Cell Biology, McGill University, Montreal, Quebec, Canada.

NEAL A. MUSTO, Department of Cell Biology, Georgetown Medical Center, Washington, D.C., USA.

DEBORAH A. O'BRIEN, The Laboratories for Reproductive Biology, Departments of Pediatrics and Cell Biology and Anatomy, University of North Carolina, Chapel Hill; and Gamete Biology Section, National Institute of Environmental Health Sciences, National Institutes of Health, Research Triangle Park, North Carolina, USA.

STEPHEN O. OGWUEGBU, Department of Cell Biology, Georgetown University Medical Center, Washington, D.C., USA.

BANKOLE O. OKE, Department of Cell Biology, Georgetown Medical Center, Washington, D.C., USA.

RICHARD J. OKO, Department of Anatomy and Cell Biology, Queen's University, Kingston, Ontario, Canada.

DAVID E. ONG, Department of Biochemistry, Vanderbilt University, Nashville, Tennessee, USA.

JESSICA H. OOSTERHUIS, Department of Medical Biochemistry, University of Calgary, Calgary, Alberta, Canada.

VASSILIOS PAPADOPOULOS, Department of Cell Biology, Georgetown University Medical Center, Washington, D.C., USA.

KEITH L. PARKER, Departments of Medicine and Pharmacology, Duke University Medical Center, Durham, North Carolina, USA.

DOMENICA PISCITELLI, Department of Public Health and Cellular Biology, University of Rome "Tor Vergata," Rome, Italy.

LAURA POZZI, Regina Elena Cancer Institute, Rome, Italy.

GAIL PRINS, Department of Obstetrics/Gynecology, Michael Reese Hospital and Medical Center, Chicago, Illinois, USA.

LAURA L. RICHARDSON, La Jolla Cancer Research Foundation, Cancer Research Center, La Jolla, California, USA.

PELLEGRINO ROSSI, Department of Public Health and Cellular Biology, University of Rome "Tor Vergata," Rome, Italy.

KOUROSH SALEHI-ASHTIANI, Department of Biochemistry, Molecular Biology and Cell Biology, Northwestern University, Evanston, Illinois, USA.

PHILIPPA T.K. SAUNDERS, Medical Research Council (MRC) Reproductive Biology Unit, Edinburgh, UK.

LI-XIN SHAN, Center for Biomedical Research, The Population Council, New York, New York, USA.

RICHARD M. SHARPE, Medical Research Council (MRC) Reproductive Biology Unit, Edinburgh, UK.

ANDREW SHENKER, Pediatric Endocrine Division, Department of Pediatrics, Northwestern University and Children's Memorial Hospital, Chicago, IL, USA.

EDWARD A. SHIPWASH, Department of Chemistry and Biochemistry, University of South Carolina, Columbia, South Carolina, USA.

VINCENZO SORRENTINO, San Raffaele Scientific Institute, Milan, Italy.

DOUGLAS M. STOCCO, Department of Cell Biology and Biochemistry, Texas Tech University Health Sciences Center, Lubbock, Texas, USA.

JEROME F. STRAUSS III, Department of Obstetrics/Gynecology, University of Pennsylvania, Philadelphia, Pennsylvania, USA.

JAY C. STRUM, Department of Molecular Cancer Biology, Duke University Medical Center, Durham, North Carolina, USA.

CARLOS A. SUAREZ-QUIAN, Department of Cell Biology, Georgetown Medical Center, Washington, D.C., USA.

TERUO SUGAWARA, Department of Obstetrics/Gynecology, University of Pennsylvania, Philadelphia, Pennsylvania, USA.

KATHERINE I. SWENSON, Department of Molecular Cancer Biology, Duke University Medical Center, Durham, North Carolina, USA.

JAMES K. TSURUTA, The Laboratories for Reproductive Biology, Department of Pediatrics, University of North Carolina, Chapel Hill, North Carolina, USA.

J. ERIC TURNER, Department of Molecular Cancer Biology, Duke University Medical Center, Durham, North Carolina, USA.

FRANS A. VAN DER HOORN, Department of Medical Biochemistry, University of Calgary, Calgary, Alberta, Canada.

BRANISLAV VIDIC, Department of Cell Biology, Georgetown University Medical Center, Washington, D.C., USA.

WILLIAM VORNBERGER, Department of Cell Biology, Georgetown Medical Center, Washington, D.C., USA.

MICHAEL R. WATERMAN, Department of Biochemistry, Vanderbilt University School of Medicine, Nashville, Tennessee, USA.

HELGE WEISSIG, La Jolla Cancer Research Foundation, Cancer Research Center, La Jolla, California, USA.

SAI XIAO, Department of Cell Biology, Georgetown Medical Center, Washington, D.C., USA.

1

Evolution of the Testis Workshop: 1972–1995

Claude Desjardins

The Testis Workshop promotes the presentation and exchange of ideas at the frontiers of research in male reproductive biology. Since its start in 1972, the workshop has flourished under a loose confederation of investigator-initiated meetings. The scientific program has evolved from a fledgling agenda involving a few participants into an internationally respected conference attracting scientists from diverse backgrounds who share a common interest in understanding the function of cells in the testis and epididymis.

This chapter documents the evolution of the Testis Workshop from 1972 to 1995. Attention is focused first on scientific interest in reproductive biology and the move to develop a special workshop devoted to male reproduction. Emphasis then shifts to the role played by Mortimer Lipsett in convening the first Testis Workshop and the organizational legacy he provided for the workshop's future. Lastly, consideration is given to the changes that have taken place in the workshop's scientific program. All three aspects of this historical overview underscore the workshop's broad mission to serve as a forum for the best new science in male reproduction without regard to disciplinary boundaries.

Banding Together

The quarter century between 1950 and 1975 brought many changes to research in reproductive biology. Federal funding for investigative work in reproduction increased steadily along with the number of investigators interested in pursuing research on the topic, the number of interested scientists increasing more or less in proportion to fiscal support. Scientists sought to gain both critique and recognition of their work in the scientific community coincident with increases in their investigative effort. Professional scientific societies responded by scheduling sessions at their annual

1

meetings for investigators whose work came to focus on topics such as ovulation, spermatogenesis, and fertilization. Diverse organizations, such as the American Association of Anatomists, the American Fertility Society (now the American Society of Reproductive Medicine), the American Society of Animal Science, and the Endocrine Society, provided investigators with an outlet to present their work.

Specialized meetings devoted entirely to reproduction were organized as early as 1944 in the United Kingdom (1) and provided the impetus to form the Society for the Study of Fertility in 1960 (1). A parallel interest in forming scientific groups focused on reproduction emerged in the United States but lagged behind those in England. Investigators interested in fundamental aspects of the reproductive process in domestic animals banded together in 1953 for the purpose of holding special conferences devoted exclusively to reproduction (2, 3). These meetings were initiated by R. Melampy of Iowa State University and were not sponsored by any particular group until they came to be affiliated with the American Society of Animal Science in 1962 (1). The Society for the Study of Reproduction was formed in 1967 through the organizational efforts of Philip Dziuk of the University of Illinois (4). This new society attracted the attention of investigators from all branches of the animal sciences, biology, and medicine by providing a common meeting ground for the presentation and discussion of scientific advances on all aspects of reproduction.

Interest in promoting the scientific study of male reproduction prompted Warren O. Nelson, then medical director of the Population Council, and Charles P. LeBlond, then chair of the Department of Anatomy at McGill University, to form a club (5). The group first met in 1968 in conjunction with the annual meeting of the American Association of Anatomists. Proposals to transform the club into a formal society were made in the early 1970s, and steps were taken to organize the American Society of Andrology during the VIIIth World Congress on Fertility and Sterility in Buenos Aires in 1974 through the efforts of Emil Steinberger, then of the University of Texas Medical School at Houston (5).

The increasingly specialized analysis of reproductive cell function prompted scientists to form alliances with peers investigating similar processes outside of the reproductive system. Scientific programs with specialized agendas expanded the opportunity to focus on specific mechanisms in all types of cells, including those of reproduction. Focused scientific meetings such as those sponsored by the Gordon Conference, starting in the 1920s, facilitated examination of the most advanced aspects of a field of interest. Such conferences avoided the distractions of a large scientific meeting while promoting intense discussion and analysis of the most novel and important aspects of topical issues.

The enthusiasm that surfaced for thematic conferences instantly appealed to scientists engaged in understanding the unique aspects of cell function in the testis. Once initiated in 1972, the Testis Workshop was

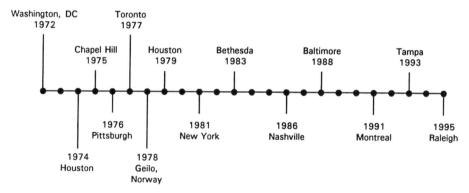

FIGURE 1.1. Time line denoting the year and location of the past meetings of the Testis Workshop. Annual workshops were held between 1974 and 1979 and then changed to biannual conferences. Gaps in the biannual schedule were occasioned by the availability of funds and the need to arrange an alternating schedule for the Testis Workshop and the European Testis Workshop.

scheduled as an annual event (Fig. 1.1), and two of the six meetings between 1974 and 1979 were held outside of the United States, evidence of the depth and breadth of interest in special topics of new and unusual interest to the field of male reproduction. Workshop organizers rapidly recognized the difficulty of generating novel and significant information about testicular cells each year and elected to reduce the frequency of workshops to biannual conferences following the 1979 meeting in Houston (Fig. 1.1).

Diversification and specialization of the workshop's scientific program were ensured by adopting a format relying on investigator-initiated meetings, each convened by a different coordinator. The range of scientific interest of past coordinators (Table 1.1) has allowed the Testis Workshop to serve the needs of scientists interested in mechanistic aspects of cell function in the testis, epididymis, and spermatozoa. Enthusiasm for the workshop's scientific programs has been sustained because organizing committees have placed a premium on inviting the best-possible speakers at the frontiers of topics relevant to male reproduction. The opportunity to interact with an audience of peer investigators and to gain attention for one's work attracts scientists who would not otherwise attend the meeting of a professional scientific society catering to broader aspects of reproductive science.

Mortimer Lipsett's Influence and Legacy

The first and second meetings of the Testis Workshop were held in 1972 and 1974 (Fig. 1.1). Mortimer Lipsett was Chief of the Reproductive Research Branch at the National Institutes of Child Health and Human Development and Associate Scientific Director for Intramural Research within the institute (Fig. 1.2). Lipsett realized the merit of focusing investigative attention on specific aspects of cell function in the testis and recognized that experts from all disciplines were needed to offer penetrating insights on such poorly understood processes, including spermatogenesis (6). The first Testis Workshop, held on Saturday, June 17, 1972, at the Shoreham Hotel in Washington D.C., immediately preceded the IVth International Congress of Endocrinology at the same location and facilitated the assembly of expert speakers. The temporal link between the first workshop and the international congress triggered the interest and attention of investigators from all parts of the world. The interface with the International Congress of Endocrinology was facilitated no doubt by Lipsett's role as the Secretary General of the International Society of Endocrinology. The preponderance of topics related to endocrine issues in the initial programs for the Testis Workshop presumably stemmed from the early involvement of workshop coordinators with the discipline of endocrinology.

Dr. Lipsett's formal involvement with the Testis Workshop ended with his move to Cleveland, Ohio, to direct the Cancer Center for Northeast Ohio in 1974 (Fig. 1.2). Leadership for the Testis Workshop remained centered at the *National Institutes of Health* (NIH) through the efforts of Lipsett's former colleagues, including Dr. Kevin Catt, Dr. Maria Dufau, Dr. Dolores Patanelli, and Dr. Richard Sherins. NIH scientists were assisted by extramural investigators such as Dr. C. Wayne Bardin, Dr. Frank French, Dr. Irving Fritz, and Dr. Anthony Means in planning and arranging the

TABLE 1.1. Coordinators, institutional affiliation, and support for the Testis Workshop.

Year[a]	Coordinator	Institutional affiliation	Primary support	Reference to published proceedings[c]
1972	M. Lipsett	NIH-NICHD[b]	NIH	—
1974	A. Means	Baylor College of Medicine	NIH	6
1975	F. French	University of North Carolina	NIH	7
1976	P. Troen	University of Pittsburgh	NIH	8
1977	I. Fritz	University of Toronto	NIH	—
1978	V. Hanson	Rikshospitalet–Oslo Karolinska Institute–Stockholm	NIH	9
1979	E. Steinberger	Unviersity of Texas Medical School at Houston	NIH	10
1981	C. Bardin	The Population Council	NIH	11
1983	K. Catt	NIH-NICHD[b]	NIH	12
1986	M. Orgebin-Crist	Vanderbilt University	NIH	13
1988	L. Ewing	Johns Hopkins University	NIH	14
1991	B. Robaire	McGill University	Corporate & NIH	15
1993	A. Bartke	American Society of Andrology	Serono & NIH	16
1995	C. Desjardins	American Society of Andrology	Serono	17

[a] Workshops held in 1979, 1991, 1993, and 1995 preceded the Annual Meeting of the American Society of Andrology.
[b] National Institutes of Health—National Institute of Child Health and Human Development.
[c] Proceedings of the 1972 and 1977 Testis Workshops were not published.

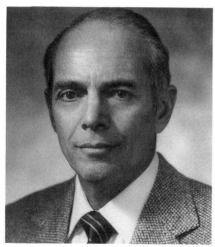

Mortimer B. Lipsett, 1921-1986

•	1943 AB	University of California - Berkeley
•	1951 MD	University of Southern California
•	1951-1952	Intern, Los Angeles County Hospital
•	1952-1954	Resident, Sautelle Hospital/ Veterans Administration, Los Angeles
•	1954- 1956	NIH Fellow, Sloan-Kettering Institute
•	1959-1966	Asst Chief, Endocrinology Branch, NCI/NIH
•	1966-1970	Chief, Endocrinology Branch, NCI/NIH
•	1970-1974	Associate Scientific Director, Intramural Research, NICHD/NIH
•	1974-1976	Director, The Cancer Center for Northeast Ohio, Cleveland
•	1976-1982	Director, The Clinical Center, NIH
•	1982-1985	Director, NICHD/NIH
•	1985-1986	Director, NIDDK/NIH

FIGURE 1.2. Mortimer B. Lipsett, circa 1984. Lipsett was a physician, scientist, educator, and public servant who provided the leadership to organize the first meeting of the Testis Workshop and played a role in facilitating early meetings. NIH, National Institutes of Health; NCI, National Cancer Institute; NICHD, National Institute of Child Health and Human Development; NIDDK, National Institute of Diabetes, Digestive, and Kidney Diseases.

early workshops. Starting with the 1974 workshop (Table 1.1), the imaginative energy needed to develop the program and gain funding for the workshop shifted to the workshop's organizing committee listed in each of the workshops' published proceedings (7–18). While the role played by Mort Lipsett in launching the Testis Workshop may seem modest from the standpoint of the brief summary presented here, it cannot be doubted that his intellectual energy, stature in the international biomedical research community, and leadership within the NIH produced a legacy that has allowed the workshop to enter its third decade. The workshop's mission remains unchanged—it is dedicated to providing the research community with a forum to present and discuss important new findings at the forefront of scientific advances made in the field of male reproduction.

Evolution of the Scientific Program and Support for the Testis Workshop

A survey of the titles of the published proceedings of past workshops (7–18) illustrates the diversity of topics explored in previous programs. Initial workshops emphasized the rapid progress made in identifying specific receptors for peptide hormones that act on cells of the testis. Clinical advances made in diagnosing and treating disorders of the testis and related tissues were topics featured at another early workshop. In the 1980s, workshop programs reflected the advances made in understanding the involvement of growth factors, cytokines, and other signaling molecules that direct specific cellular events within cells of the testis and epididymis. Although the thematic focus of the workshop has shifted with the evolution of knowledge, the program has continued to reflect the organizing committees' effort to feature the most-significant scientific developments and attract the best speakers.

Primary support for the Testis Workshop relied on funds from the NIH to defray the travel costs for speakers and to permit the organizing committees to meet and plan a workshop. Full support for the workshop was available from NIH through 1988 (Table 1.1). In 1991 the workshop was supported by multiple gifts from corporate groups and a modest award from NIH. Serono Symposia USA provided full support for the conference in 1993 and 1995 and has arranged for the publication of workshop proceedings (Table 1.1).

Planning for the next workshop program continues through the efforts of an organizing committee that is committed to the tradition of identifying important new issues at the frontier of knowledge of cells that participate in the events of male reproduction. As the Testis Workshop enters the 1990s it brings an unparalleled past together with a tradition to maintain a bold, compelling vision for the future.

Acknowledgments. The following individuals supplied information for this chapter: Dr. C. Bardin, Dr. C. Doberska, Dr. M. Dufau, Dr. P. Dziuk, Dr. F. French, Dr. I. Fritz, Dr. V. Hansson, Dr. M.-C. Orgebin-Crist, Dr. D. Patanelli, Dr. B. Robaire, Dr. F. Rommerts, Dr. R. Sherins, and Dr. E. Steinberger. Responsibility for any errors of fact or interpretation rests with the author and not with any of the individuals who contributed information for the chapter. At the University of Virginia, Ellen Barber, Meredith Beam, and Susan Hobbs provided assistance with the production of illustrations and the preparation of the manuscript.

References

1. Parks AS. The society for the study of fertility 1950–71. J Reprod Fertil 1971;25:315–27.
2. Hansel W, Dutt RH. Preface to environmental influences on reproductive processes. J Animal Sci (Suppl) 1966;25:2.
3. Amann RP, Cole HH. Preface to the symposium on male reproduction. Biol Reprod 1969; (Suppl).
4. Dziuk P. The society for the study of reproduction: 25 years in retrospect. Biol Reprod 1993;48:28.

5. Steinberger E. Presidential address. Andrologia (Suppl 1) 1976;8:11–15.
6. Lipsett MB. Foreward. In: Dufau ML, Means AR, eds. Hormone binding and target cell activation in the testis. New York: Plenum Press, 1974.
7. Hormone binding and target cell activation in the testis. In: Dufau ML, Means AR, eds. Current topics in molecular endocrinology, vol. 1. New York: Plenum Press, 1974.
8. Hormonal regulation of spermatogenesis. In: French FS, Hansson V, Ritzen EM, Nayfeh SN, eds. Current topics in molecular endocrinology, vol. 2. New York: Plenum Press, 1975.
9. Troen P, Nankin H, eds. The testis in normal and infertile men. New York: Raven Press, 1976.
10. Hansson V, Ritzen EM, Purvis K, French FS, eds. Endocrine approach to male contraception. Int J Androl 1978;2 (suppl 1).
11. Steinberger A, Steinberger E, eds. Testicular development, structure, and function. New York: Raven Press, 1980.
12. Bardin CW, Sherins RJ, eds. The cell biology of the testis. Ann NY Acad Sci 1982;383.
13. Catt KJ, Dufau ML, eds. Hormone action and testicular function. Ann NY Acad Sci 1984;438.
14. Orgebin-Crist M-C, Danzo BD, eds. Cell biology of the testis and epididymis. Ann NY Acad Sci 1987;513.
15. Ewing LL, Robaire B, eds. Regulation of testicular function: signaling molecules and cell-cell communication. Ann NY Acad Sci 1989;564.
16. Robaire B, ed. The male germ cell: spermatogonium to fertilization. Ann NY Acad Sci 1991;637.
17. Bartke A, ed. Function of somatic cells in the testis. New York: Springer-Verlag, 1994.
18. Desjardins C, ed. Cellular and molecular biology of testicular cells. New York: Springer-Verlag, 1996.

Part I

Molecular Dissection of the Cell Cycle

2

From Start to S Phase: Early Events in the Yeast Cell Cycle

MICHAEL MENDENHALL

The major events of eukaryotic cell division are coordinated by a highly conserved set of genes that center on the cyclins and the *cyclin-dependent protein kinases* (CDKs). Due to their central role in diverse processes that include signal transduction, transcription, DNA replication, DNA repair, apoptosis, differentiation, and carcinogenesis (1), the factors influencing the activity of the CDKs have come under intense scrutiny since their discovery. Not surprisingly, the regulation of the CDKs is complex. The levels of the cyclin activators of the CDKs are determined by periodic changes in transcription rates (2) and protein stability (3). Both stimulatory and inhibitory phosphorylations of the CDK catalytic subunit under the control of multiple protein kinases and phosphatases have been described (3). The subcellular localization of the CDK/cyclin complexes is also under strict controls (4–7).

In the last two years, an additional regulatory mode has been uncovered by the discovery of specific inhibitors of the CDKs, the CKIs (8–13). The CKIs are a diverse class of proteins, and although some families are now becoming apparent (14–16), many of them share very little, if any, sequence homology with others in this group. In the short time since their discovery, they have been shown to have critical roles in responses to growth factors (14, 17, 18) and DNA-damaging agents (10, 19, 20), to have tumor-suppressor properties (21–23), and to be involved in the establishment or maintenance of the differentiated state (24–26). Due to these many functions, the CKIs and their regulators are expected to be future targets for disease therapies. Additional knowledge of the means by which the CKIs are regulated is essential for the understanding of diverse cellular functions and how these functions are disrupted in the disease state. The process of dissecting these controls has proceeded most effectively when both biochemical and genetic approaches can be applied. For this reason, the budding yeast *Saccharomyces cerevisiae*, in which both of these approaches can be efficiently utilized, has been a valuable model system for studying eukaryotic cell division cycles. The structures and functions of most of the fundamental cell cycle regulators are highly conserved throughout eukaryotic evolution, so results obtained through studies of yeast cell division have been and are expected to continue to be useful predictors of mammalian processes. The yeast system has also been useful for the isolation and study of mammalian genes involved in cell cycle control.

This chapter reviews the regulatory events of the G1 phase/S phase transition in budding yeast with a focus on the function and regulation of Sic1, a CDK inhibitor that is involved in determining the timing of S-phase initiation and the fidelity with which DNA is segregated at mitosis.

The Yeast Cell Cycle

Like most eukaryotic cells, yeast cells have defined intervals for DNA replication (S phase) and chromosome segregation (M phase) separated by regulatory phases (G1 between M and S and G2 between S and M). The late G1 to early S phase interval has been especially heavily studied in budding yeast. This interval contains Start, a key decision step during which the cell commits to the mitotic cell cycle (27). After Start, other yeast "lifestyles," such as mating, G0 arrest, and meiosis/sporulation are unavailable until mitosis is completed. Start is considered to be similar to the mammalian restriction point.

Cdc28/Cyclin Complexes

Passage through Start is controlled by the activity of Cdc28 (27), one of four CDKs possessed by S. cerevisiae (28–30). The Cdc28 protein kinase is active throughout most, if not all, of the yeast cell cycle, although the level, location, and nature of the activity change in a periodic fashion (31–33). The Cdc28 protein levels do not change (31). Mutants with conditionally lethal alleles of cdc28 generally arrest at Start, indicating the relative importance of this transition with respect to Cdc28 function (34–36).

The first yeast cyclin genes, CLN1 and CLN2, were isolated as high copy suppressors of a cdc28^{ts} allele (37). That is, when present in greater than normal amounts, the CLN genes would allow the cdc28^{ts} mutant to grow at temperatures at which it normally would not. The two genes had similar sequences, and a mutant strain lacking both genes was severely defective in passage through Start, although it did retain viability. A third cyclin gene, CLN3, was discovered independently, as a mutation that conferred resistance to G1 arrest by the mating pheromone (38, 39). CLN3 is only distantly related to CLN1 and CLN2 in sequence, but a triple deletion of all three CLN genes resulted in a permanent cdc28^{ts}-like arrest in G1 (40), indicating that these genes share a common essential function. All three gene products bind and activate the Cdc28 protein kinase (32).

Additional cyclin activators of Cdc28 (CLB1 through CLB6) that were more closely related to the metazoan B cyclins were isolated by high copy suppression of a unique allele of *cdc28* that arrested in G2 (41), by high copy suppression of the triple Δ*cln1*-Δ*cln2*-Δ*Dcln3* deletion (42), and by degenerate *polymerase chain reaction* (PCR) (43, 44). These genes seem to come in pairs with the members of each pair sharing greatest sequence homology to each other and having similar transcriptional patterns and functions. The transcription of *CLB1* and *CLB2* peaks at mitosis, *CLB3* and *CLB4* peak somewhat earlier, at the S/G2 boundary, and *CLB5* and *CLB6* have a transcriptional pattern that parallels *CLN1* and *CLN2* with a peak at Start (45). Yeast strains carrying deletions of each of the *CLN* and *CLB* genes have been constructed, both singly and in almost every conceivable combination (45, 46). Defects ranging from inconsequential to fairly modest are found for most of the single deletions, while multiple deletion phenotypes range from negligible to inviable. The simple conclusion is that individual cyclins have specific functions, but that there is a great deal of overlap in the functions that cyclins can carry out in unusual conditions (such as when another cyclin gene is deleted). Dissecting out the specific functions has required a careful analysis that involves examining the timing of individual cyclin activities coupled with appropriate mutant constructions.

Cyclins and the Initiation of S Phase

An example of this sort of analysis is seen in studies of the cyclin requirement for S phase initiation. Five cyclin genes are transcribed at the G1/S boundary: *CLN1*, *CLN2*, *CLN3*, *CLB5*, and *CLB6* (32, 45). A triple deletion of the three *CLN* genes is lethal; the cells arrest at Start prior to S-phase entry (40). The greatest effect of a deletion of *CLB5*, *CLB6*, or both *CLB5* and *CLB6* is merely to delay S-phase initiation (45). These results appear to indicate that the *CLN* genes are required for S-phase initiation and that the *CLB* genes have a modest accessory role. This appearance is deceiving, however, since the S-phase delay seen in the Δ*clb5*-Δ*clb6* mutant provides time for the *CLB3* and *CLB4* genes to be transcribed. To assess the role of *CLB* gene function, a strain lacking all *CLB* genes had to be constructed (47). This strain failed to enter S-phase, but the arrested cells entered S phase synchronously when a short pulse of *CLB5* expression was provided. Apparently, any *CLB* gene will allow S-phase entry, but normally only *CLB5* and *CLB6* are expressed at the appropriate time for this function.

The current view of the function of the *CLN* gene products is that their role in S-phase initiation is indirect. Their primary function in DNA replication is to help remove an inhibitor of Clb/Cdc28 complexes called Sic1. The remainder of this chapter focuses on studies of this inhibitor.

Inhibitors of CDC28/Cyclin Complexes

The first CDK/cyclin inhibitor, Far1, was originally identified genetically as a mutation that failed to arrest cell division when cells were treated with the mating pheromone (48). Cell cycle arrest is an essential step in the process by which haploid yeast conjugates to form diploids (fungal fertilization). Chaos would result if nuclei in different phases of the cell cycle fused during karyogamy. Yeast prevents this problem by exchanging signals through peptide pheromones that cause the partner to arrest at Start (49). Cell fusion follows cell cycle arrest, so the subsequent nuclear fusion will occur between G1 nuclei. The pheromones initiate a protein kinase cascade that ultimately activates Far1 (17, 50), allowing it to inhibit Cln/cdc28 but not Clb/Cdc28 complexes (51). This differential activity is important because it allows cells that have already initiated a mitotic cycle when exposed to the mating pheromone to complete that cycle before arresting division.

The second CDK/cyclin inhibitor, Sic1, was identified biochemically as a protein that could bind to and be phosphorylated by immunoprecipitated Cdc28 complexes (52). The protein was purified (8) and shown to be an inhibitor of Cdc28/Clb, but not Cdc28/Cln complexes (47), a pattern complementary to that of Far1. These results fit neatly with observations concerning the timing of Cdc28/cyclin complexes in the period around Start. Using a Cln2 protein tagged with a hemagglutinin epitope (Cln2-HA), Schwob et al. (47) showed that the protein kinase activity associated with Cln2 rose in parallel with the transcription of the *CLN2* gene in synchronized cells. When the experiment was repeated with a similarly tagged Clb5 protein, however, the appearance of Cdc28/Clb5 protein kinase activity lagged appreciably behind that of the *CLB5 messenger RNA* (mRNA). The lag was quickly shown to be due to the presence of an inhibitory factor that was present in extracts from G1 cells but not in cell extracts taken from other phases of the cell cycle. The pattern of activity matched what was known for Sic1 (31). That Sic1 was the cause of the lag in Clb5/Cdc28 activity was demonstrated by repeating the cell synchrony experiments in a strain lacking *SIC1*. The lag was completely absent and the cells entered S phase prematurely (47). These results indicated that Sic1 had a role in the timing of S-phase initiation, a role consistent with many of the phenotypic effects possessed by Δ*sic1* cells (53) (discussed more fully below).

If Sic1 was an inhibitor of Cdc28/Clb5 in vivo, it was obvious that a way would be needed to reverse this inhibition to allow DNA replication to proceed. A mechanism has readily presented itself. Upon prolonged arrest, the strain lacking all six *CLB* genes possessed a distinctive multibudded morphology (47) that had previously been described for temperature-sensitive mutations in *cdc34* mutants at the restrictive temperature (27). A similar, though less-severe, phenotype was also seen in mutants that overexpressed the Sic1 protein (53) (Fig. 2.1). Cdc34 had previously been shown to encode a ubiquitin transferase (54), an activity that marked specific proteins for degradation. Since the failure to degrade an inhibitor of Clb function would be expected to have the same phenotype as a complete

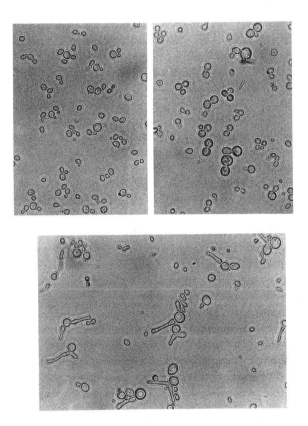

FIGURE 2.1. Photomicrographs depicting effects of Sic1 under- and overexpression. Top left: Normal mid-log phase yeast cells. Top right: Strain isogenic with strain at left but carrying a deletion of the *SIC1* gene. Note the appearance of larger than normal cells, most of which also possess a large bud. Bottom: Yeast cells overexpressing the *SIC1* gene through use of the galactose inducible *GAL1* promoter. Note the appearance of highly elongated buds in many cells and the appearance of cells with more than one bud. Reprinted with permission from Nugroho and Mendenhall (53), © 1994, American Society of Microbiology.

loss of all the *CLB* genes, it was immediately recognized that Sic1 degradation could be mediated by the Cdc34 protein. To test this, a *cdc34*[ts] Δ*sic1* double mutant was constructed and shifted to the restrictive temperature. By itself, *cdc34*[ts] mutant cells arrest cell division in the interval between Start and S phase with the multibudded morphology described above. When *sic1* is deleted, the double mutant is now able to enter and progress through S phase, demonstrating that it was the failure of *cdc34*[ts] strains to degrade Sic1 that was the cause of their inability to initiate DNA replication (47). Immunoblot analysis additionally showed that the Sic1 protein was stabilized in *cdc34*[ts] strains at the restrictive temperature as expected if Cdc34 was required for Sic1 degradation.

The involvement of the Cln/Cdc28 complexes in the determination of Sic1 stability is still preliminary. Studies of other Cdc34 substrates, such as the Cln proteins themselves, indicate that prior phosphorylation at Cdc28 consensus sites is an important determinant of Cdc34 recognition (55, 56). Sic1 is a good substrate of Cln2/Cdc28 complexes in vitro (47) and directed mutagenesis studies have indicated that at least some of the Cdc28 phosphorylation sites in Sic1 are important determinants of Sic1 stability (unpublished). Definitive proof of this hypothesis will require the demonstration in vitro that Sic1 phosphorylation is required for Cdc34 dependent ubiquitination.

A Molecular Model of the Start/s Transition

We are at a point at which we can construct a fairly detailed working model of cyclin/CDK-related events in the G1 to S phase transition (Fig. 2.2). A newborn daughter cell is born small. It must grow to a characteristic size before it can commit to the mitotic cell cycle (27). In addition, the nutritional content of the growth medium must be capable of permitting the completion of the mitotic cell cycle. When both of these conditions are met, Cln3/Cdc28 complexes (which appear to be present throughout the cell cycle) are able to activate the MBF and SBF transcription factors (57). MBF activates the transcription of a large number of genes involved in DNA replication (58) including *CLB5* and *CLB6* (20, 45, 59). Clb5 and Clb6 bind to free Cdc28 and are immediately inhibited by the binding of Sic1, which has been accumulating since *SIC1* gene transcription began at the end of the preceding mitosis (47, 60). SBF activates the transcription of *CLN1* and *CLN2* (61), the products of which immediately bind to and activate free Cdc28. If the cell is under the influence of mating pheromone, activated Far1 protein binds and inhibits the Cln/Cdc28 complexes, preventing further cell cycle progression (17).

If no mating pheromone is present, the active Cln1/Cdc28 and Cln2/Cdc28 complexes initiate the processes of budding and *spindle pole body* (SPB) duplication (47) and phosphorlyate Sic1 and the Clns. In partnership

FIGURE 2.2. Proposed
regulatory circuitry
controlling passage through
G1 and entry into S phase.
Arrows indicate stimulatory
events. Barred lines
indicate inhibitory events.
See text for further details.

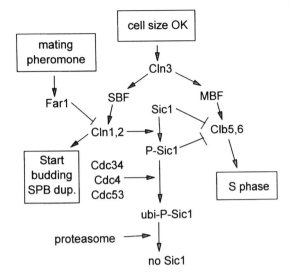

with other components, Cdc34 ubiquitinates the phosphorylated forms of
Sic1 and the Clns, causing their degradation. The loss of Sic1 activates Clb5/
Cdc28 and Clb6/Cdc28, which allows entry into S phase. The activation of
Clb/Cdc28 complexes also puts an end to G1-specific processes by turning
off SBF (62), ending the further synthesis of Cln1 and Cln2.

SIC1 as a Checkpoint Regulator

The preceding section has described the regulatory circuitry controlling the
transition from Cln-mediated growth to Clb-mediated growth, particularly
with respect to the role of Sic1. It has provided a mechanistic explanation
for the delay between mitotic commitment and S-phase initiation that is
seen in most eukaryotic cells, but it does not address the question of
the need for this delay in the cell cycle. Studies of the Sic1 deletion
phenotype (53) have produced as much shadow as light concerning this
question.

Sic1 function is not essential for viability or for the growth arrest responses to mating pheromone or nitrogen starvation (53). Cultures of Δsic1
cells have only a 50% plating efficiency compared with that of wild type,
indicating that, although not essential, Sic1 does have an important role in
promoting faithful cell division. These Δsic1 cultures have high percentages
of cells that appear to have arrested at the G2/M checkpoint (Fig. 2.1).
Chromosome loss and breakage rates are elevated 120- and 1,200-fold,
respectively, in Δscil cells. These phenotypes—reduced cellular viability
and increased chromosomal aberrations—are hallmarks of cell cycle checkpoint regulators (63).

Checkpoint regulators prevent processes from occurring at inappropriate times or under inappropriate conditions. An example of this is the dependence of mitosis on the prior completion of DNA replication. Mitotic chromosomal separation to opposite poles would be disastrous if it occurred before DNA replication was complete or if the DNA was damaged by interstrand cross-linking. Regulators that sense the replication and repair status of a cell's DNA and that prevent or delay the initiation of mitosis until the DNA is ready are checkpoint regulators. The initiation of many processes during the cell cycle is dependent upon checkpoint regulators that verify the faithful completion of an earlier process.

If Sic1 is a checkpoint regulator, what is it regulating? The Δ*sic1* cells are not sensitive to *ultraviolet* (UV) or γ-irradiation or to inhibitors of DNA synthesis or spindle formation, indicating that the cells are not involved in previously studied checkpoints. The timing of its degradation—between Start and S phase—suggests a role for processes being completed at this time. Temporal maps of the yeast cell cycle indicate the existence of at least three processes—DNA replication, SPB duplication, and bud emergence and growth—that are dependent upon the completion of Start (27) (Fig. 2.3). As discussed above, DNA replication is dependent upon the activation of Clb/Cdc28 complexes, which is in turn dependent upon the approval of the putative Sic1 checkpoint regulator. Budding and SPB duplication both initiate without the need for Clb/Cdc28 function, but both require Clb/

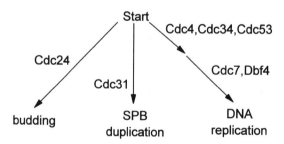

FIGURE 2.3. Semi-independent mitotic subcycles dependent upon Start completion. After passage through Start, the cells initiate budding, *spindle pole body* (SPB) duplication, and DNA replication. Representative genes involved in each of these dependent pathways are indicated near the arrows. The sequential arrows for DNA replication indicate that the *CDC4*, *CDC34*, and *CDC53* genes act prior to the action of the *CDC7* and *DBF4* genes. Normally each of these three processes only occur once per cycle, but certain mutations "decouple" these processes from the others. For example, SPB duplication is decoupled from the other cycles by the *esp1* mutation, which allows continued periodic duplication of the SPB despite the failure of the budding or DNA replication cycles. The *cdc4*, *cdc34*, and *cdc53* mutations allow continued periodic budding and SPB duplication despite the failure of the DNA replication cycle. These mutations indicate the normal existence of a checkpoint regulator that ensures each subcycle happens only once per mitotic cycle.

Cdc28 function for completion. Both of these processes therefore are good candidates for Sic1-mediated checkpoint regulation.

Spindle Pole Body Duplication

The chromosomal defects of Δ*sic1* strains and the localization of Cdc2/cyclin species to the SPBs, centrosomes, and spindles in a variety of organisms (4–7, 64) make the involvement of Sic1 in a SPB duplication checkpoint especially attractive. Furthermore, pedigree studies of dividing Δ*sic1* cells indicate that the poor viability of Δ*sci1* strains was restricted primarily to daughter cells (53) (Fig. 2.4). In any given division, the daughter cell had a roughly 50% chance of entering permanent G2 arrest but the mother cell never did. This pattern could be explained as resulting from an SPB duplication defect since it has previously been shown that SPBs duplicate conservatively and the old SPB is retained by the mother, while the new one enters the daughter (65). If the duplication were carried out improperly, the daughter cell would receive the defective SPB. The checkpoint role of Sic1 would presumably be to stop the cell cycle in response to incomplete or

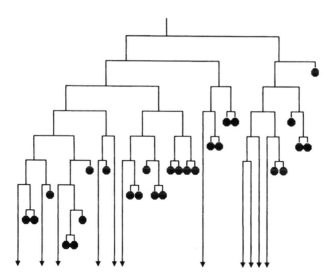

FIGURE 2.4. Pedigree analysis of dividing Δ*sic1* cells. A single cell carrying a deletion of the sic1 gene was isolated by micromanipulation. As it divided, the mother cell was separated from the daughter (mother on left, daughter on right). This was carried out for 8 generations. Octagons indicate cells that ceased dividing. In most cases these arrested with a single large bud. Arrows indicate cells that went on to form visible colonies the next day, 12 hours after the micromanipulations had ceased. Note that ~50% of all daughter cells fail to form colonies. Mother cells do not show this defect. Reprinted from Nugroho and Mendenhall (53), © 1994, American Society of Microbiology.

improper SPB duplication, allowing time for SPB completion or repair. This idea was tested by crossing numerous mutations known to be impaired for SPB duplication and function with the Δ*sic1* strain in the expectation that increasing the frequency SPB defects would increase the lethality in a Δ*sic1* background due to the lack of a checkpoint control. No such increase was seen (unpublished).

Cytoplasmic and Nuclear Asymmetry

The process of budding defines mother/daughter asymmetry. A bud site must be selected, the cell wall rearranged, and vesicular transport altered to allow the highly polarized cell growth that characterizes the budding process (20). This all occurs under the control of Cln/Cdc28 complexes. When the Clb/Cdc28 complexes take over, the cytoskeleton is rearranged and vesicular/plasma membrane fusion is no longer localized to the very tip of the daughter cell (66). While these processes could be checkpointed by Sic1, it is difficult to understand how errors in cytoplasmic structures could lead to the DNA damage seen in Δ*sic1* cells. A possible explanation comes from studies on the fate of plasmids lacking centromeres in yeast cells. These plasmids can exist in copy numbers of up to 50 per cell, yet are fairly unstable during mitotic cell division. Pedigree experiments similar to that depicted in Figure 2.4 have indicated that the plasmid loss is due to the failure of daughter cells to receive any plasmids during nuclear division (67); they are all retained by the mother. This suggests that, like the cytoskeleton, the nucleus may have a structure that is oriented relative to the mother-daughter axis. The mother/daughter asymmetry of mating type switching (68), a process by which yeast cells change their sexual identity, also indicates the existence of a specific nuclear orientation. The establishment of such an orientation may be an important prerequisite for DNA replication and thus a good candidate for Sic1 checkpoint regulation. This idea is as yet untested.

Future Directions

The primary immediate goal is to reconstruct the interactions and processes implicated by the genetic experiments in in vitro biochemical reactions. The genetic experiments identify many, perhaps all, of the players, but we can only know that by reproducing these interactions in a defined system. Using the genetics to identify the larger regulatory role played by Sic1 will also be essential to further progress in understanding how the cell coordinates the many events that are involved in constructing a faithful reproduction of the parent cell.

Looking somewhat more broadly at Figure 2.2, one is struck by how little is known about the output pathways emanating from this regulatory net. The Cln/Cdc28 complexes initiate budding and SPB duplication. The Clb/Cdc28 complexes initiate DNA synthesis and redistribute the manner in which cellular growth takes place, but the only substrates described for either of these complexes are regulators of these complexes. Virtually nothing is known about the CDK substrates that are involved in, say, S-phase initiation or SPB duplication. This is an area where yeast genetics should be able to play a role. It is known that the *CDC7* gene is required for DNA synthesis initiation and acts after *CDC34* (27). Cdc7 is a protein kinase (69) that, like the CDKs, is activated by the binding of a second subunit, Dbf4 (70). Dbf4 has been shown to bind to origins of replication and can recruit Cdc7 to these origins (71). Finally, genetic, but not physical, interactions between Cdc28 and Cdc7 have been reported (72). Thus, a weak genetic link between Cdc28 and origins of replication has been established. Strengthening this link and establishing new ones will be an important goal for future studies.

Finally, we can ask what prospects this work has for greater understanding of mammalian cell cycles. The parallels with the CDKs and cyclins are already well established. In the last two years, a host of CDK inhibitors have been reported and implicated in processes that include tumor suppression (21–23), growth factor regulation (14, 17, 18), genomic stability (73), contact inhibition (18), and differentiation (24–26). Periodic protein instability is an important part of the regulation of cyclins and of the p53 tumor suppressor. A human homologue of the Cdc34 ubiquitin transferase has recently been cloned (74), suggesting that the mechanism controlling late G1 proteolysis may have been retained throughout eukaryotic evolution. The prospects seem excellent that the dissection of the mammalian cell cycle components and how they go wrong in the disease state will be greatly enriched by the studies in model systems like *Saccharomyces cerevisiae*.

Acknowledgment. This work was supported by a grant from the American Cancer Society (CB-70B).

References

1. Hartwell LH, Kastan MB. Cell cycle control and cancer. Science 1994;266: 1821–8.
2. Sherr CJ. Mammalian G1 cyclins. Cell 1993;73:1059–65.
3. King RW, Jackson PK, Kirschner MW. Mitosis in transition. Cell 1994;79: 563–71.

4. Bailly E, Pines J, Hunter T, Bornens M. Cytoplasmic accumulation of cyclin B1 in human cells: association with a detergent-resistant compartment and with the centrosome. J Cell Sci 1992;101:529–45.
5. Ookata K, Hisanaga S-i, Okano T, Tachibana K, Kishimoto T. Relocation and distinct subcellular localization of p34^{cdc2}-cyclin B complex at meiosis reinitiation in starfish oocytes. EMBO J 1992;11:1763–72.
6. Bailly E, Dorée M, Nurse P, Bornens M. p34^{cdc2} is located in both nucleus and cytoplasm; part is centrosomally associated at G_2/M and enters vesicles at anaphase. EMBO J 1989;8:3985–95.
7. Alfa CE, Ducommun B, Beach D, Hyams JS. Distinct nuclear and spindle pole body populations of cyclin-cdc2 in fission yeast. Nature 1990;347:680–2.
8. Mendenhall MD. An inhibitor of p34^{CDC28} protein kinase activity from *Saccharomyces cerevisiae*. Science 1993;259:216–9.
9. Xiong Y, Hannon GJ, Zhang H, Casso D, Kobayashi R, Beach D. p21 is a universal inhibitor of cyclin kinases. Nature 1993;366:701–4.
10. El-Deiry WS, Tokino T, Velculescu VE, Levy DB, Parsons R, Trent JM, et al. WAF1, a potential mediator of p53 tumor suppression. Cell 1993;75:817–25.
11. Harper JW, Adami GR, Wei N, Keyomarsi K, Elledge SJ. The p21 cdk-interacting protein Cip1 is a potent inhibitor of G1 cyclin-dependent kinases. Cell 1993;75:805–16.
12. Serrano M, Hannon GJ, Beach D. A new regulatory motif in cell-cycle control causing specific inhibition of cyclin D/CDK4. Nature 1993;366:704–7.
13. Gu Y, Turck CW, Morgan DO. Inhibition of CDK2 activity in vivo by an associated 20K regulatory subunit. Nature 1993;366:707–10.
14. Hannon GJ, Beach D. p15^{INK4B} is a potential effector of TGF-β-induced cell cycle arrest. Nature 1994;371:257–61.
15. Toyoshima H, Hunter T. p27, a novel inhibitor of G1 cyclin-Cdk protein kinase activity, is related to p21. Cell 1994;78:67–74.
16. Guan K-L, Jenkins CW, Li Y, Nichols MA, Wu X, O'Keefe CL, et al. Growth suppression by p18, a p16$^{INK4/MTS1}$- and p14$^{INK4B/MTS2}$-related CDK6 inhibitor, correlates with wild-type pRb function. Genes Dev 1994;8:2939–52.
17. Peter M, Gartner A, Horecka J, Ammerer G, Herskowitz I. FAR1 links the signal transduction pathway to the cell cycle machinery in yeast. Cell 1993;73:747–60.
18. Polyak K, Kato J-y, Solomon MJ, Sherr CJ, Massague J, Roberts JM. p27^{Kip1}, a cyclin-Cdk inhibitor, links transforming growth factor-β and contact inhibition to cell cycle arrest. Genes Dev 1994;8:9–22.
19. Duliç V, Kaufmann WK, Wilson SJ, Tlsty TD, Lees E, Harper JW, et al. p53-dependent inhibition of cyclin-dependent kinase activities in human fibroblasts during radiation-induced G1 arrest. Cell 1994;76:1013–23.
20. Andrews BJ, Mason SW. Gene expression and the cell cycle: a family affair. Science 1993;261:1543–4.
21. Spruck CH III, Gonzalez-Zulueta M, Shibata A, Simoneau AR, Lin M-F, Gonzales F, et al. p16 gene in uncultured tumours. Nature 1994;370:183–4.
22. Kamb A, Gruis NA, Weaver-Feldhaus J, Liu Q, Harshman K, Tavtigian SV, et al. A cell cycle regulator potentially involved in genesis of many tumor types. Science 1994;264:436–40.

23. Nobori T, Miura K, Wu DJ, Lois A, Takabayashi K, Carson DA. Deletions of the cyclin-dependent kinase-4 inhibitor gene in multiple human cancers. Nature 1994;368:753–6.

24. Halevy O, Novitch BG, Spicer DB, Skapek SX, Rhee J, Hannon GJ, et al. Correlation of terminal cell cycle arrest of skeletal muscle with induction of p21 by MyoD. Science 1995;267:1018–21.

25. Skapek SX, Rhee J, Spicer DB, Lassar AB. Inhibition of myogenic differentiation in proliferating myoblasts by cyclin D1-dependent kinase. Science 1995;267:1022–4.

26. Parker SB, Eichele G, Zhang P, Rawls A, Sands AT, Bradley A, et al. p53-independent expression of p21[Cip1] in muscle and other terminally differentiating cells. Science 1995;267:1024–7.

27. Pringle JR, Hartwell LH. The *Saccharomyces cerevisiae* cell cycle. In: Strathern JN, Jones EW, Broach JR, eds. The molecular biology of the yeast *Saccharomyces*. Life cycle and inheritance. Cold Spring Harbor, NY: Cold Spring Harbor Laboratory, 1981:97–142.

28. Valay JG, Simon M, Faye G. The Kin28 protein kinase is associated with a cyclin in *Saccharomyces cerevisiae*. J Mol Biol 1993;234:307–10.

29. Kaffman A, Herskowitz I, Tjian R, O'Shea EK. Phosphorylation of the transcription factor PHO4 by a cyclin-CDK complex, PHO80-PHO85. Science 1994;263:1153–6.

30. Surosky RT, Strich R, Esposito RE. The yeast UME5 gene regulates the stability of meiotic mRNAs in response to glucose. Mol Cell Biol 1994;14:3446–58.

31. Mendenhall MD, Jones CA, Reed SI. Dual regulation of the yeast CDC28-p40 protein kinase complex: cell cycle, pheromone, and nutrient limitation effects. Cell 1987;50:927–35.

32. Wittenberg C, Sugimoto K, Reed SI. G1-specific cyclins of *S. cerevisiae*. Cell cycle, periodicity, regulation by mating pheromone, and association with the p34[cdc28] protein kinase. Cell 1990;62:225–37.

33. Wittenber C, Reed SI. Control of the yeast cell cycle is associated with assembly/disassembly of the Cdc28 protein kinase complex. Cell 1988;54:1061–72.

34. Hartwell LH, Culotti J, Pringle J, Reid B. Genetic control of the cell division cycle in yeast. I. Detection of mutants. Science 1974;183:46–51.

35. Mendenhall MD, Richardson HE, Reed SI. Dominant negative protein kinase mutations that confer a G_1 arrest phenotype. Proc Natl Acad Sci USA 1988;85:4426–30.

36. Reed SI. The selection of amber mutations in genes required for completion of start, the controlling event of the cell division cycle of *S. cerevisiae*. Genetics 1980;95:579–88.

37. Hadwiger JA, Wittenberg C, de Barros Lopes MA, Richardson HE, Reed SI. A family of cyclin homologs that control the G_1 phase in yeast. Proc Natl Acad Sci USA 1989;86:6255–9.

38. Cross FR. DAF1, a mutant gene affecting size control, pheromone arrest, and cell cycle kinetics of *Saccharomyces cerevisiae*. Mol Cell Biol 1988;8:4675–84.

39. Nash R, Tokiwa G, Anand S, Erickson K, Futcher AB. The WHI1[+] gene of *Saccharomyces cerevisiae* tethers cell division to cell size and is a cyclin homolog. EMBO J 1988;7:4335–46.

40. Richardson HE, Wittenberg C, Cross F, Reed SI. An essential G1 function for cyclin-like proteins in yeast. Cell 1989;59:1127–33.

41. Surana U, Robitsch H, Schuster T, Fitch I, Futcher AB, Nasmyth K. The role of CDC28 and cyclins during mitosis in the budding yeast *S. cerevisiae*. Cell 1991;65:145–61.
42. Epstein CB, Cross FR. CLB5: a novel B cyclin from budding yeast with a role in S phase. Genes Dev 1992;6:1695–706.
43. Fitch I, Dahmann C, Surana U, Amon A, Nasmyth K, Goetsch L, et al. Characterization of four B-type cyclin genes of the budding yeast *Saccharomyces cerevisiae*. Mol Biol Cell 1992;3:805–18.
44. Ghiara JB, Richardson HE, Sugimoto K, Henze M, Lew DJ, et al. A cyclin B homolog in *S. cerevisiae*: chronic activation of the Cdc28 protein kinase by cyclin prevents exit from mitosis. Cell 1991;65:163–74.
45. Schwob E, Nasmyth K. CLB5 and CLB6, a new pair of B cyclins involved in DNA replication in *Saccharomyces cerevisiae*. Genes Dev 1993;7:1160–75.
46. Richardson HE, Lew DJ, Henze M, Sugimoto K, Reed SI. Cyclin-B homologs in *Saccharomyces cerevisiae* function in S phase and in G2. Genes Dev 1992;6:2021–34.
47. Schwob E, Böhm T, Mendenhall MD, Nasmyth K. The B-type cyclin kinase inhibitor p40[SIC1] controls the G1 to S transition in *S. cerevisiae*. Cell 1994;79:233–44.
48. Chang F, Herskowitz I. Identification of a gene necessary for cell cycle arrest by a negative growth factor of yeast. FAR1 is an inhibitor of a G1 cyclin, CLN2. Cell 1990;63:999–1011.
49. Bücking-Throm E, Duntze W, Hartwell LH, Manney TR. Reversible arrest of haploid yeast cells at the initiation of DNA synthesis by a diffusible sex factor. Exp Cell Res 1973;76:99–110.
50. Elion EA, Satterberg B, Kranz JE. FUS3 phosphorylates multiple components of the mating signal transduction cascade: evidence for STE12 and FAR1. Mol Biol Cell 1993;4:495–510.
51. Peter M, Herskowitz I. Direct inhibition of the yeast cyclin-dependent kinase Cdc28-Cln by Far1. Science 1994;265:1228–31.
52. Reed SI, Hadwiger JA, Lörincz AT. Protein kinase activity associated with the product of the yeast cell division cycle gene CDC28. Proc Natl Acad Sci USA 1985;82:4055–9.
53. Nugroho TT, Mendenhall MD. An inhibitor of yeast cyclin-dependent protein kinase plays an important role in ensuring the genomic integrity of daughter cells. Mol Cell Biol 1994;14:3320–8.
54. Goebl MG, Yochem J, Jentsch S, McGrath JP, Varshavsky A, Byers B. The yeast cell cycle gene CDC34 encodes a ubiquitin-conjugating enzyme. Science 1988;241:1331–5.
55. Yaglom J, Linskens MHK, Sadis S, Rubin DM, Futcher B, Finley D. p34[cdc28]-mediated control of Cln3 cylin degradation. Mol Cell Biol 1995;15:731–41.
56. Deshaies RJ, Chau V, Kirschner M. Ubiquitination of the G_1 cyclin Cln2p by a Cdc34p-dependent pathway. EMBO J 1995;14:303–12.
57. Tyers M, Tokiwa G, Futcher B. Comparison of the *Saccharomyces cerevisiae* G1 cyclins: Cln3 may be an upstream activator of Cln1, Cln2 and other cyclins. EMBO J 1993;12:1955–68.
58. Wittenberg C, Reed SI. Control of gene expression and the yeast cell cycle. CRC Crit Rev Euk Gene Exp 1991;1:189–205.

59. Kühne C, Linder P. A new pair of B-type cyclins from *Saccharomyces cerevisiae* that function early in the cell cycle. EMBO J 1993;12:3437–47.
60. Donovan JD, Toyn JH, Johnson AL, Johnston LH. p40[SDB25], a putative CDK inhibitor, has a role in the M/G$_1$ transition in *Saccharomyces cerevisiae*. Genes Dev 1994;8:1640–53.
61. Cross FR, Tinkelenberg AH. A potential positive feedback loop controlling CLN1 and CLN2 gene expression at the start of the yeast cell cycle. Cell 1991;65:875–83.
62. Amon A, Tyers M, Futcher B, Nasmyth K. Mechanisms that help the yeast cell cycle clock tick: G2 cyclins transcriptionally activate G2 cyclins and repress G1 cyclins. Cell 1993;74:993–1007.
63. Hartwell LH, Weinert TA. Checkpoints: controls that ensure the order of cell cycle events. Science 1989;246:629–34.
64. Riabowol K, Draetta G, Brizuela L, Vandre D, Beach D. The cdc2 kinase ia nuclear protein that is essential for mitosis in mammalian cells. Cell 1989;57:393–401.
65. Vallen EA, Scherson TY, Roberts T, van Zee K, Rose MD. Asymmetric mitotic segregation of the yeast spindle pole body. Cell 1992;69:505–15.
66. Lew DJ, Reed SI. Morphogenesis in the yeast cell cycle: regulation by Cdc28 and cyclins. J Cell Biol 1993;120:1305–20.
67. Murray AW, Szostak JW. Pedigree analysis of plasmid segregation in yeast. Cell 1983;34:961–70.
68. Strathern JN, Herskowitz I. Asymmetry and directionality in production of new cell types during clonal growth: the switching pattern of homothallic yeast. Cell 1979;17:371–81.
69. Buck V, White A, Rosamond J. CDC7 protein kinase activity is required for mitosis and meiosis in *Saccharomyces cerevisiae*. Mol Gen Genet 1991;227: 452–7.
70. Jackson AL, Pahl PMB, Harrison K, Rosamond J, Sclafani RA. Cell cycle regulation of the yeast Cdc7 protein kinase by association with the Dbf4 protein. Mol Cell Biol 1993;13:2899–908.
71. Dowell SJ, Romanowski P, Diffley JFX. Interaction of Dbf4, the Cdc7 protein kinase regulatory subunit, with yeast replication origins in vivo. Science 1994;265:1243–6.
72. Sclafani RA, Jackson AL. Cdc7 protein kinase for DNA metabolism comes of age. Molec Microbiol 1994;11:805–10.
73. Hunter T, Pines J. Cyclins and cancer II: cyclin D and CDK inhibitors come of age. Cell 1994;79:573–82.
74. Plon SE, Leppig KA, Do HN, Groudine M. Cloning of the human homolog of the CDC34 cell cycle gene by complementation in yeast. Proc Natl Acad Sci USA 1993;90:10484–8.

3

Oocyte Activation and Passage Through the Meiotic Cell Cycle in *Xenopus Laevis*

JAY C. STRUM, KAREN H. MARTIN, J. ERIC TURNER,
ROBERT M. BELL, AND KATHERINE I. SWENSON

Meiotically dividing cells undergo a specialized cell cycle, wherein a cell that has replicated its DNA undergoes two successive rounds of M phase without an intervening S phase to create the haploid gametes, which are not identical in their chromosome content. These features of the meiotic cell cycle are distinctly different from those of mitotically dividing embryonic and postembryonic cells, the goal of which is to create two daughter cells, each containing an identical set of diploid chromosomes. In these mitotic cell cycles, the entry into M phase for each division depends upon the passage through a preceding S phase (reviewed in 1).

In females, entry into the meiotic divisions is triggered by the activation of quiescent oocytes, which for most species are arrested at prophase of the cell cycle. Oocyte activation and reentry into the cell cycle are induced by external cues, which are provided by hormones or, for some species, by sperm. Activation of oocytes leads to the activation of *M-phase promoting factor* (MPF), which consists of cyclin B/p34^{cdc2} kinase complexes, an event that is required in all dividing eukaryotic cells for the entry into M phase (reviewed in 2, 3). In mitotically dividing embryonic cells, passage through the cell cycle is driven by periodic activation and inactivation of these kinase complexes. Activation of these complexes is required for the entry into M phase and inactivation is required for the exit from M phase and entry into the next cell cycle. During mitosis, the activation and inactivation of these kinase complexes are driven by the synthesis and accumulation of cyclin B during S phase, which is required for p34^{cdc2} kinase activity, and the proteolysis of this cyclin, which occurs at the end of M phase in each cell cycle and leads to the loss p34^{cdc2} kinase activity. During the two meiotic divisions, the entry into M phase and exit from this stage also require the activation and inactivation, of these kinase complexes. However, during meiosis the molecular mechanisms by which the cyclin B/p34^{cdc2} complexes are activated and regulated are quite different from those that occur during mitotic divisions.

This chapter focuses on particular cellular processes and cellular components that influence or are required for oocyte activation and passage through the meiotic cell cycle of the frog, *Xenopus laevis*. The particular areas of interest that are addressed are (i) the function of the *mos* protein during the meiotic cell cycle (*mos* is a serine/threonine kinase that is found only in high levels in meiotically dividing oocytes of vertebrates and is required for the meiotic divisions in *Xenopus*); and (ii) the role of particular sphingolipids that appear to be important for oocyte activation and meiotic cell cycle progression.

The Function of *Mos* in Meiotic Cell Cycle Progression of *Xenopus* Oocytes

Quiescent, fully grown oocytes of the frog, *Xenopus laevis*, are activated and reenter the cell cycle following exposure to the natural physiological inducer, progesterone (Fig. 3.1). Within several hours of progesterone exposure, MPF is activated, which leads to *germinal vesicle breakdown* (GVBD) and entry into M phase of meiosis I. During this phase, the condensed chromosomes migrate to the plasma membrane of the darkly-pigmented animal pole, where they align on the metaphase plate of the spindle in readiness for meiosis I. Chromosome migration and formation of the spindle causes a displacement of the pigment granules in the animal pole giving rise to a characteristic white spot that can be easily detected. At the end of M phase, MPF activity declines and meiosis I occurs. This is a very unequal cell division, which gives rise to a tiny polar body. Following meiosis I, MPF is reactivated and entry into meiosis II is initiated, whereupon the still-condensed chromosomes align on the metaphase plate of the second meiotic spindle. At this point the oocyte has matured into the fertilizable gamete, the egg. The cell cycle arrests at this metaphase accompanied by high levels of MPF activity until the time of fertilization, whereupon cyclin B is proteolyzed, MPF is inactivated, meiosis II is completed to generate a second polar body, and the cell enters into S phase of the first mitotic cell cycle. The early embryo then undergoes successive rounds of mitotic divisions, each of which are driven by cyclin synthesis and its periodic proteolysis.

Unlike the mitotic divisions, activation of p34^{cdc2} kinase and entry into M phase of the meiotic divisions does not appear to require new cyclin synthesis. Cyclin B protein (B2) is present in quiescent oocytes and is found in association with p34^{cdc2} kinase in inactive complexes. The levels of this cyclin is only partially diminished at the end of meiosis I, unlike the end of

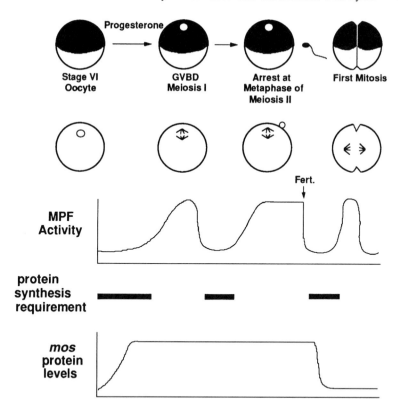

FIGURE 3.1. Meiotic cell cycle in oocytes of *Xenopus laevis* following progesterone treatment. Progesterone treatment of full-grown (stage VI) oocytes triggers GVBD, which can be detected by the formation of a white spot on the darkly pigmented animal hemisphere, and passage through meiosis 1 to generate a small polar body (top two panels). Following completion of meiosis I, these cells enter into metaphase of meiosis II (second panel), at which point they arrest in the cell cycle until the time of fertilization. Following fertilization, the mitotic divisions ensue. MPF activity, which is low in the oocyte, is stimulated to drive meiosis I. This activity transiently declines following meiosis I, is restimulated to initiate meiosis II, and is maintained at high levels until the time of fertilization, when it rapidly disappears. During each subsequent mitotic division, MPF is activated and inactivated to initiate the entry into and exit from M phase, respectively. The periods during which protein synthesis is required for the enactment of meiosis I, II, and the first mitotic division is indicated. *Mos* protein, which is not found in the oocyte, is synthesized following progesterone treatment and is maintained until the time of fertilization, when it is proteolyzed.

meiosis II following fertilization or the end of M phase during the mitotic divisions when the proteolysis of this protein appears to be more complete (4, 5). During meiosis, additional cyclins are synthesized (cyclins A1, B1, and B2) as well. That sufficient levels of cyclin protein required for p34^{cdc2}

kinase activation for both meiosis I and II are present in oocytes without further requirements for synthesis is suggested by cyclin *messenger RNA* (mRNA)-ablation studies. In these studies, cyclin antisense oligonucleotide DNAs were microinjected into oocytes to ablate the mRNAs for cyclins A1, B1, and B2, thus preventing further cyclin protein synthesis; they were found to have no effect on progesterone-induced maturation (6). While these studies cannot rule out that the synthesis of other unknown cyclin types may be important for oocyte maturation, they do indicate that the synthesis of examined cyclins are not necessary for passage through meiosis.

What then is driving the activation of MPF complexes during meiotic divisions? After exposing oocytes to progesterone, a period of protein synthesis is required for the activation of MPF complexes and the entry into meiosis I. A second period of protein synthesis is required following meiosis I for MPF activation and entry into meiosis II. One of the proteins, the synthesis of which is required during these periods for passage through the two meiotic divisions, is the product of the c-*mos* proto-oncogene (*mos*). *Mos* mRNA, but not *mos* protein, is maternally stored in *Xenopus* oocytes (7). Following progesterone treatment, *mos* protein is synthesized and maintained at high levels until the time of fertilization, when it is proteolyzed (7–10) (Fig. 3.1). *Mos* is not expressed at high levels again in any other tissue of the developing embryo or adult. If inappropriately expressed in adult tissues, *mos* can elicit cellular transformation.

The synthesis of *mos* protein and meiosis appears to be dependent upon a transient intracellular decrease in the levels of *cyclic adenosine-5'-mono-phosphate* (cAMP) occurring soon after progesterone treatment (Fig. 3.2). Pretreatment of oocytes with agents that block this decrease in cAMP levels, such as cholera toxin or forskolin, blocks progesterone-induced meiosis (reviewed in 11). Oocyte resumption of meiotic divisions, which is triggered by the drop in cAMP levels, appears to be mediated by a concomitant decrease in the activity of cAMP-dependent *protein kinase* (PKA). Microinjection studies have indicated that this decrease in the activity of PKA is necessary for progesterone-induced meiosis. The catalytic subunit of PKA (PKAc), when microinjected, blocks progesterone-induced meiosis, whereas microinjection of the regulatory subunit, or the peptide inhibitor of PKA, is sufficient to trigger meiosis in the absence of progesterone. The decrease in PKA activity appears to be necessary for the translation of *mos*, since microinjection of PKAc blocks the synthesis of *mos* protein that normally occurs following progesterone treatment (12). PKAc also appears to effect meiotic cell cycle progression at later stages following *mos* synthesis (see below).

The requirements of *mos* synthesis for the enactment of meiosis I and II has been demonstrated by *mos* mRNA ablation studies following microinjection of antisense oligonucleotide DNAs. Ablation of *mos* mRNAs in oocytes blocks the activation of MPF and meiosis I following progesterone

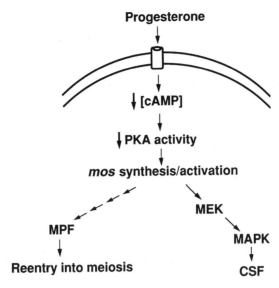

FIGURE 3.2. Signaling events in *Xenopus* oocytes treated with progesterone. Progesterone, which is thought to interact with a membrane receptor, induces a rapid, transient decrease in the intracellular levels of cAMP. This decrease in the concentration of cAMP leads to a decrease in the activity of PKA, which is necessary for the synthesis of the *mos* protein kinase. Active *mos* leads to the activation of MAPK, a mediator of *cytostatic factor* (CSF) activity, by phosphorylating and activating MEK. *Mos* also leads to the activation of MPF, which is required to drive the meiotic divisions.

treatment (7). These effects can be reversed following microinjection of recombinant *mos* protein produced in bacteria (13). The reversal of these effects by *mos* was found to occur in the presence of protein synthesis inhibitors, indicating that *mos* may be the only newly synthesized protein that is required. Work from other labs has confirmed that *mos* synthesis is required for meiosis I; whether or not it is sufficient is unconfirmed. Similar experiments have also demonstrated that *mos* is required following meiosis I for MPF activation and entry into meiosis II. Ablation of *mos* mRNA in oocytes at the time of meiosis I results in a block to both processes, which again can be abrogated following microinjection of *mos* protein (13–15). Abrogation of this block by *mos* does not occur in the presence of protein synthesis inhibitors, indicating that the synthesis of other proteins is required as well (13).

The consequences of the reactivation of MPF mediated by *mos* following meiosis I include not only the entry into meiosis II, but also the suppression of DNA replication. Maturing oocytes at the time of meiosis I, when microinjected with anti-*mos* antibodies, which were neutralizing for *mos* function, or a dominant-negative, kinase-defective p34^{cdc2} mutant protein, were found to undergo DNA replication, whereas microinjection with control antibodies or kinase-active p34^{cdc2} had no effect on the normal maturation process (16). When oocytes were microinjected with *mos* protein and then treated with protein synthesis inhibitors after meiosis I, replication also occurred, indicating that other proteins synthesized after this division were required in addition to *mos* for the suppression of DNA synthesis. The results from this study indicate that *mos* is one of the components responsible for producing the specialized features of the meiotic cell cycle, which is characterized by the absence of DNA replication between the two successive divisions, meiosis I and II.

In addition to its functions during oocyte maturation to activate MPF to drive the entry into M phase of meiosis I and II and to suppress DNA replication, *mos* also is a component of *cytostatic factor* (CSF), which is the cytoplasmic activity that is responsible for eliciting the cell cycle arrest at metaphase of meiosis II in the egg. Injection of egg cytoplasm containing CSF activity into one cell of a two-cell blastula induces a similar metaphase arrest in the injected cell, whereas cell division in the uninjected sister cell is unaffected (17). The metaphase-inducing activity of egg cytoplasm can be depleted with anti-*mos* antibodies but not with preimmune sera (8). In addition, the direct injection of *mos* mRNA or protein into one cell of a two-cell blastula will trigger a metaphase arrest (8, 18).

Once synthesized, *Mos* will lead not only to the activation of MPF, but also to the activation of a *mitogen-activated protein kinase* (MAPK) (Fig. 3.2). MAPK is activated in many cell types in response to extracellular agonists that elicit proliferation or differentiation, cellular responses that are mediated in part by the activity of this kinase (reviewed in 19). In *Xenopus* oocytes, the activation of MAPK is not required for passage through meiosis (20). However, activity of MAPK appears to mediate the CSF arrest that occurs at the end of meiosis II (21). There is evidence indicating that *mos* elicits the activation of MAPK by phosphorylating and activating MEK (22), the activator of MAPK.

Activation of Mos Protein

There is evidence that indicates that the recombinant *mos* protein must be activated to function. Kinase activity of recombinant *mos* when purified from bacteria cannot be detected (22). However, detectable kinase activity of recombinant *mos* protein, measured after immune precipitation, is acquired following its incubation in cellular lysate or microinjection into oocytes. The cellular components and mechanisms that bring about the activation of recombinant *mos* protein are not known.

Phosphatase treatment of kinase-active immunoprecipitates of recombinant *mos* protein following its incubation in cellular lysate has been reported to result in a loss of kinase activity, indicating that phosphorylation of *mos* or an associated protein may be functionally important for activation (23). Endogenous *mos*, when produced in oocytes, becomes phosphorylated on serines and this phosphorylation appears to be due to the activity of a preexisting, separate kinase rather than to autophosphorylation (7, 10, 18). However, initial studies examining the contribution of serine phosphorylation to *mos* function have suggested that this modification, at least of individual serines, may not be important for *mos* activity. In these studies, site-directed mutagenesis was used to construct point mutations of *mos*, wherein individual serine residues were converted to alanines (18). Individual mutations were made for each serine residue that is conserved among *mos* proteins of different species, all of which had been shown to function in *Xenopus* oocytes to trigger meiosis. When tested for *mos* function, all of the mutants, which had alterations of single serines that represented detectable sites of phosphorylation of nonmutant *mos*, were biologically active, indicating that phosphorylation of these conserved residues does not regulate *mos* activity (18). These studies suggest that phosphorylation of individual serines is not required for *mos* activity. It is possible that phosphorylation of more than one serine residue may contribute to *mos* activity in important ways, even though modification of any individual serine is not essential. In such a scenario, the loss of kinase activity of active *mos* immune precipitates by phosphatase treatment may result from removal of several or all of these phosphorylations. Alternatively, loss of activity following this treatment could be due to the dephosphorylation of a *mos*-associated protein, which requires phosphorylation to function as an activator of *mos*.

While it is clear that recombinant *mos* protein must undergo an activating process, the relevance of this process to active endogenous *mos* is not known. Whether or not endogenous *mos* undergoes an activation process following its synthesis has not been determined due to the technical difficulties of assaying endogenous *mos* kinase activity. Of potential bearing on this issue are recent studies of kinase-active *mos* mutants, which indicate that mutations that may induce alterations in the spatial orientation of a region of the *mos* protein that is thought to be involved in *adenosine triphosphate* (ATP) binding are sufficient to induce its activation (24). It was suggested in these studies that similar alterations may be induced during the normal activation of endogenous *mos* and that such alterations theoretically could be produced by the binding of an activator protein, analogous to the activation of the *cdc2* family of protein kinases by cyclin binding (24). However, such *mos*-associated proteins, which may functionally contribute to its activation, have not been found.

Mos *Activation of MPF*

Neither the substrates of *mos* that lead to the activation of MPF complexes nor the molecular steps in the pathway that brings about this activation required for meiosis have been identified. The activity of cyclin B/p34^{cdc2}

kinase is known to be regulated by phosphorylation and dephosphorylation due to the activity of specifically acting kinases and phosphatases (reviewed in 25). Following cyclin binding, p34^{cdc2} is phosphorylated at Thr 161, which is required for activity. This phosphorylation is carried out by *cyclin-dependent kinase-activating kinase* (CAK). Other sites of p34^{cdc2} phosphorylation, which also takes place after cyclin binding, are ones that inhibit activity of this kinase (Fig. 3.3). These include Tyr 15, a residue that is phosphorylated by the wee 1 protein kinase, and Thr 14, phosphorylated by a membrane-associated protein kinase that has not been identified. Removal of these inhibitory phosphorylations leads to the generation of an active cyclin B/p34^{cdc2} kinase complex and is mediated by the *cdc25* phosphatase.

Xenopus oocytes contain inactive complexes of cyclin B/p34^{cdc2} in which p34^{cdc2} is phosphorylated at Thr 14 and Tyr 15, both inactivating sites of phosphorylation, as well as at Thr 161 (5, 26–28). In response to the presence of active *mos* that is synthesized following progesterone treatment, p34^{cdc2} becomes dephosphorylated at Thr 14 and Tyr 15, and is activated. Dephosphorylation of the bulk of these complexes appears to be due to the activation of the *cdc25* phosphatase, which occurs at this time (29). Thus, it is possible that *mos* acts as a meiotic inducer by triggering the activation of *cdc25* in some manner.

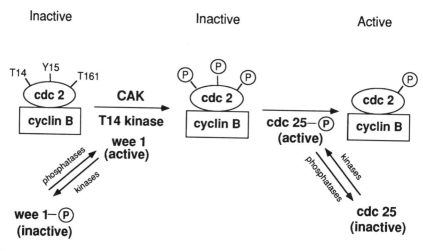

FIGURE 3.3. Activation of MPF. p34^{cdc2} kinase forms a complex with cyclin B, whereupon it becomes modified by phosphorylation at three sites. Phosphorylation at T14 and Y15, which inactivate kinase activity, is carried out by a T14 membrane-associated kinase and the wee 1 kinase, respectively. T161 phosphorylation, required for activity, is carried out by CAK. Activation of these cyclin B/p34^{cdc2} kinase complexes is elicited by the activity of the *cdc25* protein phosphatase, which removes the phosphates from both T14 and Y15. The activities of both *wee1* and *cdc25* are regulated in opposite ways by phosphorylation/dephosphorylation.

It is unlikely that *mos* leads to the activation of MPF by phosphorylating and activating *cdc25* directly. In recent studies the effects of PKA on *mos*-induced meiosis were examined. It was found that coinjection of *mos* with PKA into oocytes interfered with *mos*-induced activation of cyclin B/p34^{cdc2} kinase and passage through meiosis, whereas there was little effect on the *mos*-induced activation of MAPK (12). These results indicate that PKA does not affect the kinase function of *mos*, but rather affects, directly or indirectly, the proper enactment of the steps in the pathway leading to MPF activation. In these studies, *cdc25* was found to be dephosphorylated, suggesting that this phosphatase does not serve as a substrate for *mos*.

The determination of the biochemical step at which *mos* acts to bring about the activation of MPF is complicated by the fact that active MPF, once generated, effects the activity of both *cdc25* as well as *wee1*. The *wee1* kinase and *cdc25* phosphatase are themselves subject to regulation by phosphorylation/dephosphorylation (reviewed in 25) (Fig. 3.3). MPF is a kinase that can phosphorylate both *cdc25*, to trigger its activation, and *wee1*, to cause its inactivation. Thus, once a low level of MPF activation is achieved, it can act in a feedback manner to activate *cdc25* and inactivate *wee1*, bringing about an amplification of its own activity. The initiating event elicited by *mos* to activate MPF, then, could be through negative effects that it might have on the *wee1* pathway or through positive effects on the *cdc25* pathway. These effects of *mos* may be mediated indirectly by influencing the activity of the kinases or phosphatases that regulate *wee1* or *cdc25*. Alternatively, *mos* may not influence these pathways at all, but may effect the activity of unknown inhibitors of MPF. While these inhibitors of cyclin/cyclin-dependent kinase complexes have been found in postembryonic cells, their presence or function in oocytes has not been established.

The Role of Ceramide as a Potential Mediator of Oocyte Activation in *Xenopus* Oocytes

In the last several years it has emerged that ceramide and other sphingolipid metabolites can act as signaling components to mediate a multitude of cellular responses elicited by extracellular agonist treatments (reviewed in 30). Depending on the cell type and the specific agonist treatment, the cellular responses that have been found to be mediated by ceramide include proliferation, differentiation, and apoptosis. In many cases, the generation of ceramide following agonist treatment appears to be due to the stimulation of the phospholipase sphingomyelinase rather than to de novo synthesis (Fig. 3.4). Sphingomyelinase hydrolyzes sphingomyelin, a phospholipid present predominantly in the outer leaflet of the plasma membrane, to generate phosphocholine and ceramide, which then acts to mediate cellular

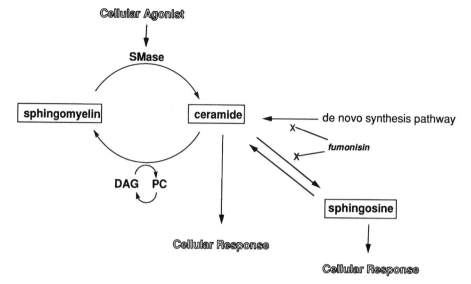

FIGURE 3.4. Biosynthesis of ceramide. Ceramide can be generated from a de novo biosynthetic pathway or from the hydrolysis of sphingomyelin, due to the activity of sphingomyelinase (SMase). In a number of cell types, sphingomyelinase activity is stimulated in response to extracellular agonist treatments to elicit cellular responses such as proliferation, differentiation, and apoptosis. The ceramide generated in these responses has been shown to be a mediator of downstream responses. Ceramide can serve as a direct effector of activities for particular enzymes (see text) or can be converted to complex sphingolipids or to sphingosine, which in some cases, have been implicated as more proximal mediators of cellular responses. The biosynthesis of ceramide, generated through the de novo pathway or from the conversion of sphingosine, can be blocked by the inhibitor, fumonisin.

responses. Thus far, two effectors of ceramide have been identified: a proline-directed serine/threonine kinase and a serine/threonine phosphatase, both activated by ceramide. The role of these effectors in further mediating the cellular responses elicited by ceramide have not yet been elucidated.

A potential role of sphingolipids in mediating oocyte activation and meiosis was first suggested by the work of Varnold and Smith (31). In these studies it was found that a brief external treatment of oocytes with sphingomyelinase or microinjection of sphingosine could trigger reentry into meiosis (31). This work has been recently extended by studies that demonstrated that oocyte activation and meiosis can be triggered following the microinjection not only of sphingosine, but of ceramide as well (32). Because ceramide and sphingosine can be interconverted inside the cell, the issue of which of these sphingolipids might be the more proximal mediator of oocyte activation was examined. It was found that sphingosine, when microinjected into oocytes, was rapidly converted to ceramide. If this conversion was blocked by coinjecting the inhibitor, fumonisin, sphingosine-induced meiosis was blocked. These results indicate that ceramide is the more proximal mediator of meiosis in oocytes microinjected with either ceramide or sphingosine.

To examine whether or not ceramide might mediate activation and meiosis following treatment with the normal physiological inducer, progesterone, bulk levels of ceramide were measured in oocytes at successive times following incubation in this hormone (Fig. 3.5). The level of ceramide rapidly increased (within 5 minutes) following progesterone treatment and was maintained in high amounts (about 3-fold higher than untreated oocytes) throughout meiosis (Fig. 3.5). The activity of endogenous sphingomyelinase in oocytes also was measured at successive times following progesterone treatment. This activity also rapidly increased (within 2 minutes) to a 3-fold level above that found in untreated oocytes (32). These results suggest that the increase in ceramide mass following progesterone treatment is due to the early activation of endogenous sphingomyelinase.

At what point in the pathway of signaling events required for progesterone-induced oocyte activation and meiosis might ceramide be mediating its effects? As a beginning step to answer this question, it was determined whether ceramide was mediating its effects to trigger meiosis at a step upstream or downstream of *mos* function. For these experiments, oocytes

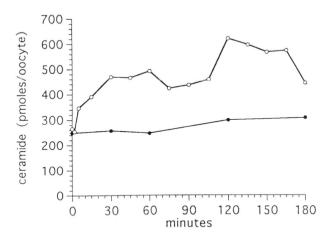

FIGURE 3.5. Ceramide levels in *Xenopus* oocytes following progesterone treatment. Groups of 20 oocytes were treated with progesterone and samples of oocytes were collected at the time intervals indicated. Ceramide was quantitated using DAG kinase. Results are expressed as pmoles ceramide/oocyte for untreated cells (filled circles), or progesterone-treated cells (open circles). These data are representative of one of three independent experiments (32).

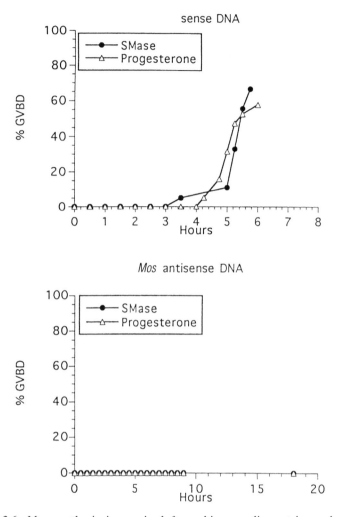

FIGURE 3.6. *Mos* synthesis is required for sphingomyelinase-triggered meiosis. Groups of 20 oocytes were microinjected either with sense oligonucleotide DNAs corresponding to 25 nucleotides present near the start of the coding region of *mos* mRNA (top panel), or with the corresponding antisense oligonucleotide (bottom panel) and incubated for 1.5 h. Injected oocytes were then treated with either progesterone (open triangles) or with sphingomyelinase (closed circles). The number of oocytes that had undergone GVBD were determined at the times indicated following these treatments and the percentages were plotted.

were first microinjected either with *mos* antisense oligonucleotide DNAs to ablate endogenous *mos* mRNAs, or with control sense oligos and then treated externally with either sphingomyelinase or progesterone (Fig. 3.6). Sense-oligo–injected oocytes underwent meiosis with either treatment, whereas those injected with antisense oligos did not. These results indicate that the effects of ceramide in oocytes generated from sphingomyelinase treatment are mediated upstream of *mos* function.

Progesterone treatment of oocytes, then, appears to activate an endogenous sphingomyelinase activity to generate ceramide and increased levels of ceramide can mediate oocyte activation and reentry into the meiotic cell cycle at a step preceding *mos* function. Important unanswered questions arising from this work include: Are the activation of sphingomyelinase and the generation of ceramide required events for progesterone-induced meiosis? What are the effectors of ceramide that function in mediating its effects to elicit oocyte activation and meiosis? The examination of these issues in *Xenopus* oocytes may provide important information regarding not only oocyte activation and reentry into the meiotic cell cycle, but also the mechanisms by which ceramide can act as a signaling component in triggering cellular responses.

Summary

Early events of *Xenopus* oocyte activation that are triggered following progesterone treatment and appear to be important for reentry into the meiotic cell cycle are a transient decrease in the levels of cAMP, accompanied by a decrease in PKA activity and an increase in ceramide mass. Experimental manipulations that artificially lower PKA activity or increase the intracellular concentration of ceramide are sufficient for activation and reentry into the meiotic cell cycle in the absence of progesterone. The effects of these events are mediated at steps preceding the synthesis of *mos*, which is required for passage through the meiotic cell cycles. A decrease in PKA activity has been shown to be required for the translation of the *mos* protein. The effectors of ceramide in this cell system have not been identified but may act to effect *mos* translation as well. Once synthesized, *mos* leads to the activation of MPF and passage through the meiotic divisions. Important unresolved issues concerning the function of *mos* during meiosis include the requirements and mechanisms of activation as a kinase and the substrates that it phosphorylates as part of the biochemical steps of *mos*-induced MPF activation.

References

1. Hartwell LH, Weinert TA. Checkpoints: controls that ensure the order of cell cycle events. Science 1989;246:629–34.
2. Murray AW, Kirschner MW. Dominoes and clocks: the union of two views of the cell cycle. Science 1989;246:614–21.
3. Nurse P. Universal control mechanism regulating onset of M-phase. Nature 1990;344:503–8.

4. Kobayashi H, Minshull J, Ford C, Golsteyn R, Poon R, Hunt T. On the synthesis and destruction of A- and B-type cyclins during oogenesis and meiotic maturation in *Xenopus laevis*. J Cell Biol 1991;114:755–65.

5. Gautier J, Maller JL. Cyclin B in *Xenopus oocytes*: implications for the mechanism of pre-MPF activation. EMBO J 1991;10:177–82.

6. Minshull J, Murray A, Colman A, Hunt T. *Xenopus* oocyte maturation does not require new cyclin synthesis. J Cell Biol 1991;114:767–72.

7. Sagata N, Oskarsson M, Copeland T, Brumbaugh J, Vande WG. Function of c-mos proto-oncogene product in meiotic maturation in *Xenopus* oocytes. Nature 1988;335:519–25.

8. Sagata N, Watanabe N, Vande Woude GF, Ikawa Y. The c-mos proto-oncogene product is a cytostatic factor responsible for meiotic arrest in vertebrate eggs. Nature 1989;342:512–18.

9. Sagata N, Daar I, Oskarsson M, Showalter SD, Vande Woude GF. The product of the mos proto-oncogene as a candidate "initiator" for oocyte maturation. Science 1989;245:643–6.

10. Watanabe N, Vande Woude GF, Ikawa Y, Sagata N. Specific proteolysis of the c-mos proto-oncogene product by calpain on fertilization of *Xenopus* eggs. Nature 1989;342:505–11.

11. Maller JL. Interaction of steroids with the cyclic nucleotide system in amphibian oocytes. Adv Cyclic Nucleotide Res 1983;15:295–336.

12. Matten W, Daar I, Vande Woude GF. Protein kinase A acts at multiple points to inhibit *Xenopus* oocyte maturation. Mol Cell Biol 1994;14:4419–26.

13. Yew N, Mellini ML, Vande Woude GF. Meiotic initiation by the mos protein in *Xenopus*. Nature 1992;355:649–52.

14. Daar I, Paules RS, Vande Woude GF. A characterization of cytostatic factor activity from *Xenopus* eggs and c-mos-transformed cells. J Cell Biol 1991;114:329–35.

15. Kanki JP, Donoghue DJ. Progression from meiosis I to meiosis II in *Xenopus* oocytes requires de novo translation of the mos[xe] protooncogene. Proc Nat Acad Sci USA 1991;88:5794–8.

16. Furuno N, Nishizawa M, Okazaki K, Tanaka H, Iwashita J, Nakajo N, Ogawa Y, Sagata N. Suppression of DNA replication via mos function during meiotic divisions in *Xenopus* oocytes. EMBO J 1994;13:2399–410.

17. Masui Y, Markert CL. Cytoplasmic control of nuclear behavior during meiotic maturation of frog oocytes. J Exp Zool 1971;177:129–45.

18. Freeman RS, Meyer AN, Li J, Donoghue DJ. Phosphorylation of conserved serine residues does not regulate the ability of mos[xe] protein kinase to induce oocyte maturation or function as cytostatic factor. J Cell Biol 1992;116:725–35.

19. Blumer KJ, Johnson GL. Diversity in function and regulation of MAP kinase pathways. Trends Biochem Sci 1994;19:236–40.

20. Fabian JR, Morrison DK, Daar IO. Requirement for Raf and MAP kinase function during the meiotic maturation of *Xenopus* oocytes. J Cell Biol 1993;122:645–52.

21. Haccard O, Sarcevic B, Lewellyn A, Hartley R, Roy L, Izumi T, Erikson E, Maller JL. Induction of metaphase arrest in cleaving *Xenopus* embryos by MAP kinase. Science 1993;262:1262–5.

22. Posada J, Yew N, Ahn NG, Vande WG, Cooper JA. Mos stimulates MAP kinase in *Xenopus* oocytes and activates a MAP kinase kinase in vitro. Mol Cell Biol 1993;13:2546–53.

23. Al-Bagdadi F, Singh B, Arlinghaus RB. Evidence for involvement of the protein kinase C pathway in the activation of p37[v-mos] protein kinase. Oncogene 1990;5:1251–7.

24. Puls A, Proikas-Cezanne T, Marquardt B, Propst F, Stabel S. Kinase activities of c-mos and v-mos proteins: a single amino acid exchange is responsible for constitutive activation of the 124 v-mos kinase. Oncogene 1995;10:623–30.

25. Coleman TR, Dunphy WG. Cdc2 regulatory factors. Curr Opin Cell Biol 1994;6:877–82.

26. Gautier J, Matsukawa T, Nurse P, Maller J. Dephosphorylation and activation of *Xenopus* p34[cdc2] protein kinase during the cell cycle. Nature 1989;339:626–9.

27. Dunphy WG, Newport JW. Fission yeast p13 blocks mitotic activation and tyrosine dephosphorylation of the *Xenopus* cdc2 protein kinase. Cell 1989; 58:181–91.

28. Brown AJ, Jones T, Shuttleworth J. Expression and activity of p40[MO15], the catalytic subunit of cdk-activating kinase, during *Xenopus* oogenesis and embryogenesis. Mol Biol Cell 1994;5:921–32.

29. Izumi T, Walker DH, Maller JL. Periodic changes in phosphorylation of the *Xenopus* cdc25 phosphatase regulate its activity. Mol Biol Cell 1992;3:927–39.

30. Hannun YA. The sphingomyelin cycle and the second messenger function of ceramide. J Biol Chem 1994;269:3125–8.

31. Varnold RL, Smith LD. The role of protein kinase C in progesterone-induced maturation. In: Davidson EH, Roderman JV, Posakony JW, eds. Developmental Biology. New York: Wiley-Liss, 1990:1–7.

32. Strum J, Swenson KI, Turner JE, Bell R. Ceramide triggers meotic cell cycle in *Xenopus* oocytes. J Biol Chem 1995;270:1354–7.

Part II

Germ-Cell Differentiation

4

Establishment of Meiotic Germ-Cell Lines and Their Use to Study Spermatogenesis In Vitro

Marie-Claude Hofmann, Donara Abramian, Helge Weissig, Laura L. Richardson, and José Luis Millán

In vertebrates, the germ-cell lineage first arises in the early embryo as a small migratory population of cells, the primordial germ cells. These cells, first identified by their high content of alkaline phosphatase in the yolk sac, near the root of the developing allantois (1, 2), proliferate and migrate to the genital ridges where they will undergo gametogenesis. Once in the gonads these primordial germ cells or gonocytes undertake markedly different pathways in the female vs. the male gonad (3–7). In the male, gonocytes undergo mitotic arrest almost immediately after colonizing the fetal testis. These arrested gonocytes will restart mitosis during puberty to proliferate and differentiate through different stages of spermatogonia, and undergo meiosis I and II to generate spermatids that differentiate into spermatozoa through the process known as spermiogenesis. The molecular signals and genetic controls that cue spermatogonia to enter the meiotic pathway, rather than to continue proliferation, remain unclear, as do the regulatory mechanisms that oversee the progression of spermatocytes through the first and second meiotic divisions and spermatid differentiation. Thus, spermatogenesis presents us with an excellent developmental model system to ask questions aimed at understanding the cellular decision between proliferation and differentiation.

From the point of view of cancer biology, understanding the mechanisms of mitotic arrest of male primordial germ cells and the molecular control of meiosis is crucial to the elucidation of the pathogenesis of germ-cell tumors. The biology of germ-cell tumors lies at the crossroads of oncology and developmental biology. These tumors have a fascinating histology, showing striking similarities with tissues found during early embryogenesis. Testicular teratomas (8–10) and embryoid bodies derived from embryonal carcinoma cells (11) in vitro have been considered "caricatures" of normal embryonic development (12–15). While germ-cell tumors are rare in women, testicular germ-cell tumors make up approximately one third of all malignancies in men aged 15 to 45 years (16). The incidence of testicular germ-cell tumors has more than tripled since 1940 (17–19), affecting both seminomas and nonseminomas, suggesting that their pathogenesis is related and that they may originate from a common precursor. Most testicular germ cell tumors are preceded by the preinvasive stage of *carcinoma in situ* (CIS) (20–22). There is evidence indicating that CIS is a congenital condition arising early during fetal life (21). These data strongly suggest that these germ-cell tumors originate from gonocytes.

In vitro studies in the areas of mammalian spermatogenesis and germ-cell tumors have been hampered by the lack of suitable cell lines. Immortalized germ-cell lines and CIS or seminoma cell lines would be extremely useful for transfection experiments aimed at dissecting the regulatory regions of germ-cell–specific genes and in testing genes believed to affect the differentiation potential of the cells or their tumorigenicity. In this chapter we describe our progress toward the goal of establishing a transfectable system useful in the study of male gametogenesis.

Establishment of Germ Cell and Somatic Testicular Cell Lines Using the SV40 Large T Antigen as Immortalizing Molecule

In our initial attempt to establish testicular cell lines, we chose to use an oncogene with wide-range specificity and with proven immortalizing properties (23). The *simian virus 40 large T antigen* (SV40 LTAg) molecule is known to bind to wild-type p53, inactivating this cell cycle control gene, thus promoting the cells to enter S phase and become immortalized. Using the SV40 LTAg molecule as an immortalizing agent, we succeeded in establishing 47 cell lines representing the major cell types of a developing seminiferous tubule in the prepubertal 10-day-old mouse testis; 16 peritubular, 22 Leydig, 8 Sertoli, and 1 germ-cell line were established (24).

Immortalized peritubular cells were identified by their spindle-like appearance, high expression of alkaline phosphatase, and the expression of the intermediate filament desmin. These cells also produce high amounts of collagen. The immortalized Leydig cells are identifiable by the accumulation of lipid droplets in their cytoplasm and the production of the enzymes 3β-ol hydroxysteroid dehydrogenase. At least three Leydig cell lines (LFG6, LAB2, and LAH7) express *luteinizing hormone* (LH) receptors on their cell surface as determined by radioactive hormone binding assays. The expression, however, is not uniform in the cell population; rather, LH receptor–positive cells are found clustered in the cultures and represent 1% to 5% of the total cell population under defined culture conditions. None of the Leydig cell lines produces any detectable levels of testosterone. Nevertheless, considering that the primary cells used for immortalization were derived from prepubertal 10-day-old mouse testis, this is not a negative finding. The immortalized Sertoli cells are able to adopt the common in vivo columnar appearance when cultured at high density (25); they display a typical indented nucleus and cytoplasmic phagosomes as revealed by electron microscopy. At least three of the Sertoli cell lines (SC5, SE121, and SF7) express *follicle-stimulating hormone* (FSH) receptors on their cell surface. Perhaps more important, we were able to establish a germ-cell line, i.e., GC-1spg (*Germ Cell-1 s*permatogonia), that, based on electron microscopy and immunocytochemistry data, appears to have type B spermatogonia and primary spermatocyte characteristics. At the ultrastructural level the GC-1spg nuclei are large and contain numerous large clumps of chromatin similar to the B-type spermatogonia and preleptotene spermatocytes. This is the first described cell line to express the germ-cell markers cytochrome c_t isoform and the *lactate dehydrogenase* (LDH) C_4 isozyme (Table 4.1) specific for spermatocytes and later stages of spermatogenesis.

These initial results (24) were very encouraging and, as presented below, these cell lines are useful in transfection experiments. However, the GC-1spg cell line did not appear to differentiate further, and since GC-1spg cells are aneuploid with a modal number of 100 chromosomes, we surmised that a high LTAg expression might have promoted chromosomal instability, preventing further differentiation of this cell line.

TABLE 4.1. Characteristics of representative testicular cell lines.

Cell line	Cell type	tsp53	Meiosis	Markers
GC-1spg	Type B spermatogonia-spermatocyte-like	No	No	LDH-C_4, Cyt. C_t
GC-2spd(ts)	Spermatocyte/spermatid-like	Yes	Yes, 37°C and 32°C; no 39°C	LDH-C_4, Cyt. C_t Acrosomal antigen Haploid DNA
GC-3spc(ts)	Spermatocyte-like	Yes	No	LDH-C_4, Cyt. C_t
SF7, SC5, and SE121	Sertoli	No	No	FSH binding, phagosomes
PG3, PE8, and PE11	Peritubular/myoid	No	No	Desmin alkaline phosphatase
LFG6, LAB2, and LAH7	Leydig	No	No	LH binding, 3β-ol-DH

Establishment of Meiotic Germ-Cell Lines Using a Combination of SV40 Large T Antigen and Temperature-Sensitive p53 as Immortalization Strategy

To attempt to modulate the immortalizing properties of the SV40 LTAg and consequently increase the probability of establishing germ-cell lines able to differentiate in vitro, we decided to use the LTAg-binding properties of p53. It had been shown that an excess of *wild-type* (WT) p53 protein is able to abolish the proliferative function of LTAg when both molecules are expressed in precrisis mouse fibroblasts (26). A temperature-sensitive mutant of p53 exists (27), [Val^{135}]p53 (tsp53), that is inactive at the nonpermissive temperature of 39°C and remains in the cytoplasm of cells stably transfected with the mutant cDNA. At the permissive temperatures of 37°C or 32°C, the mutated tsp53 protein displays a WT conformation and is localized in the nucleus. Thus, if we were to immortalize primary germ cells with a combination of LTAg and tsp53, one would predict that at 39°C the LTAg would enable the immortalization of the cells, while tsp53 would remain inactive in the cytoplasm. If the immortalized cells were switched to 37°C or 32°C, tsp53 would adopt a functional conformation, display WT characteristics in the nucleus, and counteract the effects of LTAg, thereby enabling the cells to differentiate.

Using this strategy we have established two new germ cell lines (28), i.e., GC-2spd(ts) [*Germ Cell-2 spermatid (temperature-sensitive)*] and GC-3spc(ts)[*Germ Cell-3 spermatocyte (temperature sensitive)*], after transfecting primary germ cells enriched in preleptotene spermatocytes. At 39°C the cells in both lines appear large and spherical at low density, but they become spindle-like when confluent. The cells adhere to the tissue culture dishes and grow rapidly with a doubling time of 18 hours. As expected, the tsp53 protein is confined to the cytoplasm. At this temperature the LDH-C$_4$ and cytochrome c$_t$ isoform are expressed at low or undetectable levels, respectively (29, 30). At 37°C the cells grow more slowly, with a doubling time of 24 hours. The tsp53 protein is expressed in both the cytoplasm and the nucleus, and both LDH-C$_4$ and cytochrome c$_t$ expression are enhanced. The cells show signs of morphologic differentiation visible at the light microscopy level. Particularly in GC-2spd(ts), a large dense body appears at one pole of the nucleus, whereas the cell cytoplasm at the other pole becomes elongated. The dense body stains intensely with periodic acid-Schiff and exhibits immunocytochemical staining with a monoclonal antibody against the sperm acrosome antigen MSA-63 (31). Under electron microscopic examination, this cytoplasmic body is a large, membrane-bound granule adjacent to the nucleus and sustained by the Golgi apparatus. Multivesicular bodies and small vesicles are often associated with the dense granule. The collective morphologic features indicate that this body may be a developing acrosomic granule and that these cells have some

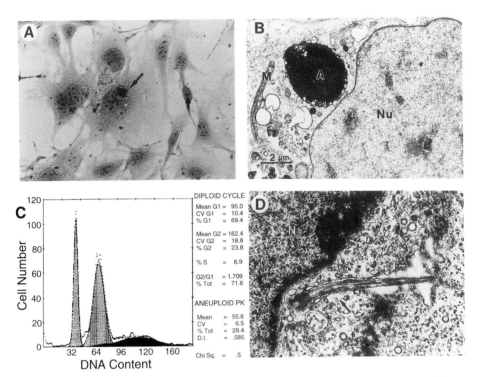

FIGURE 4.1. Morphological, immunohistochemical, and flow cytometric characteristics of the immortalized GC-2spd(ts) germ cell line. (*A*) Immunocytochemical staining of the acrosomal-like granule in a GC-2spd(ts) cell with the monoclonal antibody against MSA-63 acrosomal antigen (29). (*B*) Electron micrograph of a GC-2spd(ts) cell displaying the acrosomal-like granule (*A*), which is located adjacent to the nucleus (Nu) and appears to be derived from the Golgi apparatus. Mitochondria (M) were small round or elongated structures with distinct cristae and occasional vacuolation. (*C*) Flow cytometric analysis of the GC-2spd(ts) cell line grown at 37°C showing 28.4% of the total cell population as haploid cells. (*D*) Electron micrograph showing the initial stages of flagellar formation (arrow) in a spermatid-like cell. Axoneme microtubules extend from a centriole located adjacent to the nucleus.

characteristics of early spermatids (Fig. 4.1). Flow cytometric analysis of early generations (10th passage) of GC-2spd(ts) and GC-3spc(ts) cells cultured at 39°C and 37°C revealed a diploid and tetraploid DNA content. Upon cultivation of GC-2spd(ts) cells over 85 days at 37°C (17th passage), a third prominent haploid peak appeared that increased with time until it made up 28.4% of the cell population (30th passage). GC-3spc(ts) cells do not develop a haploid peak, and we are at this point in time uncertain as to the exact stage of immortalization of GC-3spc(ts). Chromosome spreading analysis for meiotic cells indicated a modal number of 20–21 chromosomes for the haploid stage in GC-2spd(ts). At 32°C cell proliferation slows down progressively in both the GC-2spd(ts) and GC-3spc(ts) lines, and the cells die after an average of 10 passages at this temperature. LDH-C$_4$ and cytochrome c$_t$ expression starts to increase after 2 to 3 passages (2 weeks of culture). The number of GC-2spd(ts) cells bearing the acrosomic-like granule increases from 3% at 37°C to 10% after 4 passages at 32°C. Moreover, by cultivating these cells further at 32°C in serum-free medium, at least 30% of the cells can produce this granule. Electron microscopic analysis of the GC-2spd(ts) cells at 32°C evidenced the development of a flagellar axoneme, providing additional evidence that a subset of these cells acquire characteristics of early spermatids.

To understand the kinetics of generation of the haploid and diploid GC-2spd(ts) cell populations in more detail, we separated the cells corresponding to the three DNA contents (n, 2n, 4n) (Fig. 4.2) by fluorescence-activated cell sorting (32). The haploid cell population consists of small cells of approximately 7–8 μm. The proportion of cells exhibiting a proacrosomic granule is increased from 3% in the original GC-2spd(ts) population to 45.2% in the isolated haploid fraction. This cell population consists of two subpopulations, one of adherent and the other of nonadherent cells. The adherent population is able to grow in tissue culture. After confluency, the adherent population shows an n-2n DNA cell cycle by flow cytometry (Fig. 4.2A) and the cells are LTAg and tsp53 positive. The nonadherent subpopulation, which also exhibits the acrosomic-like granule, dies within 24 hours of sorting. Semiquantitative flow cytometry analysis revealed that part of the haploid population expresses low amounts of LTAg and tsp53, while some cells are negative for both markers. These results suggest that when GC-2spd(ts) cells complete the reductive meiotic division, the integrated LTAg/tsp53 genes segregate. Cells of the sorted 2n DNA peak had an approximate diameter of 10 μm and were able to adhere rapidly in tissue culture. Flow cytometry analysis of this cell fraction revealed a diploid 2n-4n DNA cycle. Interestingly, this subpopulation of cells is able to regenerate a haploid peak that becomes visible after approximately 6 passages (Fig. 4.2B). All cells express the LTAg and tsp53 proteins. Cells with 4n DNA were also sorted and cultivated. These cells adhere rapidly and have an estimated diameter of 13–14 μm. Flow cytometry analysis revealed that they undergo a 2n-4n diploid cycle and are also able to regenerate a small haploid peak after 6 passages (Fig. 4.2C). Incorporation of bromodeoxyuridine into the S phase DNA of the total, although not synchronized, cell population shows clearly that the GC-2spd(ts) cell line consists of two cell populations undergoing overlapping but different cell cycles. One cell cycle is characterized by n/2n DNA peaks (haploid cycle), the other by 2n/4n DNA peaks (diploid cycle). Thus, the observed 2n DNA peak consists of cells in the G2 phase of the haploid cell cycle and of cells in the G1 phase of the diploid cell cycle. From the analysis of the number of chromosomes, however, it seems evident that some cells are also aneuploid

FIGURE 4.2. Flow cytometry analysis of the DNA content of sorted cells from the n, 2n, and 4n DNA populations of GC-2spd(ts), analyzed after 20 generations in culture. (A) n DNA cell population cycling through an n/2n DNA cell cycle. (B) The 2n DNA cell population reconstituting a n/2n/4n DNA pattern. (C) The 4n DNA cell population also reconstituting an n/2n/4n DNA pattern. Reprinted with permission from Hofmann et al. (32), © 1995, Wiley-Liss, Inc.

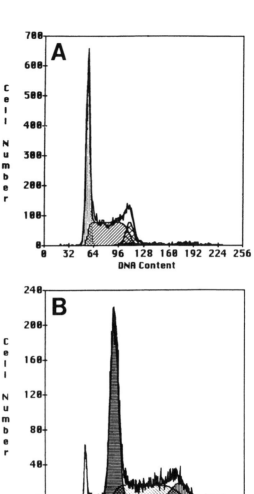

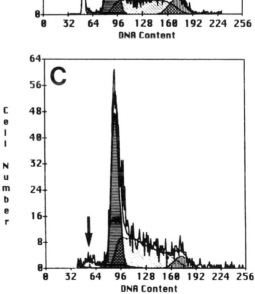

and may contain 50 to 70 chromosomes. This may be a side effect of the LTAg gene integration and activity, as reported in other studies (23, 33) and as observed in our GC-1spg cell line.

Our data and the above interpretation of our results are compatible with the following model for the cell cycle of GC-2spd(ts) in vitro (Fig. 4.3): At 37°C, a proportion of the diploid cells undergo the reductive meiotic division to form haploid cells with features of spermatids. Due to chromosomal segregation, some haploid cells inherit the LTAg/tsp53 transfected genes and are able to continue to cycle through a n/2n cell cycle. The other population of haploid cells, expressing very low levels of LTAg/tsp53 or none at all, have only a very limited life span in culture. Thus at 37°C a subpopulation of GC-2spd(ts) cells is constantly confronted with the possibility of reentering the diploid cell cycle or undergoing a reductive meiotic division. The GC-2spd(ts) cell line appears able to undergo meiosis in vitro without the interaction with Sertoli cells in culture. While the introduction of tsp53 simultaneously with LTAg was intended as a molecular trick to be able to control the proliferative effect of SV40 LTAg, this p53-mediated ability of the GC-2spd(ts) to differentiate in vitro may provide important clues as to the mechanism of induction of meiosis and the role that Sertoli cells may play in this decision. It is conceivable that one of the functions of Sertoli cells during spermatogenesis may be to initiate, through direct cell/cell contact or through paracrine factor(s), a cascade of events leading to the activation of p53 in germ cells, which enables them to complete meiosis. This GC-2spd(ts) cell line provides a valuable tool to study the molecular

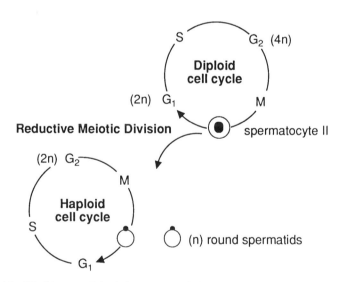

FIGURE 4.3. Working model of the GC-2spd(ts) cell cycle. Reprinted with permission from Hofmann et al. (32), © 1995, Wiley-Liss, Inc.

mechanisms involved in the cellular decision between self-renewal by mitosis and commitment to meiosis.

Use of Immortalized Testicular Cell Lines and Co-cultures to Improve the Survival of Primary Germ Cells, to Identify Paracrine Influences, and to Study Gene Regulation Using Transfection Experiments

A property of these immortalized somatic and germ-cell lines is their ability to associate and reconstitute two-dimensional tubule-like or cord-like structures (24). Tubule-like structures are formed when plating all four cell types in the relative proportions: Sertoli (16%), Leydig (16%), and peritubular (16%) cell lines together with, e.g., GC-1spg (50%) (Fig. 4.4A). GC-1spg cells always appear in the center of these formations together with some Sertoli cells. The spaces between the germ-cell islands are constituted exclusively by a mixture of the three somatic cell types. The particular localization and distribution of each cell type were identified by staining these structures with specific cyto- and immunocytochemical markers, such as desmin and alkaline phosphatase, as well as through experiments using the vital dye DiI to label individual cell types. Cord-like structures are formed by plating exclusively the somatic cell components and omitting GC-1spg (Fig. 4.4B). The cords are constituted by the Sertoli and peritubular cells, while the Leydig cells remain on the outside of the cords. These cord-like structures proved useful in maintaining freshly isolated primary pachytene spermatocytes alive for prolonged periods of time. Primary pachytene spermatocytes, isolated by the STAPUT procedure using unit gravity sedimentation, can be plated together with the Sertoli, peritubular, and Leydig cells. These primary germ cells become incorporated into the cords and remain viable for 10 to 15 days (Fig. 4.4C,D).

We have found evidence that paracrine influences from Leydig cells, peritubular cells, or both are required for the formation of three-dimensional cords. Leydig cells (LFG6, LAB2, or LAH7), peritubular cells (PE8), or a mixture of 50% Leydig and 50% peritubular cells were seeded at a total concentration of 5×10^5 cells/500 µl complete medium in each well of a 24-well plate. Twenty-four hours after seeding, a thin layer of 200 µl matrigel, diluted 1:1 with medium, was poured onto the bottom of cell culture inserts and solidified at 37°C for 1 h. The inserts were placed in the culture wells and Sertoli cells (SF7 or SC5), germ cells [GC-2spd(ts)], or a mixture of 50% Sertoli cells and 50% germ cells (total cells 5×10^5) were seeded on top of matrigel. The cells were cultivated for a maximum of 7 days. When tubules formed, they appeared after 3 days and grew well for another 4 days. As can be seen in Figure 4.5A, in the absence of LFG6/PE8-derived soluble factor(s), only three-dimensional aggregates form between SF7 and

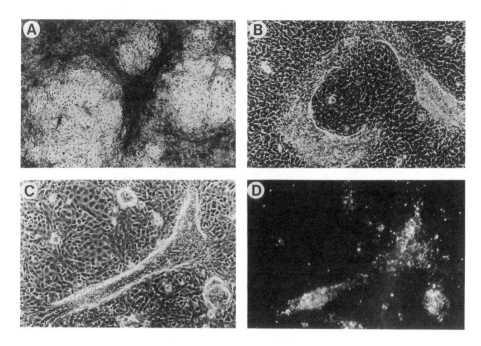

FIGURE 4.4. Typical cell aggregates formed in vitro. (*A*) Tubule-like structures formed by co-culturing a Leydig, a Sertoli, and a peritubular cell line with GC-1spg for 7 days. The Leydig and peritubular cells, both localized in the periphery of these structures, were stained for alkaline phosphatase activity to facilitate visualizing the structures. (*B*) Phase contrast micrograph of the cord-like structures formed by co-culturing only the immortalized Leydig, Sertoli, and peritubular cell lines in the absence of the germ-cell lines. (*C*) Phase contrast micrograph of cord-like structures obtained by co-culturing fluorescent-dye labeled primary pachytene spermatocytes and the immortalized Leydig, Sertoli, and peritubular cell lines. After 5 days of culture, cord-like structures appeared in which the pachytene spermatocytes were integrated. This micrograph was taken after 7 days in culture. (*D*) Same as *C*, but micrograph taken under fluorescent illumination.

GC-2spd(ts). However, in the presence of diffusible Leydig/peritubular cell-derived factor(s), large three-dimensional cords are formed (Fig. 4.5B). Immunocytochemical staining for LDH-C_4 through cross sections of these cords indicated that the germ cells were exclusively found in the center of these structures, while the negatively stained Sertoli cells formed the walls of the cords.

One strong motivation for initiating this work was the need to establish a transfectable system that could be used to analyze the structure of germ-cell–specific promoters. As demonstrated with the testis-specific *ldh-c* gene, the immortalized cell lines as well as primary germ cells in co-culture within the somatic cord-like structures can be used successfully for this purpose. The testis-specific isozyme of LDH-C_4 is present only in sperm (29) and in

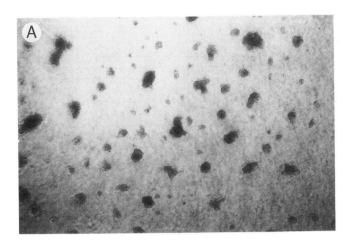

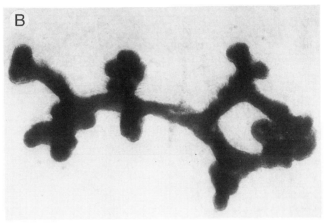

FIGURE 4.5. Co-cultures of a Sertoli cell line and GC-2spd(ts). (*A*) Co-cultures on Matrigel in the absence of soluble Leydig/peritubular cell factor(s). (*B*) Co-cultures on Matrigel in the presence of LFG6/PE8-derived soluble factor(s). Results after 7 days in culture.

the testis (34), where expression is restricted to the germinal epithelium, beginning in preleptotene spermatocytes and continuing through spermiogenesis (35). We have recently completed the cloning and characterization of the human ldh-c gene, including putative regulatory elements (36). The *ldh-c* genomic DNA upstream from exon I of the human gene is GC rich and contains no apparent TATA or CAAT-homologous sequences. A putative 180 bp regulatory 5′ sequence of the human *ldh-c* gene was inserted into a vector upstream from the LacZ reporter gene. As shown in Figure 4.6, the 180 bp *ldh-c* promoter construct was expressed very efficiently in GC-2spd(ts), followed by expression in GC-1spg and GC-3spc(ts), but showed undetectable expression in the somatic cell lines in agreement with

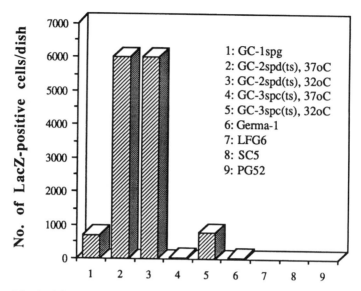

FIGURE 4.6. Activity of the *ldh-c* (180 bp)/LacZ promoter construct in immortalized germ cells and somatic cell lines. The immortalized Leydig (LFG6), Sertoli (SF7), peritubular (PG52) cell lines, the GC-1spg, GC-2spd(ts), and GC-3spc(ts) germ-cell lines, and the Germa-1 (42) human testicular cancer cell line were transfected with the *ldh-c*/LacZ construct, with an antisense negative control construct and with an SV40 promoter positive control construct. After cytochemical staining for β-galactosidase activity, the number of cells expressing the reporter protein from the *ldh-c* promoter was calculated as a percentage of the number of cells expressing β-galactosidase from the SV40 control promoter.

the in vivo expression of this gene. Expression of the *ldh-c* promoter was also demonstrated by transfecting freshly isolated primary pachytene spermatocytes maintained viable within cord-like structures formed by a combination of the somatic cell lines SF7, LFG6, and PG52. The entire cord-like structures could be transfected with control (Fig 4.7A) and test (Fig. 4.7B) promoters, providing a visual assessment of the restricted specificity of expression of the promoter in germ cells (36).

Use of the Immortalized Germ-Cell Lines to Identify Genes Expressed Differentially During Spermatogenesis

The availability of immortalized germ-cell lines able to undergo meiosis conditionally without the paracrine influence of Sertoli cells represents a particularly simple and useful system for the identification and characterization of molecules expressed differentially during spermatogenesis. Some of these molecules will very likely be involved in the important cellular choices of mitosis vs. meiosis and proliferation vs. differentiation. Experimental strategies suitable to ask these questions include resolving proteins from two cell types in two-dimensional polyacrylamide gel electrophoresis and cloning cDNAs from subtracted libraries or by subtractive hybridization. These techniques are time-consuming and technically demanding. Currently, the method of choice appears to be the *differential display–reverse transcriptase polymerase chain reaction* (DDRT-PCR) amplification of DNA (37–39). The method is based on comparisons of cDNA fragments

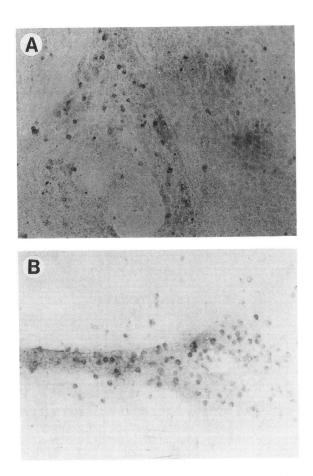

FIGURE 4.7. Activity of a *ldh-c*/LacZ promoter construct in primary pachytene spermatocytes cultured in cord-like structures in vitro. (*A*) Results of transfecting these structures with an SV40 promoter in front of LacZ as positive control. Positive β-galactosidase staining is seen in all the cell types in these structures. (*B*) Results of transfecting these structures with the *ldh-c*/LacZ construct. Positive staining is seen only in the primary pachytene spermatocytes integrated in the cord-like structures.

derived from two or more cell types on sequencing gels. By choosing suitable PCR primers, most *messenger RNAs* (mRNAs) can be displayed as 100- to 600-bp fragments. The differentially expressed bands can be identified visually upon autoradiography, cut out of the gels, subcloned, sequenced, and used for Northern blot analysis and to probe cDNA libraries to clone full-length transcripts.

We chose to optimize the DDRT-PCR approach using our germ cell lines GC-1spg, GC-2spd(ts), and GC-3spc(ts) grown at 39°C and 32°C (Fig. 4.8). The RT-PCR step was performed using RNA isolated from the germ-cell lines grown at the different temperatures and primers that were previously described (37). Thirty fragments, out of approximately 100 differentially expressed PCR bands, were sequenced (average length 270 bp; range 121 to 645 bp). By searching the nonredundant part of the GenBank database with the Blast-Algorithm (40), these cDNAs were classified as (i) sequences identical to known mouse genes, (ii) sequences homologous to but different from already cloned genes; and (iii) novel sequences without any similarity. Five of the 30 sequences were identical to mouse genes and four showed sequence similarity to known genes. Twenty-one of the cloned fragments have no homology to known genes. Table 4.2 gives some representative examples of the kinds of genes that were identified and cloned with this strategy.

While the DDRT-PCR technique is faster than subtraction libraries or subtractive hybridization to identify and clone molecules, it is critically

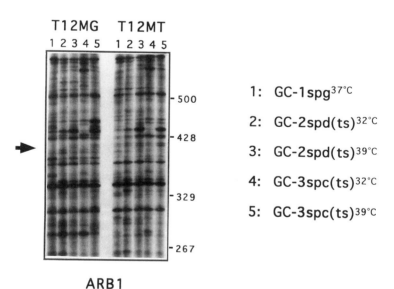

1: GC-1spg$^{37°C}$

2: GC-2spd(ts)$^{32°C}$

3: GC-2spd(ts)$^{39°C}$

4: GC-3spc(ts)$^{32°C}$

5: GC-3spc(ts)$^{39°C}$

FIGURE 4.8. Typical example of a DDRT-PCR experiment. Lane 1: GC-1spg. Lane 2: GC-2spd(ts) at 39°C. Lane 3: GC-2spd(ts) at 32°C. Lane 4: GC-3spc(ts) at 39°C. Lane 5: GC-3spc(ts) at 32°C. The arrow points to an example of a fragment present preferentially in GC-2spd(ts) at 39°C.

TABLE 4.2. Representative examples of the kinds of cDNA fragments isolated by use of the differential display polymerase chain reaction method.

Fragment	Homology found	Expression in testis			Remarks
		Diff.	Uni.	None	
1A1.26	None	•			Predominant in 14d testis; not in cell lines
1C1.26#21	None	•			Predominant in 14d; not in adult testis
1C1.26#22	3′ region of Ldh-A cDNA	•			Decreases during testis development
1C1.31#32	None	•			Increases during testis development
1C1.42#2	GTP-binding protein-related gene	•			Predominant in 14d testis
1C1.42#3	None			•	
2A1.19	None		•		
2A1.32	Zinc finger motif	•			Slightly increases during testis development
2A1.34	None			•	
2A1.48#10	None			•	
2C1.23	3′ region of cdc25M cDNA	•			Decreases during testis development
2C1.48#14	Transketolase LF1 mRNA		•		
2T1.10#6	None			•	
2T1.9/1	Repetitive sequence			•	
3A1.33#37	None			•	
4C1.24#26	Almost identical with human and bovine co-atomer proteins		•		

Data on the expression of these mRNA species by Northern blot analysis is indicated as differential (Diff.), uniform or ubiquitous (Uni.), and no expression found (None).

important to confirm by Northern blot analysis that the identified mRNAs are indeed expressed differentially. We have found that approximately 30% of the novel cDNA sequences without sequence similarity did not give a signal by Northern blot analysis. Nevertheless, we have also encountered differential expression and developmental regulation of cloned mRNAs, as will be illustrated by our identification and cloning of differentially expressed novel zinc finger proteins.

The fragment number 2A1.32 encodes a zinc finger protein (Table 4.2) that was isolated as a differentially displayed band present in GC-2spd(ts) cells at 32°C but not at 39°C or in any of the other germ-cell lines. Northern blot analysis using RNA extracted from mouse testis 7, 14, and 21 days after birth or from adult stages indicated that the expression of this zinc finger mRNA increased with age. In the process of cloning full-length cDNAs for this molecule we also isolated four additional novel zinc finger proteins and one cDNA identical to the previously described zpf-38 (41). All six mRNAs show differential patterns of expression during spermatogenesis, and the pattern is unique for each of the members of the family. This subfamily of zinc finger proteins is novel in that the predicted proteins show sequence similarity not only in the zinc finger motifs but also in the amino terminal region of the protein. The immortalized germ-cell lines should be useful in future experiments aimed at expressing these zinc finger proteins and performing functional studies to elucidate the role of these putative transcription factors during gametogenesis.

Conclusion

It should be clear from the results and studies presented in this overview that having access to immortalized germ-cell lines and somatic testicular cell lines will enable a number of experiments that are either very difficult or impossible to do with primary culture of testicular cells. It should also be clear that there are limitations and concerns with respect to other uses of this in vitro system. In particular, to what degree are the immortalized germ-cell lines able to re-create the complex genetic and structural changes that are characteristic of meiosis in vivo? And to what extent is the functional integrity of the paracrine signaling pathways between the different cell types preserved in the in vitro co-cultures? Some of these cells lines have been established permanently in culture by introducing into their genome a potent viral oncogene, SV40 LTAg, which was shown to cause chromosomal aberrations and aneuploidy in the cells. Other lines were immortalized by a combination of LTAg and tsp53 in an attempt to modulate the levels of active LTAg. However, this strategy was shown to cause disruptions in normal cell cycle regulation, well exemplified by the fact that a subpopulation of the GC2-spd(ts)–derived haploid cells can undergo an n/2n cell cycle. Nevertheless, once these limitations are understood, one can make positive use of this in vitro testicular cell system. In that light, we believe that the availability of these cells offers a powerful experimental tool that will help researchers progress faster toward the goal of understanding the molecular and cellular control of spermatogenesis.

Acknowledgments. This work was supported in part by grants CA42595, HD28384, and HD05863 from the National Institutes of Health. H.W. is supported by a DAAD HSP II/AUF graduate student scholarship. M.C.H. is supported by an institutional NIH training grant, and L.L.R. is supported by a NIH postdoctoral fellowship.

References

1. Chiquoine AD. The identification, origin, and migration of the primordial germ cells in the mouse embryo. Anat Rec 1954;118:135–46.
2. Ginsberg M, Snow MHL, McLaren A. Primordial germ cells in the mouse embryo during gastrulation. Development 1990;110:521–8.
3. Peters H. Migration of gonocytes into the mammalian gonad and their differentiation. Philos Trans R Soc Lond [Biol] 1970;259:91–101.
4. Donovan PJ, Stott D, Godin I, Heasman J, Wylie CC. Studies on the migration of mouse germ cells. J Cell Sci Suppl 1987;8:359–67.
5. Godin I, Wylie C, Heasman J. Genital ridges exert long-range effects on mouse primordial germ cell numbers and direction of migration in culture. Development 1990;108:357–63.
6. Gomperts M, Garcia-Castro M, Wylie C, Heasman J. Interactions between primordial germ cells play a role in their migration in mouse embryos. Development 1994;120:135–41.
7. Merchant-Larios H, Mendoza NM, Buehr M. The role of the mesonephros in cell differentiation and morphogenesis of the mouse fetal testis. Int J Dev Biol 1993;37:407–15.
8. Stevens LC. Experimental production of testicular teratomas in mice. Proc Natl Acad Sci USA 1964;52:654–61.
9. Stevens LC. Origin of testicular teratomas from primordial germ cells in mice. J Nat Cancer Inst 1967;38:549–52.
10. Stevens LC. Spontaneous and experimentally induced testicular teratomas in mice. Cell Differ 1984;15:69–74.
11. Evans M. Origin of mouse embryonal carcinoma cells and the possibility of their direct isolation into tissue culture. J Reprod Fertil 1981;62:625–31.
12. Mostofi FK. Tumour makers and pathology of testicular tumours. In: Kurth KH et al., eds. Progress and controversies in oncological urology. New York: A.R. Liss, 1984:69–87.
13. Mostofi FK, Sesterhenn IA, Davis CJJ. Immunopathology of germ cell tumors of the testis. Semin Diagn Pathol 1987;4:320–41.
14. Pierce GB, Abel MR. Embryonal carcinoma of the testis. Pathol Annu 1970;5:27.
15. Shevinsky LH, Knowles BB, Damjanov I, Solter D. Monoclonal antibody to murine embryos defines a stage-specific embryonic antigen expressed on mouse embryos and human teratocarcinoma cells. Cell 1982;30:697–705.
16. Pugh RCB. Combined tumours. In: Pugh RCB, ed. Pathology of the testis. Oxford: Blackwell, 1976:245–58.
17. Giwercman A, Muller J, Skakkebaek NE. Prevalence of carcinoma-in situ and other histopathological abnormalities in testes from 399 men who died suddenly and unexpectedly. J Urol 1991;145:77–80.
18. Giwercman A, Von der Maase H, Skakkebaek NE. Epidemiological and clinical aspects of carcinoma in situ of the testis. Eur Urol 1993;23:104–14.
19. Giwercman A, Skakkebaek NE. Carcinoma in situ of the testis: biology, screening and management. Eur Urol 1993;23:19–21.
20. Skakkebaek NE. Possible carcinoma-in-situ of the testis. Lancet 1972;2:515–7.
21. Skakkebaek NE, Berthelsen JG, Giwercman A, Muller J. Carcinoma-in-situ of the testis: possible origin from gonocytes and precursor from all types of germ

cell tumors except spermatocytoma. Int J Androl 1987;10:19–28.

22. Nistal M, Codesal J, Paniagua R. Carcinoma in situ of the testis in infertile men. A histological, immunocytochemical, and cytophotometric study of DNA content. J Pathol 1989;159:205–10.

23. Chang PL, Gunby JL, Tomkins DJ, Mak I, Rosa NE, Mak S. Transformation of human cultured fibroblasts with plasmids carrying dominant selection markers and immortalizing potential. Exp Cell Res 1986;167:407–16.

24. Hofmann MC, Narisawa S, Hess RA, Millán JL. Immortalization of germ cells and somatic testicular cells using the SV40 Large T antigen. Exp Cell Res 1992;201:417–35.

25. Djakiew D, Dym M. Pachytene spermatocyte proteins influence Sertoli cell function. Biol Reprod 1988;39:1193–205.

26. Fukasawa K, Sakoulas G, Pollack RE, Chen S. Excess wild-type p53 blocks initiation and maintenance of simian virus 40 transformation. Mol Cell Biol 1991;11:3472–83.

27. Michalovitz D, Halevy O, Oren M. Conditional inhibition of transformation and of cell proliferation by a temperature-sensitive mutant of p53. Cell 1990;62:671–80.

28. Hofmann MC, Hess RA, Goldberg E, Millán JL. Immortalized germ cells undergo meiosis in vitro. Proc Natl Acad Sci USA 1994;91:5533–7.

29. Goldberg E. Lactic and malic dehydrogenases in human spermatozoa. Science 1963;139:602–3.

30. Wheat TE, Hintz M, Goldberg E, Margoliash E. Analyses of stage-specific multiple forms of lactate dehydrogenase and of cytochrome c during spermatogenesis in the mouse. Differentiation 1977;9:37–41.

31. Liu M-S, Aebersold R, Fann C-H, Lee C-YG. Molecular and developmental studies of a sperm acrosome antigen recognized by HS-63 monoclonal antibody. Biol Reprod 1992;46:937–48.

32. Hofmann M-C, Abramian D, Millán JL. A hyploid and a diploid cell cycle coexist in an in vitro immortalized spermatogenic cell line. Dev Genetics 1995;16:119–27.

33. MacDonald C, Watts P, Stuart B, Kreuzburg-Duffy U, Scott DM, Kinne RKH. Studies on the phenotype and karyotype of immortalized rabbit kidney epithelial cell lines. Exp Cell Res 1991;195:458–61.

34. Blanco A, Zinkham WH. Lactate dehydrogenases in human testes. Science 1963;139:601–2.

35. Thomas K, Del Mazo J, Eversole P, Bellvé A, Hiraoka Y, Li SS-L, Simon M. Developmental regulation of expression of the lactate dehydrogenase (LDH) multigene family during mouse spermatogenesis. Development 1990;109:483–93.

36. Cooker LA, Brooke CD, Kumari M, Hofmann M-C, Millán JL, Goldberg E. Genomic structure and promoter activity of the human testis lactate dehydrogenase gene. Biol Reprod 1993;48:1309–19.

37. Bauer D, Mueller H, Reich J, Riedel H, Ahrenkiel V, Warthoe P, Strauss M. Identification of differentially expressed mRNA species by an improved display technique (DDRT-PCR). Nucleic Acids Res 1993;21:4272–80.

38. Liang P, Pardee AB. Differential display of eukaryotic messenger RNA by means of the polymerase chain reaction. Science 1992;257:967–71.

39. Sager R, Anisowicz A, Neveu M, Liang P, Sotiropoulou G. Identification by differential display of alpha 6 integrin as a candidate tumor suppressor gene.

FASEB J 1993;7:964–70.

40. Altschul SF, Gish W, Miller W, Myers EW, Lipman DJ. Basic local alignment search tool. J Mol Biol 1990;215:403–10.

41. Noce T, Fujiwara Y, Sezaki M, Fujimoto H, Higashinakagawa T. Expression of a mouse zinc finger protein gene in both spermatocytes and oocytes during meiosis. Dev Biol 1992;153:356–67.

42. Hofmann MC, Jeltsch W, Brecher J, Walt H. Alkaline phosphatase isoenzymes in human testicular germ cell tumors, their precancerous stages and three related cell lines. Cancer Res 1989;49:4696–700.

5

Mouse Spermatocyte Chromosome Cores: Protein and DNA Organization

Peter B. Moens

The results of observational and biochemical studies of meiotic chromosomes prior to 1984 have been summarized in the review of von Wettstein and colleagues (1). That date is also roughly the beginning of more extensive molecular approaches to the cytology of meiosis and meiotic chromosomes. In 1985 and 1986, Heyting et al. (2, 3) achieved a breakthrough in this field by succeeding in the production of meiosis-specific *monoclonal antibodies* (MAbs) against a variety of meiotic chromosome core proteins in the rat. This had been attempted by a number of investigators but had failed at the first necessary step of the procedure, that is, the isolation of large amounts of purified *synaptonemal complexes* (SC) (paired chromosome cores of pachytene chromosomes).

The Heyting antibodies opened the door for the identification of genes and gene products of chromosome core and pairing gene products by the screening of spermatocyte expression libraries. In a number of laboratories, the genes or portions of SC genes were cloned in expression vectors and fusion proteins raised in bacterial hosts for the production of antibodies against meiotic chromosome proteins. These are among the tools that are now being used for the dissection of chromosome structure and function at meiosis. Immunofluorescent detection of chromosome proteins in combination with fluorescent in situ hybridization of chromatin domains has been used to detect the associations between the proteinaceous chromosome components, and the DNA. This method is called *simultaneous antigen and sequence* (SAS) detection.

In an alternative approach, the genetic source of observed meiotic abnormalities was determined and the meiotic function of the gene products was resolved where possible. This methodology has been applied most successfully in the yeast *Saccharomyces cerevisiae*. The abundant information derived from that system would require a separate review and is not included here.

Phylogenetic Aspects

Meiosis-specific genes and gene products have revealed an unexpected amount of phylogenetic variation. This is surprising because superficially, meiotic functions and structures appear quite similar. The cores and the SC of meiotic chromosomes look remarkably comparable in protist, fungi, plants, and animals. This has led to the view that the SCs are highly conserved components of the sexual reproductive process. However, from informal discussions with SC investigators, it is clear that attempts to find homologous SC genes among major phylogenetic groups—fungi, plants, invertebrates, and vertebrates—have not met with much success. In my own experience, MAbs against rat SCs cross-react poorly with mouse SCs. This is unexpected, since the DNA sequences differ little, 93% identity, and the amino acid sequence even less, 98% identity (see GenBank, SCP1, Syn1). The reduction in epitope recognition suggests that even though the sequences are similar, the folding patterns and protein-protein associations may have subtle differences that differentially obscure or expose epitopes in the two species.

Polyclonal antibodies are, as expected, less selective. SCs from most mammals are recognized by polyclonal anti-hamster or anti-rat SC antibodies. The reaction is much reduced for bird SCs and is weak at best for amphibian (frog) SCs. We have seen no cross-reaction with invertebrates, plants, or fungi. Along the same lines, a polyclonal anti-hamster SC antibody recognizes an SC protein of 30 kd in the hamster, but a protein of different mass (54 kd) in rat spermatocytes. Similarly, an anti-SC antibody that recognizes one component of a rat SC recognizes a different component of the mouse SC. This then casts doubt on the idea that meiotic chromosome cores and SCs are evolutionarily conserved. Instead, core and synaptic proteins appear evolutionarily flexible, possibly responding to selective demands for low or high levels of recombination or for localization of pairing and recombinant events. In the extreme, it might be considered that meiotic mechanisms arose independently in phylogenetic lineages and that convergent requirements generated similar functions and structures.

Meiotic Chromosome Behavior, Immunocytology

The behavior of chromosomes during meiotic prophase can be monitored in part with fluorescent detection of antibodies against chromosomal components such as centromeres, chromosome cores, pairing proteins, and histones. In mouse, which has all telocentric chromosomes, the 40 centromeres are attached to the nuclear envelope, frequently in one region of the nuclear envelope (Fig. 5.1A). When the core proteins and the centromeres are visualized simultaneously, it can be seen that the cores develop at the individual centromeres and in the interior of the nucleus. The synaptic protein is detected at later stages in places where cores have initiated synapsis. Observation at this stage gives evidence that initiation

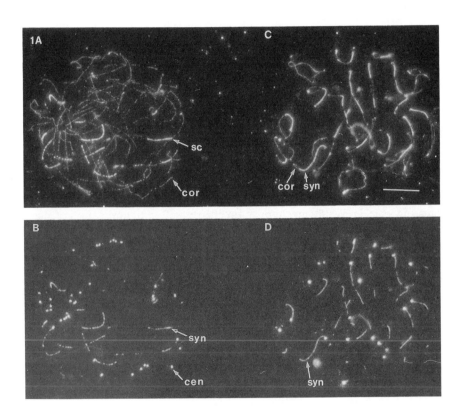

FIGURE 5.1. Immune staining of mouse spermatocyte zygotene (*A* and *B*) and at the chromosome separation stage, diplotene (*C* and *D*). In *A* and *C*, the Cor1 protein of the unpaired cores (cor) and the Syn1 protein in the paired regions (syn) are recognized by a rabbit polyclonal antibody against SCs. The secondary antibody is goat anti-rabbit conjugated to biotin followed by avidin *fluorescein isothiocyanate* (FITC). In *B* and *D*, only the Syn1 protein in the paired regions is detected by a mouse anti-Syn1 fusion protein (syn), and the centromeres (cen) by a CREST serum. The secondary antibodies are rhodamine-conjugated. In the mouse, the 40 centromeres also mark the proximal telomeres. At issue is the fact that at zygotene (*A*, *B*), chromosome pairing (sc, syn) is *not* initiated at the telomeres (*cen*). In *C* and *D* the departure of Syn1 protein from the SCs is coincident with the separation of chromosome cores at the diplotene stage of meiotic prophase. Scale bar = 10 µm.

of synapsis is not necessarily at the telomeres (Fig. 5.1A,B). This is also known from electron microscopy of serially sectioned spermatocytes but apparently needs affirmation in the view of authoritative hypotheses on the role of telomeres in meiotic chromosome pairing (4).

Synapsis of cores is rapid, so that long stretches of SCs exist concurrently with largely unpaired cores (Fig. 5.1A,B). There is evidence that SC extension need not be homologous and may thereby prevent reciprocal recombination in the vicinity of homologous pairing initiation sites. This speculation is somewhat supported by the reduction of genetic interference when SCs fail to form (5–8), but the issue of interference is a complex one that has not been resolved (9).

When the synaptic protein Syn1 dissociates from the SC, the cores of homologues can be observed to separate (Fig. 5.1C,D). When fully separated (Fig. 5.2), points of convergence correspond to the chiasmata of classical cytogenetics. Presumably non-sister chromatids cross over at those chiasma sites. Because the chromatids are still anchored to their core (see below), the chiasmata are immobilized until some later time when the anchorage is terminated, possibly by modification of the core proteins.

Immunofluorescence observations on first metaphase of meiosis show that core protein accumulates at the pairs of sister centromeres (Fig. 5.3). This suggests a possible mechanism for the reductional segregation of sister centromeres at metaphase I. Because the core protein seems to be a factor in the anchorage of sister chromatids throughout meiotic prophase, it seems reasonable to assume that it continues in that function for the sister centromeres. The disjunctional function of core protein is supported by the observation that it dissociates from the centromeres at the second meiotic division, which is the time that the sister centromeres separate from each other.

Chromatin Organization of Meiotic Prophase Chromosomes

The organization of chromatin loops in relation to the meiotic chromosome core is apparent from electron microscopy of surface-spread meiotic prophase chromosomes (10–12). To observe the details of the loop structures, we have "painted" specific DNA sequences by in situ hybridization and simultaneously visualized the chromosome cores with immunofluorescence—the SAS procedure. Major satellites were found to be attached to the SC in bouquets of loops the size of the average chromatin domain of the pachytene chromosomes. The minor satellite and the telomere sequences, on the other hand, are condensed at the synaptonemal complex, forming only short loops at best (12).

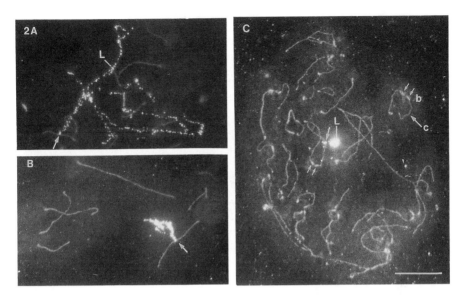

FIGURE 5.2. Evidence for continued DNA attachment to the chromosome cores at late prophase of meiosis. (A) At the early pachytene stage, the end of the 1.8-Mb λ insert (L) is attached to the SC (arrow). (B) At later pachytene stages, the insert is more condensed and still has a single attachment site to the SC (arrow). (C) At this stage, the chromosomes of the bivalents (e.g., b) have separated except for points of exchanges between non-sister chromatids, the chiasmata. The figure shows that the chromosomes still have axial cores (c) and that the DNA, exemplified here by the 1.8-Mb λ insert (L), is still attached to its core (large arrow). The core with attached DNA provides a mechanism for the hypothesized chromatid cohesion, which is necessary for chiasma maintenance and proper chromosome disjunction. The λ insert is visualized with FISH, the cores with immunofluorescence, and the DNA with propidium iodide. This mouse was heterozygous for the insert. Thus there is a single signal and the insert is attached to only one of the two cores of bivalent #4. Centromeres are marked with small arrows. Scale bar = 10 μm.

To determine the organization of a single loop relative to the SC, ideally only a single loop should be painted, but this is difficult to realize. The in situ technique requires the suppression of signals from repeated sequences and as a result the continuity of a given loop is lost, showing only an array of spotty signals that are presumably the unique sequences. However, the presence of a stably integrated foreign sequence permits visualization of the entire insert without interruptions from suppressed sequences. From a 1.8-Mb insert of 40 head-to-tail phage λ genomes, it is clear that there is a specific mode of attachment to the chromosome core (13). Hundreds of observed inserts all end exactly at the SC (Fig. 5.2), presumably anchored there by mouse sequences that flank the λ insert. It is tempting to speculate that the nucleus detects the excessively long λ loop (Fig. 5.2A) and uses the first available appropriate mouse sequence to form an SC attachment. This may not explain all aspects of the normal regulation of loop sizes, but suggests that at least one of the several interacting mechanisms may be the sensing of loop size.

Fortuitously, SAS reveals an anticipated but as yet unproven aspect of chromosome function at meiosis. Without going into the long-standing debate about the nature of chiasmata (reciprocal crossovers between non-sister chromatids), it suffices to cite the general opinion that chromosome cores to either side of the chiasma function in holding the chiasma in place, thereby promoting proper disjunction of chromosomes at first anaphase of meiosis. This hypothesis is predicated on the assumption that there are chromosome cores at the diplotene stage and that the chromatids are still attached to the cores when homologous chromosomes separate at diplotene and metaphase I. With SAS, we have been able to show that the core proteins are axial to the chromosomes at those later prophase stages and the DNA is still attached to the core, as demonstrated by the attachment of the λ insert to the core (Fig. 5.2A) (13).

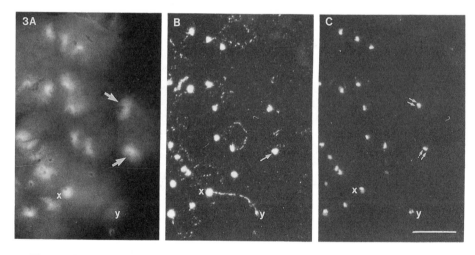

FIGURE 5.3. Evidence for the association of Cor1 protein with pairs of sister centromeres at metaphase I. (A) The large arrows mark the centromeric heterochromatin of a bivalent. (B) The arrows mark the Cor1 protein, which is concentrated at the centromeres. There also remain small amounts of Cor1 protein axial to the chromosomes, particularly in the X-Y bivalent (x, y). (C) Embedded in the Cor1 protein are the pairs of sister centromeres (small arrows). This observation suggests that the reductional division of sister chromatids may be regulated by the Cor1 protein. In A the DNA is stained with DAPI; B is immunostained for Cor1 protein, and C is immunostained with CREST serum for centromeres. Scale bar = 10 μm.

Future Avenues

The expectations for the future of this type of research are numerous. It seems unlikely that the repertoire of meiotic chromosome proteins has been exhausted. With the available genes and gene products it may be possible to screen cDNA libraries for additional proteins by in vivo two-hybrid or in vitro systems. One hopes the interaction of the proteins with each other and with the associated DNA will be clarified. The modifications of SC proteins at various stages of meiotic prophase should reveal more about their functions. Attempts are under way to do knockouts of SC genes in the mouse. Major progress should be made in the identification of plant meiotic chromosome proteins where only one is reported so far. The numerous meiotic mutants in plants may provide a handle on the characterization of responsible genes, gene products, and SC functions. Still no SC proteins have been reported in insects, or *Caenorhabditis elegans*, where the genetics and molecular biology can give access to the functions of the SCs. The area of research that is far ahead in this work at present is the analysis of structure-function of meiotic chromosomes in *Saccharomyces cerevisiae*. The results will continue to serve as a model for function in other organisms.

Acknowledgments. The research done at York University is financially supported by NSERC and MRC of Canada to P.B.M.

The results discussed here were obtained with the kind assistance and collaboration of Melanie Dobson, John Heddle, Henry Heng, Christa Heyting, Ron Pearlman, Emanuel Rosonina, Xiao-Mei Shi, and Barbara Spyropoulos. For the contents of this discussion, however, I am responsible.

References

1. von Wettstein D, Rasmussen SW, Holm PB. The synaptonemal complex in genetic segregation. Annu Rev Genet 1984; 18:331–431.
2. Heyting C, Dietrich AJJ, Redeker EJW, Vink ACG. Structure and composition of the synaptonemal complexes, isolated from rat spermatocytes. Eur J Cell Biol 1985;36:307–14.
3. Heyting C, Moens PB, van Raamsdonk W, Dietrich AJJ, Vink ACG, Redeker EJW. Identification of the lateral elements of synaptonemal complexes of the rat. Eur J Cell Biol 1987;43:148–54.
4. Sen D, Gilbert W. Formation of parallel four-stranded complexes by guanine-rich motifs in DNA and its implications for meiosis. Nature 1988;334:364–6.
5. Moens PB. Molecular perspectives of chromosome pairing at meiosis. Bioessays 1993;16:101–6.
6. Sym M, Roeder GS. Crossover interference is abolished in the absence of a synaptonemal complex protein. Cell 1994;79:283–92.

7. Kohli J, Bahler J. Homologous recombination in fission yeast: absence of cross-over interference and synaptonemal complex. Experientia 1994;50:295–306.
8. Munz P. An analysis of interference in the yeast *Schizosaccaromyces pombe*. Genetics 1994;137:701–7.
9. Stahl FW, Lande R. Estimating interference and linkage map distance from two-factor tetrad data. Genetics 1995;139:1449–54.
10. Rattner JB, Goldsmith MR, Hamkalo BA. Chromosome organization during male meiosis in Bombyx mori. Chromosoma 1981;82:341–51.
11. Weith A, Traut W. Synaptonemal complexes with associated chromatin in a moth, Ephistia kuehniella Z. Chromosoma 1980;78:275–91.
12. Moens PB, Pearlman RE. Chromatin organization at meiosis. Bioessays 1988;9:151–3.
13. Heng HHQ, Tsui L-C, Moens PB. Organization of heterologous DNA inserts on the mouse meiotic chromosome core. Chromosoma 1994;103:401–7.

6

CREMτ Activates the Spermatid-Specific RT7 and Mouse Protamine 1 Promoters

JESSICA H. OOSTERHUIS AND FRANS A. VAN DER HOORN

The differentiation of round spermatids to spermatozoa is accompanied by extensive changes in gene expression. A distinct set of genes is exclusively transcribed in round spermatids at high levels and encodes a number of chromosomal proteins involved in nuclear condensation, a set of proteins involved in acrosome formation and formation of sperm tails, and testis-specific isoforms of various enzymes. The switch in gene expression that accompanies the transition from spermatocytes to spermatids results mainly from changes in transcription (1), although RNA processing (2) and translational control (3) are also implicated in some instances. Evidence for the importance of transcriptional control comes from transgenic mouse experiments, which show that a number of spermatid-specific promoters (mP1, mP2, tACE, RT7) confer correct spatial and temporal expression onto reporter genes (4–7). Examination of promoter sequences suggest that various small sequences are conserved among spermatid-specific promoters (8). One of these resembles the *adenosine 3':5'-cyclic monophosphate (cAMP) response element* (CRE) and is found in approximately the same relative position in these promoters (9). CRE elements interact with members of the CREB and CREM families of transcription factors. The CREM gene encodes several nuclear factors that differ as a result of differential splicing, differential polyadenylation, and alternative translation start sites (10, 11). It was shown that most cells produce CREM isoforms that antagonize transcription because they contain the DNA binding domain but lack transactivating domains (12). In the testis differential polyadenylation and splicing lead to production of the antagonists in somatic cells and in germ cells up to and including spermatocytes. Spermatids express the strong positive transactivator CREMτ (13), translated from a *messenger RNA* (mRNA) that has increased stability due to the use of an alternative polyadenylation site (11). We recently showed that nuclear

CREMτ binds to the RT7 promoter (14). RT7 encodes a 27-kd spermatid-specific protein that localizes to sperm tails (15). Various lines of evidence strongly suggest that RT7 encodes the major, 27-kd, outer dense fiber protein (15–17). The RT7 promoter harbors two testis-specific nuclear factor binding sites: one at −120, which interacts with TTF-D, and one at −50, which resembles the CRE and can bind CREMτ (18). The RT7 promoter drives expression of the lacZ and c-*mos* reporter genes in transgenic mice in spermatids, but not in spermatocytes or any other tissue or organ examined (7). Thus, integrated copies of RT7-lacZ are transcriptionally silent. Transient co-transfections of CREMτ expression plasmids and a vector containing a dimer of the RT7 CRE linked to a minimal tk promoter and the CAT reporter gene show that CREMτ can transactivate nonintegrated copies of the RT7 promoter sequence in a *protein kinase A* (PKA)-dependent fashion (14). However, this situation is not directly comparable to that in RT7-lacZ transgenic spermatids, where transgenes are stably integrated in low copy number (the copy number during transient transfections is estimated in the thousands in positively transfected cells) and subject to regulation by chromatin structure. We therefore set out to reproduce the transgenic situation in stable transfections to show that CREMτ can transactivate integrated, silent copies of RT7-lacZ. In addition, we investigated whether a bacterially produced GST-CREMτ fusion gene can bind the RT7 CRE and whether CREMτ present in nuclear extracts prepared from seminiferous tubules activates the RT7 and mP1 promoters.

Procedures

Bacterial GST-CREMτ Protein

To express GST-CREMτ in bacteria, the CREMτ coding region was produced by *polymerase chain reaction* (PCR) using the pBS-CREMτ plasmid (12) and primers that introduced BamHI and XbaI sites. BamHI-XbaI–restricted products were ligated in restricted pGEX-KG plasmid DNA generating pGEX-CREMτ. This vector was introduced in XL1-Blue bacteria. Crude bacterial extracts were prepared after induction by *isopropylthiogalactoside* (IPTG), and GST-CREMτ was denatured and renatured (19). GST-CREMτ was purified using glutathione-agarose beads (Sigma) as described (20). Phosphorylation of GST-CREMτ was done using 1 μg/ml PKA (gift of Dr. M. Walsh) and 0.1 mM [^{32}P-γ] *adenosine triphosphate* (ATP) in 20 mM Tris.HCl, pH 7.4, 1 mM *ethyleneglycoltetraacetic acid* (EGTA), 5 mM MgCl$_2$, 10 nM okadaic acid. Proteins were analyzed on 10% SDS-polyacrylamide gels by staining with Coomassie Blue or by autoradiography.

Gel Retardation Assays

Gel retardation assays were carried out as described above (21) using double-strand oligonucleotides RT7-CREM (5' AATTGGGTGAGTCAC 3') and SMS-8 (5' GATCCTTGGCTGACGTCAGAGAGAG 3') end-labeled with Klenow DNA polymerase. Reaction mixtures contained 1 ng probe, 1 μg poly(dI-dC)(dI-dC), GST-CREMτ. In indicated cases GST-CREMτ was incubated with PKA in 20 mM Tris.HCl, pH 7.4, 1 mM EGTA, 5 mM MgCl$_2$, 10 nM okadaic acid, 0.1 mM ATP. In some experiments 400 ng of oligonucleotides RT7-CREM, SMS-8, or ΔT (5' AATTACAGAACACAA 3') was added as competitor. Reaction products were separated on 6% nondenaturing polyacrylamide gels and visualized by autoradiography.

In Vitro Transcription

Nuclear extracts were prepared from isolated rat *seminiferous tubules* (ST) as described previously (18). Protein concentrations of ST extracts range from 5 to 10 μg/μl. Transcription reactions were carried out for 45 min at 30°C as described (18), using approximately 40 μg protein, 1 μg pRT7-CAP0.2, which contains a 0.16-kb RT7 promoter fragment linked to a 390-bp G-free cassette (18), and 0.1 μg pAdMLP, which contains the *adenovirus major late promoter* fragment linked to a 190 bp G-free cassette. Reaction products were analyzed on 6% urea-polyacrylamide gels. In indicated instances 100 ng of competitor oligonucleotides were added representing the RT7-CREM (5' AATTGGGTGAGGTCAC 3') or somatostatin CRE SMS-8 (5' GATCCTTGGCTGACGTCAGAGAGAG 3').

Cell Lines and Transfections

C3H10T½ cells were transfected with plasmids pRT7-lacZ, which had been used to generate transgenic mice previously (7), and pRSV-neo by the calcium-phosphate co-precipitation method as described before (22). Twenty-four hours after transfection, cells were split 1:5 and grown in DMEM/10% newborn calf serum supplemented with 150 μg/ml G418. After 3 weeks colonies were individually trypsinized and propagated in medium containing G418. Derived cell lines were analyzed by PCR for the presence of the RT7-lacZ DNA. RT7-lacZ DNA-positive cell lines were frozen and later used in transfection assays. None of these cell lines expressed detectable β-galactosidase activity.

C3H-RT7-lacZ cells were transfected transiently with pSVCREMτ (gift of Dr. Sassone-Corsi), which contains the SV40 early promoter linked to the CREMτ coding region, or with pMT1a-CREMτ, which contains the sheep metallothionein 1a promoter (23) linked to the CREMτ coding region. Forty-eight to sixty hours after transfection, β-galactosidase activity was measured in cell-free extracts derived from the transfected cells as described (24). In the case of the MT1a promoter transfected cells were grown with or without 75 μM ZnSO₄.

Results and Discussion

Phosphorylated GST-CREMτ Fusion Protein Binds to the RT7 Promoter

The RT7 promoter contains a CRE and binds a testis-specific nuclear factor that may be identical to CREMτ (14). CREMτ is a strong, spermatid-specific transactivator encoded by the CREM gene (12). By differential splicing and use of alternative translation starts, this gene produces a complex array of CREM-like proteins, several of which (CREM-α,-β, -γ, and S) are antagonists of CRE-mediated transactivation (11). These forms, which are present in somatic cells and in premeiotic male germ cells, lack the glutamine-rich transactivation domains. However, the predominant species produced in spermatids is CREMτ, which is a strong, positive transactivator (12). To obtain CREMτ protein for RT7 promoter-protein interaction studies, we chose the GST expression system to produce GST-CREMτ fusion protein. The CREMτ coding region DNA was produced by PCR and linked to the GST portion present in vector pGEX-KG. XL1-Blue bacteria were transformed with this construct and produced the 67-kd GST-CREMτ protein after induction with IPTG (Fig. 6.1, lanes *c* and *d*). Using gel retardation assays we show in Figure 6.1 that the unmodified GST-CREMτ protein, but not GST (lane *n*), binds to either the RT7 CRE (lane *o*) or the somatostatin CRE (lane *g*). The formation of these complexes is efficiently competed by somatostatin CRE oligonucleotides (lanes *j*, *k*, and *p*) but not by the ΔT oligonucleotide, which contains a CRE-half site (lanes *l* and *q*). Unrelated oligonucleotides did not compete either, as was expected (not shown). Next we used PKA to phosphorylate the GST-CREMτ protein; previous results had demonstrated that CREMτ is a target for nuclear PKA in spermatids (25). Figure 6.1 shows that GST-CREMτ protein (lane *f*), but not GST (lane *e*), is efficiently phosphorylated by PKA in vitro. Binding of GST-CREMτ to the CRE is enhanced by phosphorylation, as evidenced by increased amounts of retarded complex (compare lanes *t* and *v*). Phosphorylation of GST has no effect on binding (lanes *s* and *u*). Thus the interaction of GST-CREMτ protein with the RT7 CRE is specific and efficient.

We next investigated the potential of CREMτ protein to activate the RT7 and *mouse protamine 1* (mP1) promoters in vitro. The RT7 promoter is active in transcription assays employing ST-derived nuclear extracts (18).

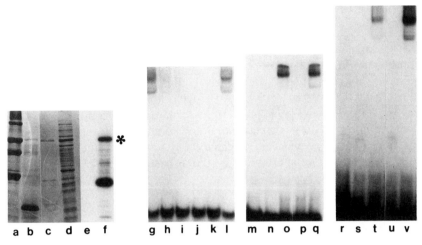

FIGURE 6.1. Interaction of GST-CREMτ with the RT7 CRE. GST-CREMτ (67 kd; indicated by star) was induced in bacteria with IPTG (lanes *c* and *d*: column-purified and crude extract, respectively) and used in gel retardation experiments using the somatostatin CRE (lanes *g–l*) and the RT7 CRE (lanes *o–q*, *t*, and *v*) as probes. RT7 CRE alone (lanes *m* and *r*) and RT7 CRE incubated with GST (lanes *n*, *s*, and *u*) were included as controls. Competitions included an excess of 200 and 400 ng RT7 CRE (lanes *h* and *i*, respectively), 200 ng somatostatin CRE (lane *j*), 400 ng of somatostatin CRE (lanes *k* and *p*), and 400 ng ΔT (lanes *l* and *q*). GST and GST-CREMτ were phosphorylated in vitro with PKA (lanes *e* and *f*). Lanes *s* and *u*: RT7 CRE incubated with unmodified or phosphorylated GST; lanes *t* and *v*: RT7 CRE incubated with unmodified or phosphorylated GST-CREMτ. Molecular weight markers are shown in lane *a* (116, 96, 68, 57, and 40 kd) and lane *b* (30 kd).

The RT7 promoter linked to the G-free cassette reporter gene, used previously to identify essential transcriptional *cis*-acting elements, and the mP1 promoter linked to a G-free cassette were incubated in ST extracts with or without addition of different amounts of RT7-CREM oligonucleotide, which acts as competitor for the binding of endogenous CREMτ to these promoters. Figure 6.2 shows that the addition of 150 ng of this oligo reduces RT7 promoter activity (lanes *a* and *b*) and mP1 promoter activity (lanes *c* and *d*) to undetectable levels. The addition of 50 ng RT7-CREM oligonucleotide indicates that this decrease depends on the excess of RT7 CRE added (lanes *e–h*). The oligo has no effect on the activity of the AdMLP (lanes *a–h*), which is present in all transcription reactions as internal control (the AdMLP lacks a CRE). This demonstrates that CREMτ is a major player in the transcription of both the mP1 and RT7 promoters, since an excess of CRE oligo essentially abolishes transcription.

Transactivation of an Integrated, Transcriptionally Inactive RT7 Promoter

We recently generated lines of transgenic mice carrying the following transgenes: RT7-lacZ and RT7-c-*mos*. The transgenes contain the RT7 promoter linked to the β-galactosidase coding region and the c-*mos* gene, respectively (7). In transgenic mice the lacZ gene and the c-*mos* gene are exclusively and efficiently expressed in spermatids, demonstrating that the RT7 promoter confers correct spatial and temporal transcription on two different reporter genes. This specificity may result from the regulation of the RT7 promoter in spermatids by the spermatid-specific transactivator CREMτ.

To investigate the activation by CREMτ of the transgene RT7 promoter, which is transcriptionally silent in any cell other than spermatids, we set out to try to reproduce the conditions (RT7-lacZ DNA stably integrated in chromatin in low copy number) present in the transgenic mice by producing C3H10T½ mouse fibroblast cell lines carrying copies of the same RT7-lacZ DNA employed in the transgenic experiments. Derived cell lines were analyzed for detectable β-galactosidase expression either by staining with Xgal and detection of blue-colored cells under the microscope or by measurement of β-galactosidase activity in cell-free extracts as described (24).

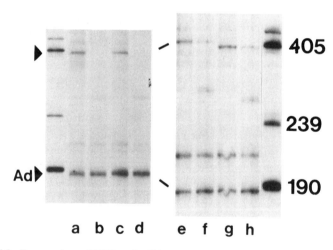

FIGURE 6.2. Repression of RT7 and mP1 promoter activity by RT7 CRE. Promoter activities were assayed in vitro using ST nuclear extracts. All reactions contained pAdMLP as internal control, which produces a 190-nucleotide transcript. Lanes *a* and *b*: pRT7-C$_2$AT without or with 150 ng RT7 CRE; lanes *c* and *d*: mP1-C$_2$AT without or with 150 ng RT7 CRE; lanes *e* and *f*: pRT7-CAP0.2 without or with 50 ng RT7 CRE; lanes *g* and *h*: mP1-C$_2$AT without or with 50 ng RT7 CRE. The arrow indicates the test-promoter driven transcript.

None of the C3H-RT7-lacZ cell lines expressed β-galactosidase (see below). Therefore, the situation in C3H-RT7-lacZ cells appears similar to that of cells other than spermatids in RT7-lacZ transgenic mice.

To try to induce lacZ expression we next transfected C3H-RT7-lacZ cells with pSVCREMτ, which constitutively expresses CREMτ, with pBS-CREMτ, which contains the CREMτ coding region but lacks a promoter, with pBS, the vector used in plasmid constructions, and with pCH110, which expresses lacZ under the control of the herpes simplex virus thymidine kinase promoter. After transfection, cell-free extracts were prepared and β-galactosidase activity was measured. The results shown in Figure 6.3 demonstrate that CREMτ expression from the SV40 promoter induces β-galactosidase expression in C3H-RT7-lacZ cells. As expected, neither pBS-CREMτ nor pBS induced β-galactosidase expression.

We next transfected C3H-RT7-lacZ cells with pMT1a-CREMτ, which contains the sheep metallothionein promoter linked to CREMτ and drives expression of CREMτ after induction of the MT1a promoter by zinc. This particular metallothionein promoter had been shown previously to be readily inducible by zinc both in cell lines (23) and in transgenic mice (26). Figure 6.3 shows that β-galactosidase expression is induced only in the presence of zinc. Thus these transfection studies show that CREMτ efficiently activates transcriptionally inactive, integrated copies of the sperma-

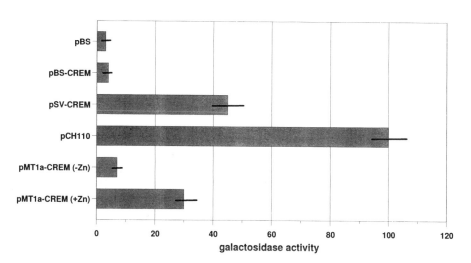

FIGURE 6.3. Induction of an integrated RT7 promoter by CREMτ. C3H-RT7-lacZ mouse fibroblasts were transfected with pBS KSII+, pBS-CREMτ, pSV-CREMτ, pCH110, pMT1a-CREMτ without zinc added, and pMT1a-CREMτ in the presence of zinc. After 48 h cell extracts were prepared and β-galactosidase activity was measured. Data are expressed on an arbitrary scale (pCH110-induced β-galactosidase activity was set to 100) and error bars indicate the observed variation among 5 transfections.

tid-specific RT7 promoter in mouse fibroblasts. Our preliminary results (not shown) indicate that β-galactosidase activity can also be induced in C3H-RT7-lacZ cells by microinjection of GST-CREMτ protein. These data extend our previous results (14), which suggested that CREMτ is an activator of the RT7 promoter in spermatids. It has been noted before that a number of spermatid-specific genes (the protamine genes, TP1, RT7, tACE) appear to contain a CRE at approximately the same position in their promoter (9).

Since transgenic experiments employing these promoters demonstrate that spermatid-specific transcription accounts for the cell-specific expression (4–7), it appears very likely that each of these promoters is activated by CREMτ. Our results of the in vitro transcription assays demonstrate directly that indeed the RT7 and the mouse protamine 1 promoters are regulated by CREMτ. Other recent data suggest that the TP1 promoter is also activated by CREMτ (27). Thus CREMτ may act as a master switch in the initial stages of spermiogenesis, exerting control over a large number of highly specific genes.

Acknowledgments. The work described in this chapter was supported by grants from the National Cancer Institute of Canada and the Medical Research Council of Canada to F.A.vdH. We thank Drs. P. Sassone-Corsi, M. Walsh, and F. Sierra for gifts of reagents. J.H.O. is the recipient of an Alberta Cancer Board Studentship.

References

1. Willison K, Ashworth A. Mammalian spermatogenic gene expression. Trends Genet 1987;3:351–5.
2. Oppi C, Shore SK, Reddy EP. Nucleotide sequence of testis-derived c-abl cDNAs: implications for testis-specific transcription and abl oncogene activation. Proc Natl Acad Sci USA 1987;84:8200–4.
3. Braun RE, Peschon JJ, Behringer RR, Brinster RL, Palmiter RD. Protamine 3' untranslated sequences regulate temporal translational control and subcellular localization of growth hormone in spermatids of transgenic mice. Genes Dev 1989;3:793–802.
4. Peschon JJ, Behringer RR, Palmiter RD, Brinster RL. Expression of mouse protamine 1 genes in transgenic mice. Ann NY Acad Sci 1989;564:186–97.
5. Stewart TA, Hecht NB, Hollingshead PG, Johnson PA, Leong JC, Pitts SL. Haploid-specific transcription of protamine-myc and protamine-T-antigen fusion genes in transgenic mice. Mol Cell Biol 1988;8:1748–55.
6. Howard T, Balogh R, Overbeek P, Bernstein KE. Sperm-specific expression of angiotensin-converting enzyme (ACE) is mediated by a 91-base-pair promoter containing a CRE-like element. Mol Cell Biol 1993;13:18–27.
7. Higgy NA, Zackson SL, van der Hoorn FA. Cell interactions in testis develop-

ment: overexpression of C-mos in spermatocytes leads to increased germ cell proliferation. Dev Genet 1995;16:190–200.

8. Johnson PA, Peschon JJ, Yelick PC, Palmiter RD, Hecht NB. Sequence homologies in the mouse protamine 1 and 2 genes. Biochem Biophys Acta 1988;950:45–53.

9. Oliva R, Dixon GH. Vertebrate protamine genes and the histone-to-protamine replacement reaction. Prog Nucleic Acid Res 1991;40:25–94.

10. Foulkes NS, Sassone-Corsi P. More is better: activators and repressors from the same gene. Cell 1992;68:411–4.

11. Foulkes NS, Schlotter F, Pévet P, Sassone-Corsi P. Pituitary hormone FS directs the CREM functional switch during spermatogenesis. Nature 1993;362:264–7.

12. Foulkes NS, Borrelli E, Sassone-Corsi P. CREM gene: use of alternative DNA binding domains generates multiple antagonists of cAMP-induced transcription. Cell 1991;64:739–49.

13. Foulkes NS, Mellström B, Benusiglio E, Sassone-Corsi P. Developmental switch of CREM function during spermatogenesis: from antagonist to activator. Nature 1992;355:80–4.

14. Delmas V, van der Hoorn FA, Mellström B, Jégou B, Sassone-Corsi P. Induction of CREM activator proteins in spermatids: down-stream targets and implications for haploid germ cell differentiation. Mol Endocrinol 1993;7:1502–14.

15. Higgy NA, Pastoor T, Renz C, Tarnasky HA, van der Hoorn FA. Testis-specific RT7 protein localizes to the sperm tail and associates with itself. Biol Reprod 1994;50:1357–66.

16. Burfeind P, Hoyer-Fender S. Sequence and developmental expression of a mRNA encoding a putative protein of rat outer dense fibers. Dev Biol 1991;148:195–204.

17. Morales CR, Oko R, Clermont Y. Molecular cloning and developmental expression of an mRNA encoding the 27 kDa outer dense fiber protein of rat spermatozoa. Mol Reprod Dev 1994;37:229–40.

18. van der Hoorn FA, Tarnasky HA. Factors involved in regulation of the RT7 promoter in a male germ cell-derived in vitro transcription system. Proc Natl Acad Sci USA 1992;89:703–7.

19. Harada R, Bérubé G, Tamplin OJ, Denis-Larose D, Nepveu A. DNA-binding of the Cut repeats from the human Cut-like protein. Mol Cell Biol 1995;15:129–40.

20. Frangioni JV, Neel BG. Solubilization and purification of enzymatically active glutathione S-transferase (pGEX) fusion proteins. Anal Biochem 1993;210:179–87.

21. van der Hoorn FA. Identification of the testis c-mos promoter: specific activity in a seminiferous tubule-derived extract and binding of a testis-specific nuclear factor. Oncogene 1992;7:1093–9.

22. van der Hoorn FA, Müller V. Differential transformation of C3H10T½ cells by v-mos: sequential expression of transformation parameters. Mol Cell Biol 1985;5:2204–11.

23. Peterson G, Mercer JFB. Differential expression of four linked sheep metallothionein genes. Eur J Biochem 1988;174:425–9.

24. Sambrook J, Fritsch EF, Maniatis T. Molecular cloning: a laboratory manual, 2nd ed. New York: Cold Spring Harbor Laboratory Press, 1989.

25. De Groot RP, den Hertog J, Vandenheede JR, Goris J, Sassone-Corsi P. Mul-

tiple and cooperative phosphorylation events regulate the CREM activator function. EMBO J 1993;12:3903–11.

26. Shanahan CM, Rigby NW, Murry JD, Marshall JT, Townrow CA, Nancarrow CD, et al. Regulation of expression of a sheep metallothionein 1a-sheep growth hormone fusion gene in transgenic mice. Mol Cell Biol 1989;9:5473–9.

27. Kistler MK, Sassone-Corsi P, Kistler WS. Identification of a functional cyclic adenosine 3′,5′-monophosphate response element in the 5′ flanking region of the gene for transition protein 1 (TP1), a basic chromosomal protein of mammalian spermatids. Biol Reprod 1994;51:1322–9.

7

Role of Vitamin A in Male Germ-Cell Development

Kwan Hee Kim and Karin M. Akmal

It has been known since the 1920s that vitamin A is required for normal spermatogenesis (1, 2). Depletion of vitamin A from the diet was shown to cause spermatogenic arrest and testicular atrophy, whereas the replenishment of retinol, the principal form of vitamin A, to the *vitamin A–deficient* (VAD) animals restored spermatogenesis (3). Since then, numerous investigators have analyzed the cell types that are present in the VAD testis (4–8) and described various spermatogenic depletion and retinol replenishment processes resulting in synchronization of spermatogenic stages in the replenished testes (9–15). However, to date, the molecular mechanism by which vitamin A is obligatory for spermatogenesis has not been elucidated. In fact, which cell types in the testis respond directly to the vitamin A signal is not completely clear. The challenge is to define which individual cells in the testis are the direct target of vitamin A and to understand how these cells interact with other cells to determine whether they proliferate, differentiate, survive, or degenerate. Recently, it has been established that nuclear retinoid receptors, members of the steroid/thyroid superfamily of receptors, which are now accepted as the transcription factors that mediate the retinoic acid signal in most tissues (16), are also important mediators of the vitamin A signals in testis (17–22). As such, *retinoic acid receptor-α* (RAR-α) transcripts can be used as biochemical markers to elucidate the cellular sites and the sequential pathways of vitamin A action in the testis.

Vitamin A–Deficient Rat Testis

In the VAD testis that can be reinitiated with retinol replenishment, the tight junctions between adjacent Sertoli cells creating the blood-testis barrier (23) have been demonstrated to remain largely intact (24). Even so, meiosis seems inhibited, and the meiotic and haploid germ cells residing on the adluminal side of the tight junctions have completely disappeared (4–6).

Typically, two synergistic events are responsible for these results: degeneration of spermatocytes and spermatids, and maturation depletion of the differentiated spermatogonial population (24). On the basal side of the tight junctions, the principal remaining cells are the type A_1 spermatogonia and preleptotene spermatocytes, although there are only about 30% of the normal number. In addition, a small number of the stem cell A_0 spermatogonia and pre–type A spermatogonia (intermediate between the type A_0 and A_1 spermatogonia) are present (7, 8). The other mitotic and differentiated spermatogonia, the type A_2, A_3, A_4, In, and B spermatonia, that are in the direct lineage of the type A_1 spermatogonia, in between A_1 and the preleptotene spermatocytes, have entirely degenerated. As a consequence, the remaining germ cells seem to be arrested at stages VII and VIII of the spermatogenic cycle.

No mitosis is observed in the type A_1 spermatogonia, although mitosis itself is not inhibited. A slightly higher number of mitotic figures are detected in the stem cell A_0 spermatogonia in the VAD condition than in the normal testis (8). Also noteworthy and thought provoking is the accumulation ("trapping") of pre–type A spermatogonia, an intermediate type between the A_0 spermatogonia and the A_1 spermatogonia. The number of these cells is about 20% of the number for the A_1 spermatogonia in the VAD condition, but interestingly, they do not occur in normal testis (7).

Onset of Spermatogenesis After VAD Regression in Rat Testis

After regression of spermatogenesis in VAD rats has been established, spermatogenesis can be initiated in a synchronous manner by injection of retinol into VAD rats (9). The reinstated spermatogenesis attains synchrony such that only a few stages of the cycle of the seminiferous epithelium are represented at any given time in the regenerated testis, instead of the normal 14 stages found in rats (7, 9–15, 25). Spermatogenesis is shown to resume from the remaining germ-cell types, especially from the type A_1 spermatogonia and preleptotene spermatocytes that constitute the two major populations in the VAD testis (8, 26).

More specifically, Ismail et al. (8) demonstrated that the germ cells that repopulate the regenerated testis are derived mainly from the type A_1 spermatogonia and not from the preleptotene spermatocytes. Only about 15% of the preleptotene spermatocytes in the VAD testis have advanced to the pachytene phase of meiosis 7 days after retinol injection. The others seemed to have degenerated. However, the mitotic figures in germ cells were detected 3h after retinol injection into VAD rats. This led them to conclude that the type A_1 spermatogonia and the preleptotene spermatocytes are arrested at the G2 phase of the cell cycle.

Similarly, when biochemical assays of cdc2 kinase, which is only active for 2 h between the G2/M phase transition and the metaphase/anaphase transition of mitosis (27), were carried out, they demonstrated that the cells enter into mitosis as early as 4 h and up to about 24 h after the retinol replenishment of VAD rats, with the peak at 12 h (28). This timing before mitosis is consistent with the A_1 spermatogonia and preleptotene spermatocytes arrested at the end of S phase, before the G2 phase of the cell cycle.

In contrast, de Rooij et al. (29) have proposed that the germ cells that are present in the regenerated testis are derived from the stem cell A_0 spermatogonia. Supporting this, tritiated thymidine incorporation was highest at 24 h after retinol acetate injection, and the mitotic index was highest at 48 h after injections of Wistar rats (26). Since the G2 phase is about 11 h long and the S phase about 19.5 h long (30, 31), the timing is consistent with the stem cell A_0 spermatogonia arrested at a resting state, the G0/G1 phase transition of the cell cycle, in the VAD testis.

The apparent differences found in the arrest point of the cell cycle in the remaining germ cells may partially reflect the technical difficulty in predicting the degree of regression in live animals. In fact, it is not trivial to predict precisely the time window (usually about a week) when the testes are still capable of regeneration with the retinol injection, yet vitamin A deficiency in the testes is as complete as one can predict by palpation. Moreover, it is known that if vitamin A deficiency proceeds too long, even more of the germ cells may die (10). When this happens, the more advanced germ cells degenerate first—the preleptotene spermatocytes, the type A_1 spermatogonia, and the stem cell A_0 spermatogonia, in this order—until eventually no regeneration can occur within the VAD tubules even after retinol injection. In this scenario, if the VAD tubules are left with only the A_0 spermatogonia, then they would proliferate first to replenish the type A_1 spermatogonia. But this type of proliferation would happen anyway or even increase in the absence of vitamin A, as has been observed for the A_0 spermatogonia in VAD tubules. On the other hand, if the VAD tubules still contain the type A_1 spermatogonia, it would not be necessary to move the A_0 spermatogonia out of the resting phase first, but the type A_1 could undergo mitosis between 3 and 24 h, peaking at 12 h after retinol injection. According to this line of reasoning, the spermatogenesis in the VAD testis is mostly reinitiated from the most advanced germ cells that survive VAD conditions. For a time window of about 1 week in Sprague-Dawley rats, the most advanced germ cells are the type A_1 spermatogonia and preleptene spermatocytes.

Retinoic Acid Is Active During Onset and Maintenance of Spermatogenesis

Although nearly all of the other systemic effects of vitamin A deficiency can be relieved by the feeding of retinoic acid, the oxidative derivative of retinol, it does not restore spermatogenesis after VAD regression (5, 32). Recently, a partial explanation was provided when it was demonstrated that ^{3}H-retinoic acid from the bloodstream did not effectively enter the testis (33). However, enough retinoic acid must reach the basal compartment of the tubules to qualitatively maintain the spermatogonial population (34). The VAD rats maintained on retinoic acid diet exhibited normal mitotic indices of A, In, and B spermatogonia and a normal number of A_0 spermatogonia, although the total number of A spermatogonia was half of normal, and the numbers of B spermatogonia and preleptotene spermatocytes were severely reduced. Additionally, in organ cultures of cryptorchid mouse testis explant, retinoic acid was shown to stimulate development of In and B type spermatogonia in the presence of *adenosine 3':5'-cyclic monophosphate* (cAMP) for a limited time (35). These results together support the notion that retinoic acid and its derivatives are one of the active factors that stimulate development of germ cells in the basal compartment of the seminiferous tubules.

In contrast, the adluminal germ-cell development does not occur with retinoic acid feeding of the VAD rats. It appears that the adluminal germ cells require a different pool of retinoids (derivatives of vitamin A), such as retinol and retinyl esters found abundantly in Sertoli cells (36, 37). It has been speculated that this large reservoir of retinol and retinyl esters may be required for some mechanisms of retinoid storage and transfer between Sertoli cells and the germ cells on the adluminal side of the tubules. Recently, a repeated regimen of 2 times/week administrations of retinoic acid for 7 weeks was shown to restore spermatogenesis fully in VAD rats (38). It is apparent from the success of this experiment that repeated large dosages of retinoic acid could somehow overcome inefficient entry of retinoic acid into the adluminal compartment of seminiferous tubules, bypassing the requirement for an intermediate step of storage in Sertoli cells and delivery of retinoids to the adluminal germ cells. More important, the experiment clearly shows that retinoic acid and its derivatives can serve as biologically active factors in the development of germ cells in the adluminal compartment of the seminiferous tubules.

Proteins Involved in the Mediation of Vitamin A Signals in Testis

Although the lipid-soluble nature of retinoids, derivatives of vitamin A, suggests simple diffusion as a mode of transport across membranes, a large body of evidence supports the notion that retinol and retinoic acid are not available as free molecules in the bloodstream or in cells. Instead, these are bound by a varied array of proteins for the purpose of transport across membranes or within the cell, cellular storage and metabolism, and eventually transcriptional regulation in the nucleus. The requirement of a multiple number of proteins that bind retinoids at one time or another may reflect a need for tightly controlling the concentration of free retinoids in a cell. That is thought to be due to a dual effect of retinoids on most cells, dependent on the concentration, being toxic to cells at a higher level but beneficial for cell differentiation or proliferation at a lower level.

In testis, a recent report (39) delineated a delivery mechanism for retinol to Sertoli cells through peritubular cells. Retinol is first delivered to peritubular cells by *retinol-binding protein* (RBP) and *transthyretin* (TTR) in an equal molar ratio. The peritubular cells, in turn, synthesize their own RBP, which is then secreted with retinol and delivered to the Sertoli cell membranes.

Inside the seminiferous tubules, *cellular retinol-binding protein I* (CRBP I) appears to localize exclusively to Sertoli cell cytoplasm, whereas *cellular retinoic acid–binding protein I* (CRABP I) localizes predominantly to the cytoplasm of pachytene spermatocytes of stages IX to XI, diplotene spermatocytes, and all spermatids (40). The reason for this mutually exclusive pattern of expression is not clear, but CRBP I and CRABP I are known to function in a slightly different manner (41). CRBP I binds retinol and is thought to function mostly in the metabolism of retinol. In contrast, CRABP I binds retinoid acid and is thought not only to participate in retinoic acid metabolism but also to sequester retinoic acid, regulating its availability for interaction with the nuclear receptors. Thus, an increased level of CRABP may result in reduced sensitivity of some cells to retinoic acid and, at the same time, may increase retinoic acid metabolism to more polar metabolites. In VAD testis, the level of CRBP I is substantially decreased at the protein and mRNA levels (40, 42). Following retinol replacement, the level of CRBP I mRNA was observed to increase about 2- to 3-fold (43), which is compatible with the more recent finding of a retinoic acid responsive element located on the CRBP I gene (44).

Furthermore, there is now substantial evidence that several subtypes of the retinoid receptors are distributed in Sertoli cells and germ cells of testis (18–22). One family of receptors, the RARs, are known to bind all-*trans retinoic acid* (RA) and 9-*cis* RA, a derivative of RA, whereas the other family of receptors, the *retinoid X receptors* (RXRs), preferentially bind 9-*cis* RA (45). The effects of RA on a wide variety of genes are mediated by the numerous isoforms of these receptors and by formation of heterodimers between RARs and RXRs. Furthermore, RXRs have been shown to heterodimerize with other members of the nuclear hormone receptor family, such as the vitamin D receptor and the thyroid hormone receptors, providing a mechanism of cross talk between hormone signaling pathways (16). Through these receptors, RA has the ability to regulate transcription of genes and to dramatically alter the differentiation state of a particular cell.

In testis, the fact that injection of RA alone, albeit in repeated and large doses, can reinitiate and maintain spermatogenesis after VAD regression (38) argues that transcriptional regulation of specific genes by the retinoid receptors is likely to be the principal molecular mechanism by which vitamin A controls spermatogenesis. The results from the recent transgenic mice work similarly demonstrated that retinoid receptors are critical for spermatogenesis, especially the subtype RAR-α (46). The only identifiable phenotypic lesion in the all-isoform RAR-α–null mice was testis degeneration due to depletion of germ cells. The testicular morphology in the RAR-α–null mice mostly resembled that observed in males kept on VAD diet. This was not observed in the RAR-β2 isoform or the all-isoform RAR-γ–null mice (47, 48).

Primary Site of Vitamin A Action During Reinitiation of Spermatogenesis After VAD Regression

It is clear that RARs, especially the subtype RAR-α, are important mediators of vitamin A action during spermatogenesis in the testis. As such, RAR-α is an especially good biochemical marker to determine which cells respond directly to the vitamin A signal in testis. The localization pattern of RAR-α *messenger RNA* (mRNA) in testis would point to the cells that utilize the nuclear mechanism involving the transcriptional regulation of RA-responsive genes to control spermatogenesis.

In VAD testis, the in situ hybridization of RAR-α cRNA to testis sections revealed hybridization above the background level in the Sertoli cells (Fig. 7.1). Four hours after retinol replenishment, the hybridization was again predominantly over Sertoli cells, but at increased levels (Fig. 7.1). It was interesting that the hybridization was not clustered over germ cells, as depicted for a germ-cell–specific *mak* transcript (49) expressed in the VAD testis (Fig. 7.1). Twenty-four hours after retinol injection, the number of silver grains has decreased to the VAD level (data not shown). These results are consistent with the previous results obtained by Northern blot analysis using mRNA populations from the VAD testis and 0.5, 2, 4, 7, and 12h after retinol administration of the VAD rats (18). The RAR-α mRNA level increased 2.5-fold within 0.5h of retinol injection into the VAD rats and reached a 3-fold increase at its peak. It remained at the peak level for at least 7h and then decreased to the level found in the VAD rats by 12h. However, the in situ hybridization experiments here revealed the crucial information that the increase in the level of RAR-α mRNA is predominantly in the Sertoli cells, and not in the germ cells. This indicates that the primary site of retinoid-mediated regulation for reinitiation occurs in Sertoli cells instead of germ cells remaining in the VAD testis.

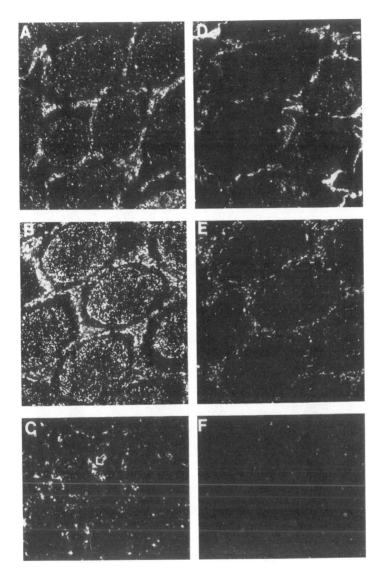

FIGURE 7.1. In situ hybridization of rat RAR-α cRNA to VAD testis sections and to sections of 4-h retinol-replenished testis. The testes were fixed with a 4% paraformaldehyde/0.25% glutaraldehyde fixative, embedded in paraffin, and cut into 3-μm sections onto slides. Sequential tissue sections of the VAD testis (A, D) and 4-h retinol-replenished testis (B, E) were hybridized with the ³⁵S-radiolabeled antisense (A, B) or sense (D, E) rat RAR-α cRNA probes. The VAD testis sections were also probed with ³⁵S-radiolabeled antisense (C) or sense (F) rat mak-1 cRNA probes. Expression of mak mRNA was shown to be germ cell-specific (49). After hybridization and washing, slides were dipped in Kodak NTB-2 nuclear tracking emulsion (Eastman Kodak, Rochester, NY) and exposed at 4°C. Slides were then developed and counterstained with hematoxylin and eosin. The dark-field photomicrographs were taken through a 10× objective; magnification, ×125.

Proposed Model of Vitamin A Action During Reinitiation of Spermatogenesis After VAD Regression

The potential RA-mediated interactions among remaining cells in the VAD testis after the initial vitamin A signal to Sertoli cells are shown in a proposed model (Fig. 7.2). Although the proposed model depicts only bare essential interactions, the main feature of this model is that vitamin A acts directly on Sertoli cells. Then, gene products regulated by RA via nuclear RARs are most likely responsible for providing factors to the preleptotene spermatocytes and the A spermatogonia. These factors may signal the A type to survive and proliferate, and the preleptotene spermatocytes to initiate the prophase of meiosis. This series of events has to be triggered within a specific time period, as implicated by the high level of RAR-α mRNA for about 7h after retinol administration followed by a decline to

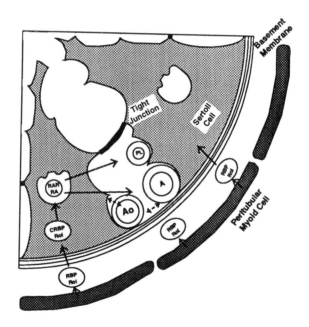

FIGURE 7.2. Schematic diagram of the proposed model for retinol action during reinitiation of spermatogenesis in the VAD testis. The diagram shows a portion of the retinol-replenished seminiferous tubule cross section after VAD regression. The solid arrow indicates the direction of a signal. The dotted arrows indicate cross talk between cells. Rol, retinol; RBP, retinol binding protein; CRBP, cellular retinol binding protein; RA, retinoic acid; RAR, retinoic acid receptors; A_0, stem cell A_0 spermatogonia; A, A spermatogonia; PL, preleptotene spermatocytes. The diagram was drawn using the Adobe illustrator program.

the VAD level. The second feature of this model includes mechanisms in which A_0 spermatogonia communicate (cross-talk) with A type or Sertoli cells, so that the number of germ cells differentiating would be continually adjusted. According to these mechanisms, if the number of differentiating spermatogonia decline, the relatively quiescent stem cell A_0 spermatogonia would enter into active mitosis to give rise to type A_1 spermatogonia, thus restoring the spermatogonial population. These mechanisms are consistent with the stem cell A_0 types continuing to undergo mitosis or even increasing mitosis in the VAD condition.

Ten-Day-Old Rat Sertoli Cells

The developing prepubertal testes, before 20 days of age for rats, are where new germ cells derived from gonocytes and stem-cell A_0 spermatogonia emerge for the first time (50). In situ hybridization of RAR-α cRNA probe to 5-, 10-, and 20-day-old rat testis sections revealed that the level of RAR-α mRNA was expressed mainly in Sertoli cells and developmentally regulated (Fig. 7.3). The level of the RAR-α mRNA was highest in the 10-day-old Sertoli cells. Since the number of Sertoli cells continues to increase to 20 days of age (51), the level of mRNA being highest in the 10-day-old testis sections is probably unrelated to the number of Sertoli cells. In fact, when Northern blot analyses were conducted and the amount of hybridization normalized to the number of Sertoli cells, the level of RAR-α mRNA was higher in the 10-day-old testis than in the 20-day-old testis (data not shown). The result suggests that the Sertoli cells of 10-day-old testis are more sensitive to RA than the 5-day or 20-day Sertoli cells. Further experimentation that is under way with developing testes between the ages of 10 and 20 days may better define when Sertoli cells are most sensitive to RA.

What is special about Sertoli cells in the 10-day-old testis? Structurally, the 10-day-old testis cross sections show the presence of gonocytes; Sertoli cells, some of them undergoing mitosis; the type A spermatogonia; and a few B spermatogonia or preleptotene spermatocytes (data not shown). The tight junctions between adjacent Sertoli cells, which form later at about 20 days of age, have not formed yet in the 10-day-old testis (23). At the level of regulation, it is postulated that selective proliferation and degeneration of germ cells begins at this time, with just those located in close association with the basement membrane surviving (50). More important, related to the retinol regulation, the mitotic proliferation of Sertoli cells is coming to an end and Sertoli cells are differentiating (51). We can speculate that RA is one of the required differentiation signals for the Sertoli cells in the 10-day-old testis. This is in line with the accepted notion that RA is a differentiating signal in many cells (16).

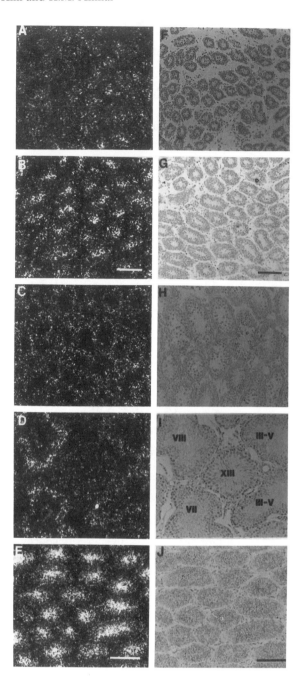

Round Spermatids Are the Other Site of Vitamin A Action in Adult Testes

In situ hybridization of RAR-α cRNA probe to the adult testis revealed the expression of RAR-α mRNA to be stage-specific in the cycle of the seminiferous epithelium (Fig. 7.3). The level was highest in stage VIII and decreased rapidly to a low level in stage IX, reaching the lowest levels in stages XI to XIV, and intermediate levels in stages I to VI (Fig. 7.4). This is mostly in agreement with previous Northern blot analyses using mRNAs from the synchronized testes (18). More specifically, in situ hybridization showed that the expression was most prominent over the round spermatids compared with other cell types, but highest over round spermatids (steps 7 and 8) in the stages VII and VIII. There was some expression detected in the pachytene spermatocytes, but virtually no silver grains were detected over the elongated spermatids (data not shown). The silver grains were detected over Sertoli cells in adults, but the number was far smaller than that found over the round spermatids (data not shown).

Proposed Model of Vitamin A Action in Normal Rat Testis

The data presented above support a proposed model in which vitamin A directly signals round spermatids (Fig. 7.5). In this model, retinol signals Sertoli cells first, but then retinol or its derivatives from the Sertoli cells are transferred to the round spermatids, where RA or its derivatives regulate transcription of retinoid-responsive genes that may trigger the beginning of spermiogenesis involving nuclear condensation, acrosome remodeling, and flagellum formation. Additionally, the proposed model incorporates the possibility that the gene products regulated by RA in Sertoli cells are

---

FIGURE 7.3. In situ hybridization of rat RAR-α cRNA to 5-day, 10-day, 20-day, and adult rat testis sections. Testes were fixed in 4% paraformaldehyde and glutaraldehyde solution, embedded in paraffin, and sectioned onto slides. Tissue sections from 5-day (*A, F*), 10-day (*B, G, E, J*), 20-day (*C, H*), and adult (*D, I*) were hybridized with ^{35}S-radiolabeled antisense rat RAR-α cRNA (*A–D, F–I*) or SGP-2 cRNA (*E, J*). Expression of SGP-2 mRNA has been shown to occur predominantly in Sertoli cells (52). The slides were treated as indicated in Figure 7.1. The dark-field (*A–E*) and light-field (*F–J*) photomicrographs were taken through a 10× objective. Magnifications for *E* and *J* are different from *A–D* and *F–I* magnifications. Bars in *B, E, G, J* = 100 μM. Numbers inside the tubule cross sections indicate their respective stages in the spermatogenic cycle.

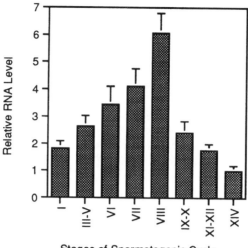

FIGURE 7.4. Quantitation of silver grains representing RAR-α transcripts across the stages of the seminiferous epithelium in adult testis. The silver grains were counted with the aid of Bioquant system IV (R & M Biometrics, Inc.). Essentially, a rectangular grid was overlaid on a sector of the seminiferous tubule under microscope and the numbers of silver grains for 10 grids were averaged; each grid was counted three times and for three distinct tubule cross sections representing stages indicated on the x-axis. The relative RNA level was calculated by setting the lowest level at stage XIV to 1. Error bars represent the standard deviation of the sample.

secreted into the adluminal side of the seminiferous tubule and are then recognized by the round spermatids and perhaps by pachytene spermatocytes. All aspects of this model are obviously based on the widely accepted view that the blood-testis barrier effectively blocks transfer of factors like retinol, so retinol or derivatives have to pass through the Sertoli cells (23).

In summary, Sertoli cells are the primary target cells of vitamin A signal in the retinol-replenished VAD testis, in the developing testis, and in adult testis. Vitamin A may be a differentiation signal for Sertoli cells. The other main target cells of vitamin A signal are the round spermatids. The level of RAR-α mRNA increases steadily in round spermatids from stage I to VIII of the spermatogenic cycle, until it is at its highest at stage VIII. At the stage VIII, Sertoli cells may orchestrate production of the RA-regulated secretory factors that can be recognized by the A spermatogonia, preleptotene spermatocytes, and round spermatids. Additionally, Sertoli cells have the ability to transfer retinol or its derivatives directly to round spermatids, where RAR-α may function to regulate transcription of genes involved in the differentiation of round spermatids. Effectively, the Sertoli cell seems to

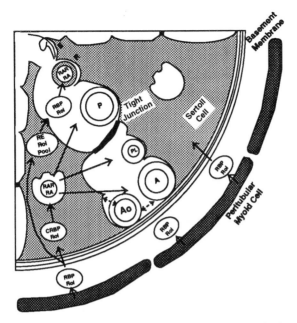

FIGURE 7.5. Schematic diagram of the proposed model for retinol action at stage VIII of the normal rat testis. The diagram shows a sector of the stage VIII seminiferous tubule cross section. The solid arrow indicates the direction of a signal. The dotted arrows indicate cross talk between cells. RE, retinyl esters; P, pachytene spermatocytes; R, round spermatids; E, elongated spermatids; also see Figure 7.2.

act as a "master" cell that balances the proliferation of A spermatogonia, the onset of meiosis of preleptotene spermatocytes (viewed both as a process of cell differentiation and as a modification of the mitotic proliferation), and the differentiation of round spermatids to elongated spermatids.

Future Work

The obvious future task is to identify vitamin A–regulated signals from the Sertoli cells that control the survival and proliferation of A spermatogonia, the onset of meiosis of preleptotene spermatocytes, and the differentiation of round spermatids. At the same time, it is important to understand how the responding cells integrate these vitamin A–regulated signals to decide whether to proliferate, die, undergo meiosis, or differentiate, for example, by a receptor-mediated phosphorylation cycle.

Acknowledgments. The authors are grateful to Ms. Morgan Mizoguchi for preparing the drawings. The work was supported by NIH grant HD 25094.

References

1. Wolbach SB, Howe PR. Tissue changes following deprivation of fat-soluble vitamin A. J Exp Med 1925;42:753–77.
2. Mason KE. Differences in testes injury and repair after vitamin A deficiency, vitamin E deficiency and inanition. Am J Anat 1933;52:153–239.
3. Thompson JN, Howell JMcC, Pitt GAJ. Vitamin A and reproduction in rats. Proc R Soc 1964;159:510–35.
4. Mitranond V, Sobhon P, Tosukhowong P, Chindaduangrat W. Cytological changes in the testes of vitamin A deficient rats. I. Quantitation of germinal cells in the seminiferous tubules. Acta Anat 1979;103:159–68.
5. Huang HFS, Hembree WC. Spermatogenic response to vitamin A in vitamin A deficient rats. Biol Reprod 1979;21:891–904.
6. Unni E, Rao MR, Ganguly J. Histological and ultrastructural studies on the effect of vitamin A depletion and subsequent repletion with vitamin A on germ cells and Sertoli cells in rat testis. Indian J Exp Biol 1983;21:180–92.
7. Griswold MD, Bishop PD, Kim KH, Ren P, Siiteri KE, Morales C. Function of vitamin A in normal and synchronized seminiferous tubules. Ann NY Acad Sci 1989;564:154–72.
8. Ismail N, Morales C, Clermont Y. Role of spermatogonia in the stage-synchronization of the seminiferous epithelium in vitamin A–deficient rats. Am J Anat 1990;188:57–63.
9. Morales CR, Griswold MD. Retinol-induced stage synchronization in seminiferous tubules of the rat. Endocrinology 1987;121:432–4.
10. Siiteri JE, Karl AF, Linder CC, Griswold MD. Testicular synchrony: evaluation and analysis of different protocols. Biol Reprod 1991;46:284–9.
11. Bartlett JM, Weinbauer GF, Nieschlag E. Stability of spermatogenic synchronization achieved by depletion and restoration of vitamin A in rats. Biol Reprod 1990;42:603–12.
12. Huang HFS, Marshall GR, Nieschlag E. Enrichment of the stages of the seminiferous epithelium in vitamin A–replaced vitamin A–deficient rats. J Reprod Fertil 1990;85:51–60.
13. van Beek MEAB, Meistrich ML. A method for quantifying synchrony in testes of rats treated with vitamin A deprivation and readministration. Biol Reprod 1990;42:424–31.
14. van Beek MEAB, Meistrich ML. Stage-synchronized seminiferous epithelium in rats after manipulation of retinol levels. Biol Reprod 1991;45:235–44.
15. van Pelt AMM, de Rooij DG. Synchronization of the seminiferous epithelium after vitamin A replacement in vitamin A–deficient mice. Biol Reprod 1990;43:363–7.
16. Giguère V. Retinoic acid receptors and cellular retinoid binding proteins: complex interplay in retinoid signaling. Endocr Rev 1994;15:61–79.

17. Kim KH, Wang ZQ. Action of vitamin A on testis: role of the Sertoli cell. In: Griswold MD, Russell L, eds. The sertoli cell. Clearwater, FL: Cache River Press, 1993:514–35.
18. Kim KH, Griswold MD. The regulation of retinoic acid receptor mRNA levels during spermatogenesis. Mol Endocrinol 1990;4:1679–88.
19. Eskild W, Ree AH, Levy FO, Jahnsen T, Hansson V. Cellular localization of mRNAs for retinoic acid receptor α, cellular retinol-binding protein, and cellular retinoic acid-binding protein in rat testis: evidence for germ cell-specific mRNA. Biol Reprod 1991;44:53–61.
20. van Pelt AMM, van den Brink CE, de Rooij DG, van der Saag PT. Changes in retinoic acid receptor messenger ribonucleic acid levels in the vitamin A–deficient rat testis after administration of retinoids. Endocrinology 1992;131:344–50.
21. Wan YJ, Wang L, Wu TC. Detection of retinoic acid receptor mRNA in rat tissues by reverse transcriptase-polymerase chain reaction. J Mol Endocrinol 1992;9:291–4.
22. Huang HFS, Li MT, Pogach LM, Qian L. Messenger ribonucleic acid of rat testicular retinoic acid receptors: developmental pattern, cellular distribution, and testosterone effect. Biol Reprod 1994;51:541–50.
23. Setchell BP, Waites GMH. The blood-testis barrier. In: Hamilton DW, Greep RP, eds. Handbook of physiology, sect. 7: Endocrinology, vol. 5. Male reproductive system. Washington, DC: American Physiological Society, 1975: 143–72.
24. Ismail N, Morales CR. Effects of vitamin A deficiency on the inter-Sertoli junctions and on the germ cell population. Microsc Res Tech 1992;20(1):43–9.
25. Leblond CP, Clermont Y. Definition of the stages of the cycle of the seminiferous epithelium in the rat. Ann NY Acad Sci 1952;55:548–73.
26. van Pelt AMM, de Rooij DG. The origin of the synchronization of the seminiferous epithelium in vitamin A–deficient rats after vitamin A replacement. Biol Reprod 1990;42:677–82.
27. Strausfeld U, Labbé JC, Fesquet D, Cavadore JC, Picard A, Sadhu K, Russell P, Dorée M. Dephosphorylation and activation of a p34^{cdc2}/cyclin B complex in vitro by human CDC25 protein. Nature 1991;351:242–5.
28. Wang ZQ, Kim KH. Vitamin A–deficient testis germ cells are arrested at the end of S phase of the cell cycle: a molecular study of the origin of synchronous spermatogenesis in regenerated seminiferous tubules. Biol Reprod 1993; 48:1157–65.
29. de Rooij DG, van Dissel-Emiliani FMF, van Pelt AMM. Regulation of spermatogonial proliferation. Ann NY Acad Sci 1989;564:140–53.
30. Hilscher W. DNA synthesis: proliferation and regeneration of the spermatogonia in the rat. Arch Anat Microsc Morphol Exp 1967; 56:75–84.
31. Huckins C. The spermatogonial stem cell population in adult rats. I. Their morphology, proliferation and maturation. Anat Res 1971;169:533–58.
32. Howell JMcC, Thompson JN, Pitt GAJ. Histology of the lesions produced in the reproductive tract of animals fed a diet deficient in vitamin A alcohol but containing vitamin A acid. I. The male rat. J Reprod Fertil 1963;5:159–67.
33. Blaner WS, Olson JA. Retinol and retinoid acid metabolism. In: Sporn MB, Roberts AB, Goodman DS, eds. The retinoids, 2nd ed. New York: Raven Press, 1994:244–5.
34. van Beek MEAB, Meistrich ML. Spermatogenesis in retinol-deficient rats maintained on retinoic acid. J Reprod Fertil 1992;94:327–36.

35. Haneji T, Koide SS, Nishimune Y, Oota Y. Dibutyryl adenosine cyclic mono-phosphate regulates differentiation of type A spermatogonia with vitamin A in adult mouse cryptorchid testis in vitro. Endocrinology 1986;119:2490–6.
36. Bishop PD, Griswold MD. Uptake and metabolism of retinol in cultured Sertoli cells: evidence for a kinetic model. Biochemistry 1987;26:7511–8.
37. Shingleton JL, Skinner MK, Ong DE. Retinol esterification in Sertoli cells by lecithin-retinol acyltransferase. Biochemistry 1989;28:9647–53.
38. van Pelt AMM, de Rooij DG. Retinoic acid is able to reinitiate spermatogenesis in vitamin A–deficient rats and high replicate doses support the full development of spermatogenic cells. Endocrinology 1991;128:697–704.
39. Davis JT, Ong DE. Retinol processing by the peritubular cell from rat testis. Biol Reprod 1995;52:356–64.
40. Porter SB, Ong DE, Chytil F, Orgebin-Crist M-C. Localization of cellular retinol-binding protein and cellular retinoic acid binding-protein in the rat testis and epididymis. J Androl 1985;6:197–212.
41. Ong DE, Newcomer ME, Chytil F. Cellular retinoid-binding proteins. In: Sporn MB, Roberts AB, Goodman DS, eds. The retinoids, 2nd ed. New York: Raven Press, 1994: 283–318.
42. Rajan N, Blaner WS, Soprano DR, Suhara A, Goodman DS. Cellular retinol-binding protein messenger RNA levels in normal and retinoid-deficient rats. J Lipid Res 1990;31:821–9.
43. Eskild W, Oyen O, Beebe S, Jahnsen T, Hasson V. Regulation of mRNA levels for cellular retinol binding protein in rat Sertoli cells by cyclic AMP and retinol. Biochem Biophy Res Commun 1988;152:1504–10.
44. Husmann M, Hoffmann B, Stump DG, Chytil F, Pfahl M. A retinoic acid responsive element from the rat CRBPI promoter is activated by an RAR/RXR heterodimer. Biochem Biophys Res Commun 1992;187:1558–64.
45. Heyman RA, Mangelsdorf DJ, Dyck JA, Stein RB, Eichele G, Evans RM, Thaller C. 9-cis retinoic acid is a high affinity ligand for retinoid X receptor. Cell 1992;68:397–406.
46. Lufkin T, Lohnes D, Mark M, Dierich A, Gorry P, Gaub M-P, et al. High postnatal lethality and testis degeneration in retinoic acid receptor α mutant mice. Proc Natl Acad Sci USA 1993;90:7225–9.
47. Mendelsohn C, Mark M, Dolle P, Dierich A, Gaub MP, Krust A, et al. Retinoic acid receptor β2 (RARβ2) null mutant mice appear normal. Dev Biol 1994; 166:246–58.
48. Lohnes D, Kastner P, Dierich A, Mark M, Lemeur M, Chambon P. Function of retinoic acid receptor γ in the mouse. Cell 1993;73:643–58.
49. Wang ZQ, Kim KH. Retinol differentially regulates male germ cell-associated kinase (mak) messenger ribonucleic acid expression during spermatogenesis. Biol Reprod 1993;49:951–64.
50. Zhengwei Y, Wreford NG, de Kretser DM. A quantitative study of spermatogenesis in the developing rat testis. Biol Reprod 1990;43:629–35.
51. Orth J. Proliferation of Sertoli cells in fetal and postnatal rats: a quantitative autoradiographic study. Anat Rec 1982;203:485–92.
52. Collard MW, Griswold MD. Biosynthesis and molecular cloning of sulfated glycoprotein 2 secreted by rat Sertoli cells. Biochemistry 1987;26:3297–303.

8

Alternative Forms and Functions of the c-*kit* Receptor and Its Ligand During Spermatogenesis

Pellegrino Rossi, Cristina Albanesi, Susanna Dolci,
Marco Giorgio, Paola Grimaldi, Domenica Piscitelli,
Laura Pozzi, Vincenzo Sorrentino, and Raffaele Geremia

In both W and SI mice mutants, one major symptom, together with anemy and pigmentation defects, is sterility. In W mutants the defect is intrinsic to stem cells of the affected lineage, whereas in SI mutants the defect lies in the microenvironment where stem cells migrate, grow, and differentiate (1). W locus encodes the c-*kit* transmembrane receptor tyrosine- kinase (2). The c-*kit* receptor is a ~150-kd protein consisting of an immunoglobulin-like extracellular domain, a transmembrane domain, and an intracellular tyrosine kinase domain, characteristically split into an *adenosine triphosphate* (ATP)-binding site and a phosphotransferase catalytic site, which are divided by an intervening sequence (3). SI locus encodes the c-*kit* ligand (4), which has been named *Steel factor* (SLF), *stem-cell factor* (SCF), or *mast-cell growth factor* (MGF). SLF can exist under both a soluble and a transmembrane form, encoded by distinct *messenger RNAs* (mRNAs), produced by alternative splicing (5).

Many independent mutations of the W and the Sl locus have been identified that vary in their degree of severity in affecting different cell lineages. Two of these mutations, W and W^v, are particularly interesting, since they indicate that c-*kit* plays a role in development of the male germ-cell line both pre- and postnatally. Deletion of the transmembrane domain of the c-*kit* receptor in the classical W mutation (6) is accompanied by complete absence of germ cells within the postnatal testis, due to lack of migration and/or proliferation of primordial germ cells in the embryonal gonad (7). A point mutation in the ATP-binding site of the intracellular domain of c-*kit* in W^v mutants (6) is accompanied by the presence of spermatogonia and few meiotic germ cells after birth, but spermatogenesis is completely arrested after these stages (7). Thus, it can be inferred that the expression of c-*kit* and Steel gene products is required not only in germ cells in the early stages of development in the embryo, but also in the completion of spermatogenesis after birth.

Interaction of the c-*kit* Receptor in Mitotic Germ Cells and Alternative Forms of SLF Produced by Sertoli Cells

Expression of c-kit and SLF in the Mouse Testis

The c-*kit* mRNA is expressed both in primordial germ cells of the embryonal gonad (8) and, at high levels, in type A spermatogonia of the postnatal testis (9). Immunoblotting and immunoprecipitation experiments confirm the presence in type A spermatogonia of the normal 150-kd c-*kit* receptor, which has autophosphorylative activity (unpublished observations).

SLF mRNAs for both the soluble and the transmembrane forms are produced in the testis by Sertoli cells (10, 11). The ratio between mRNAs for the soluble and the transmembrane form of SLF increases during postnatal testicular development, suggesting that the c-*kit* ligand is produced by postnatal Sertoli cells mainly as a soluble factor (11). The mRNA for the soluble SLF is also the form that increases most following in vitro stimulation of Sertoli cells with *follicle-stimulating hormone* (FSH) or its intracellular mediator *adenosine 3':5'-cyclic monophosphate* (cAMP) (11).

Stimulation of DNA Synthesis in Spermatogonia by the Soluble Form of SLF

We have shown that addition of the recombinant soluble form of SLF to highly enriched cultures of postnatal germ cells at the mitotic stages stimulates DNA synthesis selectively in type A spermatogonia (11), in agreement with the presence of a functional c-*kit* receptor in these cells. This DNA synthesis is of replicative type, since it is drastically reduced by addition to the culture of aphidicolin (12), an inhibitor of DNA–polymerase-α, and it is accompanied by increased activity of a specific stimulator of DNA-dependent DNA primase activity involved in DNA replication, which has been previously identified in spermatogonia (13). FSH induction of the soluble form of SLF in Sertoli cells and stimulation of DNA synthesis in type A spermatogonia by the soluble form of the factor represent the first example of a direct correlation between gonadotropin action on the somatic compartment of the testis and release of a growth factor that directly promotes germ-cell proliferation.

We also found that the soluble form of SLF stimulates in cultured spermatogonial cells an increase of DNA–polymerase-β activity (12), which is involved in DNA repair synthesis. An increase in DNA–polymerase-β activity could be related to an increase in survival of mitotic germ cells in the in vitro culture conditions, and we are currently studying whether there is a correlation between action of SLF on spermatogonia and suppression of apoptosis, together with stimulation of proliferation. Alternatively, since DNA–polymerase-β is needed for DNA repair during crossing-over in the subsequent meiotic stages of spermatogenesis and is expressed mainly in spermatocytes (14), the soluble form of SLF could also play a role as a growth factor that regulates progression of germ cells into further differentiative steps of spermatogenesis.

Role of the Transmembrane Form of SLF in the Male Gonad

The transmembrane form of SLF stimulates survival, but not proliferation, of primordial germ cells in the embryonal gonad (15), and it has been shown to be important for adhesion of postnatal spermatogonia to cultured Sertoli cell monolayers (16). Possibly, the two forms of the c-*kit* ligand could have different roles in their interaction with developing germ cells, the transmembrane form being mainly a factor involved in their survival and/or migration and adhesion, and the soluble form being an inducer of proliferation and/or differentiation. It will be interesting to verify whether the ratio between the two forms varies in different stages of the seminiferous epithelium, according to the well-known variation of sensitivity to FSH stimulation (17). If this is the case, local regulation of the balance between the two forms could be one of the still poorly understood mechanisms for the establishment of the wave of the seminiferous epithelium itself.

Additional Evidence for a Role of the c-kit/SLF System in Spermatogenesis

Further evidence that the c-*kit*/SLF system plays an important role in mitotic stages of spermatogenesis after birth is provided by the observation that injection of antibodies directed against the extracellular domain of the c-*kit* receptor selectively depletes seminiferous tubules from type A spermatogonia (18), and that spermatogenesis can be reestablished in W mutant mice after transplantation within the seminiferous tubules of type A spermatogonia from normal animals (19).

Alternative Gene Products of the c-*kit* Proto-Oncogene Are Expressed During Spermiogenesis

Expression of a Truncated Form of c-kit *in Spermiogenesis*

We originally found that in the meiotic stages of spermatogenesis c-*kit* expression ceases, but in the subsequent haploid stages an alternative short transcript is present (9). This transcript encodes a truncated form of the receptor in which the extracellular and transmembrane domains, together with the first box of the split kinase domain, including the ATP-binding site, are missing, and only the second box of the split kinase is present (20). A 30-kd protein, corresponding to the size predicted through molecular cloning of the alternative c-*kit* transcript (20), can be identified at low levels in round spermatids (stages 1–9 of spermiogenesis), but not in spermatogonial cells (unpublished observations), by Western blotting, using antibodies directed against the carboxyterminal part of the c-*kit* polypeptide. Surprisingly, preliminary experiments show that a 30-kd protein in round spermatids is also detectable by immunoprecipitation followed by in vitro phosphorylation. Since this protein lacks the ATP-binding site, and thence should also lack intrinsic kinase activity, we can interpret this result as a phosphorylation event performed by coprecipitating different kinase activities.

W Mutations Affecting Spermiogenesis

The observation that in the W^v mutation, spermatogonia and even meiotic cells can be found in seminiferous tubules (7), and that spermatogenesis is arrested in more advanced stages, sustains the hypothesis of a function for the c-*kit* gene in the haploid stages of spermatogenesis. This mutation, however, affects the ATP-binding site located in the intracellular domain of the c-*kit* receptor (6), which is absent in the truncated c-*kit* protein expressed in spermatids, containing only the phosphotransferase catalytic site and the carboxyterminus of the c-*kit* receptor. Mutations in the phosphotransferase domain of the c-*kit* protein have been identified, and, probably due to a different degree of impairment of tyrosine-kinase function (6), they are associated either with a severe phenotype, such as in W^{42}, or with mild effects on male fertility, such as in W^{41}. It cannot be excluded that other, still unknown, mutations in the carboxyterminal domain of the c-*kit* receptor selectively impair spermiogenesis without affecting mitotic germ cells or stem cells of other lineages; such mutants, not presenting pigmentation defects, would escape an easy phenotypic identification. Such mutations could interfere with a function of the truncated c-*kit* protein in haploid germ cells not necessarily related to tyrosine-kinase activity. A tyrosin kinase-independent function has also been suggested for the carboxyterminal domain of *Drosophila* c-*abl* proto-oncogene, which would play an essential role in axonal outgrowth during neurogenesis (21).

Search for a Function of the Truncated c-kit

The relatively low amount of the truncated c-*kit* protein detected in round spermatids, together with the lack of a suitable purification protocol, hampers its biochemical studies, which would be a necessary step in assigning a function to this protein during spermiogenesis. As an alternative approach to the characterization of this protein product, we have tried to dissect the mechanisms underlying its specific expression during the haploid stages of spermatogenesis.

Identification of a Presumptive Promoter for the Expression of the Truncated c-kit

We had previously found by RNAse mapping that the 5′ end of the alternative c-*kit* transcript maps within an intron that separates the exon encoding the interkinase domain from the first exon encoding the phosphotransferase domain (20). According to the published structure of the murine c-*kit* gene (22), these sequences correspond to the 16th intron. In vitro transcription experiments using nuclear extracts from round spermatids (Fig. 8.1) suggest that the alternative c-*kit* transcript during spermiogenesis is generated by a cryptic promoter present within this intron. This promoter appears not to be active using nuclear extracts from meiotic germ cells or Sertoli cells (unpublished observations), suggesting that it is active exclusively in round spermatids.

Sequence analysis of the mouse c-*kit* 16th intron showed no canonical TATA-, nor CAAT-, nor GC-boxes, which are typical elements of eukaryotic promoters active in somatic cell lineages. Other potential binding sites for known transcription factors, such as AP1 (*jun-fos*), ATF-CREB-CREMτ, NFkB, AP3, C-EBP, and PRDI-BF1, were present (see the sequence published in ref. 20).

The Presumptive Promoter Has Binding Sites for Spermatid Nuclear Proteins

DNA-binding experiments show that nuclear factors present in extracts from spermatids, but not from spermatocytes or Sertoli cells, bind discrete sequences within the c-*kit* intron. Figure 8.2 shows schematically that, using

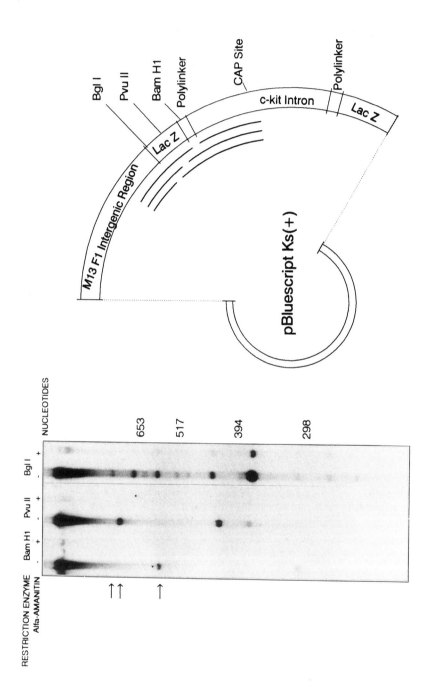

electrophoretic mobility shift assays, we have been able to map two small regions within this presumptive promoter that are essential for binding of spermatid-specific nuclear factors, at positions −485/−404 (the 82-bp fragment between two EcoRI sites in the figure) and −68/−50 (the 19-bp fragment between MboII and HpaII sites in the figure), respectively, from the transcriptional start site.

Experiments using a synthetic oligonucleotide spanning the −471/−437 region show that at least one of these factors binds a perfect "enhancer core" element, which can bind transcription factors such as AP-3 and C-EBP (23), since it can be competed by SV40 enhancer sequences. A PRDI-BF1 (23) potential binding site is present a few base pair downstream from this area within this oligonucleotide (Fig. 8.3). Southwestern experiments show that a series of polypeptides present in nuclear extracts from round spermatids, but not from spermatocytes or Sertoli cells, are specifically recognized by the same oligonucleotide (unpublished observations). Another sequence similar to the binding site of transcription factor PRDI-BF1 (22) is present also in the −68/−50 region (Fig. 8.3), which is more proximal to the transcriptional start site, suggesting that similar factors could also bind in this area. All this preliminary information strongly supports the hypothesis that a promoter specifically activated in the haploid stages of spermatogenesis is present within the 16th intron of the mouse c-*kit* gene.

The Intronic c-kit Promoter Is Active in Spermatids of Transgenic Mice

To confirm in vivo the activity of the intronic promoter, we have generated transgenic mice in which about 1 kb of these sequences are linked to the

FIGURE 8.1. Sequences within the 16th intron of the mouse c-*kit* gene act as a transcriptional promoter in vitro. In vitro run off transcription experiments using nuclear extracts from mouse round spermatids (stage 1–9 of spermiogenesis) in the presence of labeled ribonucleotide precursors. As a template for in vitro RNA synthesis we used the plasmid shown on the right, containing the 16th intron of the mouse c-*kit* gene. The plasmid had been digested with the indicated restriction enzymes, which cut downstream from the presumptive transcriptional (CAP) site present within this genomic sequence. If promoter sequences were present within the intron, labeled RNA fragments of discrete size (540, 700, and 730 nt, respectively) should be generated, as indicated by bars within the scheme of the template starting from the CAP site. The predicted RNA bands are effectively present in the autoradiography shown on the left (arrows). Other bands represent aspecific transcription starting from the M13 F1 intergenic region and are also indicated by bars in the scheme. Transcription is RNA polymerase-II dependent, since it is completely abolished by using as a specific inhibitor α-amanitin (+ lanes).

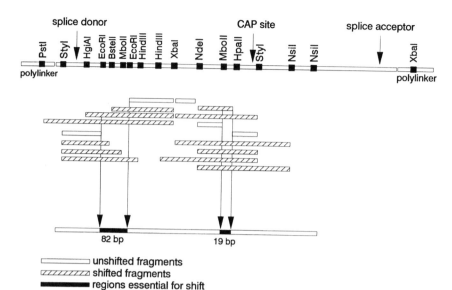

FIGURE 8.2. Discrete sequences within the 16th intron of the mouse c-*kit* gene specifically bind DNA-binding factors present in mouse spermatid nuclei. Summary of the results of autoradiographies of electrophoretic mobility shift assays with nuclear extracts from mouse round spermatids (stages 1–9 of spermiogenesis) using as probes several labeled restriction fragments of the DNA region encompassing the 16th intron of the mouse c-*kit* gene. The restriction map of the intron is reported above, whereas a schematic representation of the areas that are critical for specific binding of nuclear factors is drawn below. CAP site indicates the presumptive start of transcription of the truncated c-*kit* mRNA expressed during mouse spermiogenesis.

reporter *Escherichia coli* LacZ gene. The transgene was correctly integrated into the mouse genome and transmitted in a mendelian fashion (unpublished observations). We found that in the transgenic offspring of two separate founders β-galactosidase activity was specifically expressed only within seminiferous tubules, within the cytoplasm of haploid germ cells at stages 8–9 of spermiogenesis (Fig. 8.4). No expression was found in other organs (such as brain, liver, kidney, spleen, and heart), and the copy number of the integrated transgene did not appear to affect the degree of its expression in spermatids, whereas position effects due to random integration in the genome can influence its expression in male haploid germ cells (unpublished observations). These data indicate that the intronic promoter is active only in the latest transcriptional stages of round spermatids, and that the truncated form of the c-*kit* receptor should be produced during the first stages of elongation of haploid cells (from stage 10 of spermiogenesis), thus explaining the fact that relatively low levels of the truncated c-*kit* protein were detected in round spermatids.

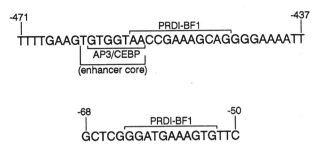

```
-471                                    PRDI-BF1                      -437
  |                          ┌─────────────────────┐                  |
TTTTGAAGTGTGGTAACCGAAAGCAGGGGAAAATT
              └────────────┘
               AP3/CEBP
              (enhancer core)


              -68              PRDI-BF1              -50
               |      ┌─────────────────────┐       |
              GCTCGGGGATGAAAGTGTTC
```

FIGURE 8.3. Minimal sequences within the 16th intron of the c-*kit* gene required for the binding of nuclear factors from round spermatids. The sequences shown are those of (top) an oligonucleotide corresponding to position −471/−437 from the presumptive transcriptional start site for the truncated c-*kit* mRNA, which contains an "enhancer core" and a PRDI-BF1 potential binding site; (bottom) a discrete area close to the presumptive transcriptional start site (−68/−50), which also contains a PRDI-BF1 potential binding site. Both these sequences are required for binding of nuclear factors from round spermatids. The −471/−437 oligonucleotide probably binds factors related to AP3 or CEBP in the area of the "enhancer core," since its binding can be competed by SV40 enhancer sequences.

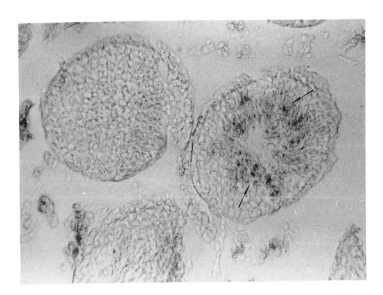

FIGURE 8.4. Sequences within the 16th intron of the mouse c-*kit* gene drive specific expression of the *E.Coli* LacZ reporter gene in male haploid germ cells in vivo. Light photograph of a 30-μm cryostatic section of testis from an adult F_3 heterozygous transgenic mouse carrying multiple copies of a fusion construct between the c-*kit* intronic region and the LacZ sequences, after staining of the whole fixed organ with X-gal. Expression of β-galactosidase is revealed by a blue-green precipitate (the dark crystals indicated by the arrows). Dark crystals are present in haploid germ cells immediately surrounding the lumen of ∼20% of seminiferous tubules, all at stages VIII–IX of the cycle of the seminiferous epithelium, when spermiation occurs and round spermatids begin the phase of elongation. Precipitates, which can be observed in interstitial cells, represent endogenous β-galactosidase activity, since it is observed with equal frequency and intensity in cryostatic section from testes of nontransgenic adult animals, as also observed by others (25).

Future Perspectives

Expression of the truncated c-*kit* transcript at the beginning of spermatid elongation could imply a tyrosine-kinase–independent role for the carboxyterminus of the c-*kit* protein in the formation of the sperm tail, which would recall the tyrosine-kinase–independent role played by *Drosophila abl* in axonal outgrowth (21). We are currently trying to purify subfractions of elongating spermatids to establish the exact moment of maximal accumulation of the c-*kit* gene product during spermiogenesis. Transgenic experiments indicate that the cryptic haploid-specific promoter present within the 16th intron of the c-*kit* gene could be an ideal target for homologous recombination (24), in order to establish the functional meaning of the truncated receptor in spermatids without altering the structure of the normal receptor expressed in the mitotic stages of spermatogenesis. We are planning to replace in embryonic stem cells the intronic sequences, which recognize spermatid-specific nuclear factors, with the *neo* marker gene, saving the splice donor and acceptor sequences (see Fig. 8.2). In this way we would generate chimeric mice possibly transmitting the knockout c-*kit* haploid-specific promoter through the germ-cell line. Analysis of the effect on spermiogenesis of altered transcription of the truncated c-*kit* protein will be possible on homozygous recombinant mice.

References

1. Russell ES. Hereditary anemias of the mouse: a review for geneticists. Adv Genet 1979;20:357–459.
2. Chabot B, Stephenson DA, Chapman VM, Besmer P, Bernstein A. The protooncogene c-*kit* encoding a transmembrane tyrosine kinase receptor maps to the mouse W locus. Nature 1988;335:88–9.
3. Qiu F, Ray P, Barker PE, Jhanwar S, Ruddle FH, Besmer P. Primary structure of c-*kit*: relationship with the CSF-1/PDGF receptor kinase family–oncogenic activation of v-*kit* involves deletion of extracellular domain and C terminus. EMBO J 1988;7:1003–11.
4. Besmer P. The *kit* ligand encoded at the murine Steel locus: a pleiotropic growth and differentiation factor. Curr Opin Cell Biol 1991;3:939–46.
5. Flanagan JF, Chan DC, Leder P. Transmembrane form of the *kit* ligand growth factor is determined by alternative splicing and is missing in the SI^d mutant. Cell 1991;64:1025–35.
6. Nocka K, Tan JC, Chiu E, Chu TY, Ray P, Traktman P, Besmer P. Molecular bases of dominant negative and loss of function mutations at the murine c-*kit*/white spotting locus: W^{37}, W^v, W^{41} and W. EMBO J 1990;9:1805–13.
7. Coulombre JL, Russell ES. Analysis of the pleiotropism at the W-locus in the mouse. J Exp Zool 1954;126:4277–95.

8. Manova K, Bachvarova RF. Expression of c-*kit* encoded at the W locus of mice in developing embryonic germ cells and presumptive melanoblasts. Dev Biol 1991;146:312–24.

9. Sorrentino V, Giorgi M, Geremia R, Besmer P, Rossi P. Expression of the c-*kit* proto-oncogene in the murine male germ cells. Oncogene 1991;6:149–51.

10. Rossi P, Albanesi C, Grimaldi P, Geremia R. Expression of the mRNA for the ligand of c-*kit* in mouse Sertoli cells. Biochem Biophys Res Commun 1991;176:910–4.

11. Rossi P, Dolci S, Albanesi C, Grimaldi P, Ricca R, Geremia R. Follicle-stimulating hormone induction of Steel Factor (SLF) mRNA in mouse Sertoli cells and stimulation of DNA synthesis in spermatogonia by soluble SLF. Dev Biol 1993;155:68–74.

12. Geremia R, Albanesi C, Dolci S, Giustizieri L, Grimaldi P, Grippo P, Orlando PA, Piscitelli D, Rossi P. c-*kit* receptor function and regulation by SLF in the postnatal testis. In: Dufau ML, Fabbri A, Isidori A, eds. Cell and molecular biology of the testis. Frontiers in endocrinology. Rome, Italy: Ares Serono Symposia 1994;5:189–98.

13. Orlando P, Geremia R, Frusciante C, Grippo P. Replicating pre-meiotic germ cells of the mouse contain a novel DNA primase stimulatory factor. Cell Differ 1989;27:129–36.

14. Grippo P, Geremia R, Locorotondo G, Monesi V. DNA-dependent DNA polymerase species in male germ cells of the mouse. Cell Differ 1978;7:237–48.

15. Dolci S, Williams DE, Ernst MK, Resnick JL, Brannan CI, Lock LF, Lyman SD, Boswell HS, Donovan PJ. Requirement for mast cell growth factor for primordial germ cell survival in culture. Nature 1991;352:809–11.

16. Marziali G, Lazzaro D, Sorrentino V. Binding of germ cells to mutant Sl^d Sertoli cells is defective and is rescued by expression of the transmembrane form of the c-*kit* ligand. Dev Biol 1993;157:182–90.

17. Parvinen M. Regulation of the seminiferous epithelium. Endocr Rev 1982; 3:404–17.

18. Yoshinaga K, Nishikawa S, Ogawa M, Hayashi S, Kunisada T, Fujimoto T, Nishikawa S-I. Role of c-*kit* in mouse spermatogenesis: identification of spermatogonia as a specific site of c-*kit* expression and function. Development 1991;113:689–99.

19. Brinster RL, Avarbock MR. Germline transmission of donor haplotype following spermatogonial transplantation. Proc Natl Acad Sci USA 1994;91:11303–7.

20. Rossi P, Marziali G, Albanesi C, Charlesworth A, Geremia R, Sorrentino V. A novel c-*kit* transcript, potentially encoding a truncated receptor, originates within a *kit* gene intron in mouse spermatids. Dev Biol 1992;152:203–7.

21. Henkemeyer M, West SR, Gertler FB, Hoffmann FM. A novel tyrosine-kinase-independent function of *Drosophila abl* correlates with proper subcellular localization. Cell 1990;63:949–60.

22. Gokkel E, Grossman Z, Ramot B, Yarden Y, Rechavi G, Givol D. Structural organization of the murine c-*kit* proto-oncogene. Oncogene 1992;7:1423–9.

23. Faisst S, Meyer S. Compilation of vertebrate-encoded transcription factors. Nucleic Acids Res 1992;20:3–26.

24. Capecchi MR. Altering the genome by homologous recombination. Science 1989;244:1288–92.

25. Behringer RR, Crotty DA, Tennyson VM, Brinster RL, Palmiter RD, Wolgemuth DJ. Sequences 5′ of the homeobox of the Hox-1.4 gene direct tissue-specific expression of lacZ during mouse development. Development 1993;117:823–33.

9

The IGF-II/Cation-Independent Mannose 6-Phosphate Receptor Mediates Changes in Spermatogenic Cell Gene Expression

James K. Tsuruta and Deborah A. O'Brien

Cell-cell interactions are acknowledged to play a crucial role during the normal progression of germinal cells through the process of spermatogenesis (reviewed in 1, 2). However, surprisingly little is known about the specific mechanisms underlying these interactions. A number of growth factors secreted by Sertoli cells including *insulin-like growth factor-I* (IGF-I), *transforming growth factor-β* (TGF-β), and interleukin-1 are proposed to influence germ-cell functions by interacting with their cognate receptors on the plasma membranes of germ cells. Although the site of synthesis of these factors has been investigated, their actions on germ cells have not been characterized (reviewed in 2). The soluble form of steel factor stimulates DNA synthesis in spermatogonia (3). Similarly, activin increases ^{3}H-thymidine incorporation in cocultures of Sertoli cells and germ cells, consistent with stimulation of the division of spermatogonia and/or spermatocytes (4), and IGF-II stimulates spermatogonial incorporation of ^{3}H-thymidine in cultures of seminiferous tubule segments (5). While Sertoli cell effects upon spermatogenic cell DNA synthesis have been investigated, little work has been published on changes in spermatogenic cell gene expression mediated by factors secreted by Sertoli cells. Rivarola et al. (6) demonstrated that co-culture with Sertoli cells increased total RNA synthesis in spermatogenic cells. However, few specific genes have been identified that undergo changes in expression in spermatogenic cells in response to the binding of factors secreted by Sertoli cells.

Our studies have focused on the IGF-II/*cation-independent mannose 6-phosphate receptor* (IGF-II/CI-MPR) and its role in mediating Sertoli cell–germ cell interactions. As described in this chapter, we have determined that this receptor is differentially expressed in the cells of the seminiferous epithelium, that Sertoli cells secrete IGF-II/CI-MPR ligands, and that this receptor-ligand system is capable of altering the expression of at least two specific genes in spermatogenic cells.

Germ Cell–Sertoli Cell Interactions Regulate Spermatogenesis

There is substantial evidence that interactions between Sertoli cells and germ cells are important for the regulation of spermatogenesis. Extensive junctions between Sertoli cells form the blood-testis barrier, dividing the seminiferous epithelium into two compartments. In the basal compartment, spermatogonia undergo a series of mitotic divisions. They produce preleptotene spermatocytes, which replicate DNA in the last S phase during spermatogenesis. Spermatocytes begin a prolonged meiotic prophase and then enter the adluminal compartment, where meiosis and the subsequent haploid period of spermatogenesis are completed (reviewed in 7).

Sertoli cells secrete a wide array of proteins and several growth factors. This secretory activity largely defines the milieu in which spermatogenic cells develop and differentiate into spermatozoa in the adluminal compartment. In vitro studies indicate that spermatogenic cells survive for longer periods in the presence of Sertoli cells and retain a limited capacity for differentiation (8–10). Sertoli cell production of metabolic substrates such as lactate and pyruvate, which are used preferentially by spermatogenic cells in culture, may be one component of this interaction (11). In addition, Sertoli cells secrete several growth factors that typically exert their effects through specific receptors (12, 13). These include insulin-like growth factors (14), as well as high affinity *IGF-binding proteins* (IGFBPs) that modulate the bioavailability and actions of these factors (15, 16).

In addition to establishing the specialized environment in the adluminal compartment of the seminiferous epithelium, recent studies indicate that Sertoli cells exert paracrine effects on early spermatogenic cells in the basal compartment. In testicular organ cultures from immature rats, *follicle-stimulating hormone* (FSH) is essential for the differentiation of type A spermatogonia to the pachytene stage of meiotic prophase, while testosterone, *luteinizing hormone* (LH), and vitamins A, C, and E are ineffective (17). Similarly, FSH maintains the number of spermatogonia and preleptotene spermatocytes at or above control levels in rats treated with a *gonadotropin-releasing hormone* (GnRH) antagonist (18), providing evidence that FSH also affects early spermatogenic cells in adult rats. Since FSH receptors appear to be restricted to Sertoli cells (1), these effects on early spermatogenic cells result from modulation of Sertoli cell function.

Several studies indicate that IGF-II and the IGF-II/CI-MPR may be particularly important during differentiation. IGF-II, but not IGF-I, stimulates the differentiation of PCC3 embryonic carcinoma cells (19). In myoblasts IGF-II is an autocrine factor that stimulates differentiation and the expression of a muscle-specific transcription factor (20). Additional studies have shown that this effect is mediated by the IGF-II/CI-MPR (21) and can be inhibited with IGFBP-6, a binding protein that binds selectively to IGF-II (22). Expression of IGF-II and IGF-II/CI-MPR *messenger RNAs* (mRNAs) also undergoes specific changes during spontaneous differentiation of colon epithelial cells (23). Our studies provide evidence that germ-cell differentiation in the testis may also be regulated by the IGF-II/CI-MPR and its ligands.

The IGF-II/CI-MPR Is a Multifunctional Receptor

The cation-independent *mannose 6-phosphate* (M6P) receptor was found to be identical to the IGF-II receptor when the nucleotide sequences of these two receptor mRNAs were compared (24, 25). Separate binding sites for IGF-II and M6P are present within the large extracytoplasmic domain of this multifunctional receptor (reviewed in 26, 27). The IGF-II/CI-MPRs, along with the smaller *cation-dependent MPR* (CD-MPR), are capable of targeting acidic hydrolases to lysosomes. Lysosomal hydrolases acquire M6P on their asparagine-linked oligosaccharides during posttranslational processing, serving as a highly specific recognition marker for the MPRs. The IGF-II/CI-MPR binds M6P glycoproteins without requiring divalent cations, both intracellularly for lysosomal trafficking and at the cell surface where it mediates signal transduction as well as endocytosis. In contrast, the smaller CD-MPR requires divalent cations for optimal ligand binding in some species, generally does not mediate the endocytosis of M6P glycoproteins, and does not bind IGF-II (26, 27). Interestingly, the IGF-II/CI-MPR and IGF-II genes are reciprocally imprinted, resulting in preferential expression from the maternal (IGF-II/CI-MPR) or paternal alleles (IGF-II) (27).

The IGF-II/CI-MPR is structurally distinct from other growth factor receptors, since it does not have the seven transmembrane segments characteristic of many G protein–linked receptors or the intrinsic tyrosine kinase activity found in IGF-I and insulin receptors (25). However, a casein kinase-II–type enzyme is capable of phosphorylating the short cytoplasmic tail of this receptor on specific serine residues (28). The IGF-II/CI-MPR is linked to signal transduction pathways in multiple systems (29). Binding of IGF-II (30, 31) or M6P-bearing peptides (32) to this receptor activates phospholipase C, producing inositol trisphosphate (IP_3) and diacylglycerol in basolateral kidney membranes. IGF-II binding also couples the IGF-II/CI-MPR to a G_{i2} guanine nucleotide-binding protein (G protein), which subsequently activates a calcium channel to allow a flux of calcium into primed-competent BALB/c 3T3 cells (33, 34). Specific cellular activation processes may be required to elicit this response since similar coupling of IGF-II/CI-MPR to G proteins was not demonstrated in mouse L-cells (35). A domain for G_{i2} interaction and activation has been identified as a specific 14-amino acid sequence in the cytoplasmic portion of the IGF-II/CI-MPR (36, 37).

The TGF-β precursors (38, 39) and a prolactin-related glycoprotein called proliferin (40) are growth factors that have M6P on their N-linked oligosaccharides. Consequently, these growth factors also bind to IGF-II/CI-MPRs. Like IGF-II, these growth factors activate phospholipase C in kidney membranes, an effect that cannot be reproduced with M6P alone or M6P-bearing lysosomal hydrolases (32). Rifkin et al. (41) have proposed that IGF-II/CI-MPRs also play a role in the activation of the latent TGF-β precursors, since addition of M6P to co-cultures blocks the formation of active TGF-βs. It is interesting to note that expression of IGF-II/CI-MPR and the TGF-β1 precursor increases coordinately during liver regeneration (42) as well as during monoterpene-induced regression of mammary tumors (43). Thus, the IGF-II/CI-MPR is a multifunctional receptor; it functions in targeting lysosomal enzymes, may mediate activation of TGF-β precursors, and has been shown to mediate signaling of IGF-II and M6P-bearing growth factors.

Distribution of IGF-II/CI-MPRs in the Seminiferous Epithelium

IGF-II/CI-MPRs are present in mouse spermatogenic cells and Sertoli cells, although there are substantial differences in the amount and location of the receptors in different cell types in the seminiferous epithelium. In vitro studies indicate that Sertoli cells synthesize abundant IGF-II/CI-MPRs that are localized predominantly on intracellular membranes (44). Pachytene spermatocytes and round spermatids synthesize much lower levels of IGF-II/CI-MPR but express a significant proportion of these receptors on the cell surface (44, 45).

The expression of IGF-II/CI-MPR mRNA was examined by Northern blot analysis of poly(A)$^+$ RNAs from Sertoli cells and from germ cells at defined stages of spermatogenesis (46). The CI-MPR mRNA (~10 kb) is detected in pachytene spermatocytes, round spermatids, condensing spermatids, Sertoli cells, and somatic tissues (brain, liver). The steady-state level of this transcript in Sertoli cells is not altered when FSH is added to the culture medium. As anticipated from our previous studies of MPR protein synthesis in testicular cells (44), IGF-II/CI-MPR mRNAs are less abundant in pachytene spermatocytes and round spermatids than in Sertoli cells. In addition, CI-MPR mRNAs persist in condensing spermatids, suggesting that synthesis of this receptor may continue in the late haploid phase of spermatogenesis after transcription ceases.

The distribution of IGF-II/CI-MPR proteins in the testis was determined by immunohistochemistry (47), using a rabbit antibody raised against purified rat IGF-II/CI-MPR (provided by Dr. C. Scott, Royal Prince Alfred Hospital, Australia). This antibody binds specifically to rat and mouse IGF-II/CI-MPRs, as demonstrated by radioimmunoassay, immunoblotting, and competition assays (48, 49). In the adult testis, the IGF-II/CI-MPR is abundant in Sertoli cells and less pronounced in pachytene spermatocytes and spermatids (47), consistent with our previous results (44, 46). In pachytene spermatocytes the IGF-II/CI-MPR is concentrated in a spherical structure in the cytoplasm, most likely the Golgi apparatus, which is prominent during this period of spermatogenesis.

Our recent studies have determined that IGF-II/CI-MPR mRNA and protein levels are markedly higher in spermatogonia and early spermatocytes than in pachytene spermatocytes and spermatids (47). Studies in the rat (50) and mouse (51) indicate that lysosomes are rare in spermatogonia and primary spermatocytes and increase in number during the haploid spermatid stages. Therefore, it is unlikely that the IGF-II/CI-MPR serves only a lysosomal targeting function during early spermatogenesis. We hypothesize that the IGF-II/CI-MPR functions as a growth factor receptor during the proliferative and early meiotic phases of germ-cell development.

Ligands for the IGF-II/CI-MPR Are Present in the Seminiferous Epithelium

The IGF-II/CI-MPR can function as a mediator of germ cell–Sertoli cell interactions only if ligands for this receptor are present in the seminiferous epithelium. Our studies have shown that Sertoli cells secrete multiple M6P glycoproteins (45). Using IGF-II/CI-MPR receptor affinity chromatography, we routinely isolate at least ten M6P glycoproteins from *Sertoli cell–conditioned medium* (SCM). These glycoproteins are specifically eluted from the column with M6P, which does not alter binding of IGF-II to the purified receptor (52). We have identified several constituents of this fraction and shown that Sertoli M6P glycoproteins are endocytosed by pachytene spermatocytes or round spermatids (45). Assays of lysosomal enzyme activities indicate that Sertoli cells selectively secrete β-N-acetylhexosaminidase and α-mannosidase, but not β-galactosidase or β-glucuronidase. We also demonstrated that the β-N-acetylhexosaminidase activity is confined to the high-affinity M6P-glycoprotein fraction (peak C) isolated from SCM.

Procathepsin L, another lysosomal enzyme precursor that is secreted by Sertoli cells (53), is present in both the low-affinity (peak B) and high-affinity (peak C) fractions isolated from SCM by IGF-II/CI-MPR affinity chromatography. This lower affinity for the IGF-II/CI-MPR is characteristic of procathepsin L (54). Both procathepsin L (53) and the cystatin C inhibitor of this enzyme (55) are expressed at distinct stages of the cycle of the seminiferous epithelium, suggesting that this protease has important roles during specific periods of germ-cell development.

Since the IGF-II growth factor is an important ligand for the IGF-II/CI-MPR, Northern blot analysis was used to determine whether cells from the seminiferous epithelium express IGF-II mRNA. A 4-kb IGF-II transcript is detected in poly(A)$^+$ RNAs from mouse Sertoli cells, mixed spermatogenic cells from adult testes, and brain (56). A recent in situ hybridization study indicates that IGF-II mRNAs are also present in the seminiferous epithelium of the adult rat (57). Preliminary studies using radioimmunoassay and immunohistochemistry have detected the IGF-II growth factor in the mouse testis and in Sertoli cell–conditioned medium.

These results demonstrate that multiple ligands for the IGF-II/CI-MPR are secreted by Sertoli cells. In culture these cells express low levels of IGF-II/CI-MPR on their cell surface, even though intracellular levels of this receptor are quite high (44). In contrast, pachytene spermatocytes and round spermatids express a larger proportion of their IGF-II/CI-MPRs on their plasma membranes. Thus, Sertoli cells secrete IGF-II/CI-MPR ligands that are able to function as regulators of germ-cell development after binding to IGF-II/CI-MPRs present on the plasma membranes of spermatogenic cells.

Effects of IGF-II/CI-MPR Ligands on Spermatogenic Cells

Our studies demonstrate that Sertoli IGF-II/CI-MPR ligands increase steady-state levels of c-*fos* mRNA and ribosomal RNA in spermatogenic cells, providing important evidence that signal transduction pathways can be stimulated by these ligands.

To determine whether Sertoli M6P glycoproteins or IGF-II modulates gene expression in spermatogenic cells, we first used a specific RNase protection assay to monitor increases in c-*fos* mRNA levels. C-*fos*, an early response gene, encodes a constituent of the AP-1 transcription factor, which in turn modulates the specific transcription of AP-1–responsive genes (58). Elevation of c-*fos* mRNA synthesis has been used as a sensitive indicator of transcriptional activation by growth factors and other stimuli (59). Low levels of c-*fos* mRNA have been detected in mouse spermatogenic cells (60, 61), although modulation of c-*fos* gene expression in these cells has not been reported previously.

Our initial studies of c-*fos* expression focused on pachytene spermatocytes and round spermatids since we previously demonstrated that these germ cells have surface IGF-II/CI-MPRs (44, 45). We found that steady-state levels of c-*fos* mRNA are elevated by our enzymatic dissociation procedure (62), similar to the elevation of c-*jun* and junB mRNAs observed in germ cells isolated by these methods (63). However, we determined that these increases in c-*fos* mRNA are transient, declining to low levels after 5 h in culture. Therefore, prior to treatment we routinely cultured germ cells overnight in MEM$_{GC}$ (MEM with Earle's salts, 15 mM HEPES, 1 mM pyruvate, 6 mM lactate) with 5% fetal bovine serum (64), followed by serum-free culture in the same medium for 1 h. The overnight culture period also allows regeneration of surface receptors and the removal of Sertoli cells, which adhere to the tissue culture dishes (56). Unfractionated SCM and IGF-II stimulate dose-dependent increases in c-*fos* mRNA in adult spermatogenic cells (predominantly pachytene spermatocytes and spermatids), and maximum mRNA levels are reached after 60 min of treatment (56). Furthermore, M6P glycoproteins purified from SCM by receptor affinity chromatography stimulate a similar response at a much lower concentration than unfractionated SCM (65). The changes in c-*fos* mRNA levels resulting from treatment with SCM appear to be mediated primarily by the binding of M6P glycoproteins to the IGF-II/CI-MPR, since these effects were largely abolished when spermatogenic cells were treated in the presence of 5 mM M6P. To our knowledge, this is the first direct demonstration that proteins secreted by Sertoli cells can modulate the expression of a *specific* germ-cell gene.

We found that phorbol esters such as phorbol 12-myristate 13-acetate (TPA) and the calcium ionophore A23187 also induce c-*fos* expression in spermatogenic cells. This indicates that signal transduction pathways involving protein kinase C and calcium are active in spermatogenic cells and may participate in IGF-II/MPR–mediated stimulation of c-*fos* expression (56, 65–67).

We are currently using a quantitative *reverse-transcription–polymerase chain reaction* (RT-PCR) assay to monitor changes in the steady-state levels of c-*fos* mRNA induced by IGF-II/CI-MPR ligands (56, 68). In addition to being quantitative, this assay is very sensitive. Reliable data are obtained from samples of 1×10^6 cells in 0.2 ml culture medium, reducing the number of cells and IGF-II/CI-MPR ligands needed by a factor of 50 compared with the amounts needed for our previous Northern blot and RNase protection assays (56, 65, 66).

SCM Increases Steady-State Levels of 18S Ribosomal RNA in Germ Cells

While establishing the quantitative RT-PCR assay, we observed that addition of SCM stimulates dose-dependent increases in the steady-state levels of 18S *ribosomal RNA* (rRNA) in round spermatids. This stimulation is completely blocked by the addition of 5 mM M6P, providing evidence that Sertoli M6P glycoproteins modulate rRNA transcription or processing in spermatogenic cells (56). The 18S rRNA levels also increase in pachytene spermatocytes treated with SCM, although the increase above basal levels is approximately half of that observed in round spermatids (56, 67). In previous studies we found that pachytene spermatocytes and round spermatids endocytose equal amounts of M6P glycoproteins, even though pachytene spermatocytes are larger cells with ~2.5 times more surface area (44). These observations suggest that the density of surface IGF-II/CI-MPRs may be higher on round spermatids than on pachytene spermatocytes.

Like germ cells at later periods of differentiation, spermatogonia isolated from 8-day-old mice display elevated c-*fos* mRNA and 18S rRNA levels after treatment with IGF-II/CI-MPR ligands. After treatment with SCM for 1 h, the relative increase in steady-state levels of 18S rRNA in spermatogonia is approximately 3-fold higher than in round spermatids (67), consistent with the higher levels of IGF-II/CI-MPRs detected in early spermatogenic cells. We have also used IGF-II analogues (69) to confirm that IGF-II stimulation of c-*fos* mRNA and 18S rRNA levels in spermatogonia is specifically mediated by the IGF-II/CI-MPR (67).

In summary, these studies provide substantial evidence that IGF-II/CI-MPR ligands present in the seminiferous epithelium can modulate gene expression in spermatogenic cells via receptor-mediated signal transduction pathways.

Acknowledgments. This work was supported by the Mellon Foundation (J.K.T.) and NIH grants HD26485, (D.A.O.), P30-HD18968, P32T-HD07315 (the Laboratories for Reproductive Biology) and CA16086 (Lineberger Comprehensive Cancer Center).

References

1. Griswold MD. Interactions between germ cells and Sertoli cells in the testis. Biol Reprod 1995;52:211–6.
2. Skinner MK, Norton JN, Mullaney BP, Rosselli M, Whaley PD, Anthony CT. Cell-cell interactions and the regulation of testis function. Ann NY Acad Sci 1991;637:354–63.
3. Rossi P, Dolci S, Albanesi C, Grimaldi P, Ricca R, Geremia R. Follicle-stimulating hormone induction of steel factor (SLF) mRNA in mouse Sertoli cells and stimulation of DNA synthesis in spermatogonia by soluble SLF. Dev Biol 1993;155:68–74.
4. Mather JP, Roberts PE, Krummen LA. Signaling molecules and their receptors. In: Bartke A, ed. Functions of somatic cells in the testis. Proceedings in the Serono Symposia, USA Series. New York: Springer-Verlag, 1994:245–52.

5. Soder O, Bang P, Wahab A, Parvinen M. Insulin-like growth factors selectively stimulate spermatogonial, but not meiotic, deoxyribonucleic acid synthesis during rat spermatogenesis. Endocrinology 1992;131(5):2344–50.

6. Rivarola MA, Sanchez P, Saez JM. Stimulation of ribonucleic acid and deoxyribonucleic acid synthesis in spermatogenic cells by their coculture with Sertoli cells. Endocrinology 1985;117(5):1796–802.

7. Russell LD, Ettlin RA, Sinha Hikim AP, Clegg ED. Histological and histopathological evaluation of the testis. Clearwater, FL: Cache River Press, 1990:286.

8. Tres LL, Kierszenbaum AL. Viability of rat spermatogenic cells in vitro is facilitated by their coculture with Sertoli cells in serum-free hormone-supplemented medium. Proc Natl Acad Sci USA 1983;80:3377–81.

9. Hadley MA, Byers SW, Suarez-Quian CA, Kleinman HK, Dym M. Extracellular matrix regulates Sertoli cell differentiation, testicular cord formation, and germ cell development in vitro. J Cell Biol 1985;101:1511–22.

10. Rassoulzadegan M, Paquis-Flucklinger V, Bertino B, Sage J, Jansin M, Miyagawa K, van Heyningen V, Besmer P, Cuzin F. Transmeiotic differentiation of male germ cells in culture. Cell 1993;75:997–1006.

11. Grootegoed JA, Jansen R, Van Der Molen HJ. The role of glucose, pyruvate and lactate in ATP production by rat spermatocytes and spermatids. Biochim Biophys Acta 1984;767:248–56.

12. Bellve AR, Zheng W. Growth factors as autocrine and paracrine modulators of male gonadal functions. J Reprod Fertil 1989;85:771–93.

13. O'Brien DA, Gabel CA, Welch JE, Eddy EM. Mannose 6-phosphate receptors: potential mediators of germ cell-Sertoli cell interactions. Ann NY Acad Sci 1991;637:327–39.

14. Smith EP, Svoboda MJ, Van Wyk JJ, Kierszenbaum AL, Tres LL. Partial characterization of a somatomedin-like peptide from the medium of cultured rat Sertoli cells. Endocrinology 1987;120:186–93.

15. Smith EP, Dickson BA, Chernausek SD. Insulin-like growth factor binding protein-3 secretion from cultured rat Sertoli cells: dual regulation by follicle stimulating hormone and insulin-like growth factor-I. Endocrinology 1990; 127:2744–51.

16. Rappaport MS, Smith EP. Insulin-like growth factor (IGF) binding protein 3 in the rat testis: follicle-stimulating hormone dependence of mRNA expression and inhibition of IGF-I action on cultured Sertoli cells. Biol Reprod 1995;52:419–25.

17. Boitani C, Politi MG, Menna T. Spermatogonial cell proliferation in organ culture of immature rat testes. Biol Reprod 1993;48:761–7.

18. Sinha Hikim AP, Swerdloff RS. Temporal and stage-specific effects of recombinant human follicle-stimulating hormone on the maintenance of spermatogenesis in gonadatropin-releasing hormone antagonist-treated rat. Endocrinology 1995;136:253–61.

19. Trojan J, Johnson TR, Rudin SD, Blossey BK, Kelley KM, Shevelev A, Abdul-Karim FW, Anthony DD, Tykocinski ML, Ilan J. Gene therapy of murine teratocarcinoma: separate functions for insulin-like growth factors I and II in immunogenicity and differentiation. Proc Natl Acad Sci USA 1994;91:6088–92.

20. Florini JR, Magri KA, Ewton DZ, James PL, Grindstaff K, Rotwein PS. "Spontaneous" differentiation of skeletal myoblasts is dependent upon autocrine

secretion of insulin-like growth factor-II. J Biol Chem 1991;266:15917–23.
21. Rosenthal SM, Hsiao D, Silverman LA. An insulin-like growth factor-II (IGF-II) analog with highly selective affinity for IGF-II receptors stimulates differentiation, but not IGF-I receptor down-regulation in muscle cells. Endocrinology 1994;135:38–44.
22. Bach LA, Hsieh S, Brown AL, Rechler MM. Recombinant human insulin-like growth factor (IGF)-binding protein-6 inhibits IGF-II-induced differentiation of L6A1 myoblasts. Endocrinology 1994;135:2168–76.
23. Kiess W, Yang Y, Kessler U, Hoeflich A. Insulin-like growth factor II (IGF-II) and the IGF-II/mannose 6-phosphate receptor: the myth continues. Horm Res 1994;41(suppl 2):66–73.
24. Lobel P, Dahms NM, Breitmeyer J, Chirgwin JM, Kornfeld S. Cloning of the bovine 215-kDa cation-independent mannose 6-phosphate receptor. Proc Natl Acad Sci USA 1987;84:2233–7.
25. Morgan DO, Edman JC, Standring DN, Fried VA, Smith MC, Roth RA, Rutter WJ. Insulin-like growth factor II receptor as a multifunctional binding protein. Nature 1987;329:301–7.
26. Kornfeld S. Structure and function of the mannose 6-phosphate/insulin-like growth factor II receptors. Annu Rev Biochem 1992;61:307–30.
27. von Figura K. Molecular recognition and targeting of lysosomal proteins. Curr Opin Cell Biol 1991;3:642–6.
28. Rosorius O, Mieskes G, Issinger O, Korner C, Schmidt B, von Figura K, Braulke T. Characterization of phosphorylation sites in the cytoplasmic domain of the 300 kDa mannose-6-phosphate receptor. Biochem J 1993;292:833–8.
29. Vignon F, Rochefort H. Interactions of pro-cathepsin D and IGF-II on the mannose-6-phosphate/IGF-II receptor. Breast Cancer Res Treat 1992;22:47–57.
30. Rogers SA, Hammerman MR. Insulin-like growth factor II stimulates production of inositol trisphosphate in proximal tubular basolateral membranes from canine kidney. Proc Natl Acad Sci USA 1988;85:4037–41.
31. Rogers SA, Hammerman MR. Mannose 6-phosphate potentiates insulin-like growth factor II-stimulated inositol trisphosphate production in proximal tubular basolateral membranes. J Biol Chem 1989;264:4273–6.
32. Rogers SA, Purchio AF, Hammerman MR. Mannose 6-phosphate-containing peptides activate phospholipase C in proximal tubular basolateral membranes from canine kidney. J Biol Chem 1990;265:9722–7.
33. Murayama Y, Okamoto T, Ogata E, Asano T, Iiri T, Katada T, Ui M, Grubb JH, Sly WS, Nishimoto I. Distinctive regulation of the functional linkage between the human cation-independent mannose 6-phosphate receptor and GTP-binding proteins by insulin-like growth factor II and mannose 6-phosphate. J Biol Chem 1990;265:17456–62.
34. Nishimoto I. The IGF-II receptor system: a G protein-linked mechanism. Mol Reprod Dev 1993;35:398–407.
35. Korner K, Nurnberg B, Uhde M, Braulke T. Mannose 6-phosphate/insulin-like growth factor II receptor fails to interact with G-proteins. J Biol Chem 1995;270:287–95.
36. Okamoto T, Nishimoto I, Murayama Y, Ohkuni Y, Ogata E. Insulin-like growth factor-II/mannose 6-phosphate receptor is incapable of activating GTP-binding proteins in response to mannose 6-phosphate, but capable in response to insu-

lin-like growth factor-II. Biochem Biophys Res Commun 1990;168:1201–10.

37. Takahashi K, Murayama Y, Okamoto T, Yokota T, Ikezu T, Takahashi S, Giambarella U, Ogata E, Nishimoto I. Conversion of G-protein specificity of insulin-like growth factor II/mannose 6-phosphate receptor by exchanging of a short region with β-adrenergic receptor. Proc Natl Acad Sci USA 1993;90:11772–6.

38. Purchio AF, Cooper JA, Brunner AM, Lioubin MN, Gentry LE, Kovacina KS, Roth RS, Marquardt H. Identification of mannose 6-phosphate in two asparagine-linked sugar chains of recombinant transforming growth factor-β1 precursor. J Biol Chem 1988;263:14211–5.

39. Brunner AM, Lioubin MN, Marquardt H, Malacko AR, Wang W, Shapiro RA, Neubauer M, Cook J, Madisen L, Purchio AF. Site-directed mutagenesis of glycosylation sites in the transforming growth factor-β1 (TGFβ1) and TGFβ2 (414) precursors and of cysteine residues within mature TGFβ1: effects on secretion and bioactivity. Mol Endocrinol 1992;6:1691–700.

40. Lee S, Nathans D. Proliferin secreted by cultured cells binds to mannose 6-phosphate receptors. J Biol Chem 1988;263:3521–7.

41. Rifkin DB, Kojima S, Abe M, Harpel JG. TGF-β: structure, function, and formation. Thromb Haemost 1993;70:177–9.

42. Jirtle RL, Carr LI, Scott CD. Modulation of insulin-like growth factor-II/mannose 6-phosphate receptors and transforming growth factor-β1 during liver regeneration. J Biol Chem 1991;266:22444–50.

43. Jirtle RL, Haag JD, Ariazi EA, Gould MN. Increased mannose 6-phosphate/insulin-like growth factor II receptor and transforming growth factor β1 levels during monoterpene-induced regression of mammary tumors. Cancer Res 1993;53:3849–52.

44. O'Brien DA, Gabel CA, Rockett DL, Eddy EM. Receptor-mediated endocytosis and differential synthesis of mannose 6-phosphate receptors in isolated spermatogenic and Sertoli cells. Endocrinology 1989;125:2973–84.

45. O'Brien DA, Gabel CA, Eddy EM. Mouse Sertoli cells secrete mannose 6-phosphate containing glycoproteins that are endocytosed by spermatogenic cells. Biol Reprod 1993;49:1055–65.

46. O'Brien DA, Welch JE, Fulcher KD, Eddy EM. Expression of mannose 6-phosphate receptor mRNAs in mouse spermatogenic and Sertoli cells. Biol Reprod 1994;50:429–35.

47. O'Brien DA, Magyar PL, Hanes RN, Tsuruta JK. Expression of the IGF-II/cation-independent mannose 6-phosphate receptor in the mouse seminiferous epithelium. Mol Biol Cell 1993;4:137a.

48. Scott CD, Baxter RC. Purification and immunological characterization of the rat liver insulin-like growth factor-II receptor. Endocrinology 1987;120:1–9.

49. Hartshorn MA, Scott CD, Baxter RC. Immunofluorescent localization of type II insulin-like growth factor receptor in rat liver and hepatoma cells. J Endocrinol 1989;121:221–7.

50. Chemes H. The phagocytic function of Sertoli cells: a morphological, biochemical, and endocrinological study of lysosomes and acid phosphatase localization in the rat testis. Endocrinology 1986;119:1673–81.

51. O'Brien DA, Magyar PL, Sleat DE, Lobel P. Mannose 6-phosphate-bearing glycoproteins are abundant in mouse testis and brain. Mol Biol Cell 1994;5:221.

52. Tong PY, Tollefsen SE, Kornfeld S. The cation-independent mannose 6-phosphate receptor binds insulin-like growth factor II. J Biol Chem 1988;263: 2585–8.

53. Erickson-Lawrence M, Zabludoff SD, Wright WW. Cyclic protein-2, a secretory product of rat Sertoli cells, is the proenzyme form of cathepsin L. Mol Endocrinol 1991;5(12):1789–98.

54. Lazzarino DA, Gabel CA. Protein determinants impair recognition of procathepsin L phosphorylated oligosaccharides by the cation-independent mannose 6-phosphate receptor. J Biol Chem 1990;265:11864–71.

55. Tsuruta JK, O'Brien DA, Griswold MD. Sertoli cell and germ cell cystatin C: stage-dependent expression of two distinct messenger ribonucleic acid transcripts in rat testes. Biol Reprod 1993;49(5):1045–54.

56. Tsuruta JK, O'Brien DA. Sertoli cell-spermatogenic cell interaction: the IGF-II/cation-independent mannose 6-phosphate receptor mediates changes in spermatogenic cell gene expression. Biol Reprod 1995;53:1454–64.

57. Bondy CA, Zhou J, Chin E, Reinhardt RR, Ding L, Roth RA. Cellular distribution of insulin-degrading enzyme gene expression: comparison with insulin and insulin-like growth factor receptors. J Clin Invest 1994;93:966–73.

58. Angel P, Karin M. The role of Jun, Fos and the AP-1 complex in cell-proliferation and transformation. Biochim Biophys Acta 1991;1072:129–57.

59. Smith EP, Hall SH, Monaco L, French FS, Wilson EM, Conti M. A rat Sertoli cell factor similar to basic fibroblast growth factor increases c-*fos* messenger ribonucleic acid in cultured Sertoli cells. Mol Endocrinol 1989;3: 954–61.

60. Sorrentino V, McKinney MD, Giorgi M, Geremia R, Fleissner E. Expression of cellular protooncogenes in the mouse male germ line: a distinctive 2.4-kilobase pim-1 transcript is expressed in haploid postmeiotic cells. Proc Natl Acad Sci USA 1988;85:2191–5.

61. Wolfes H, Kogawa K, Millette CF, Cooper GM. Specific expression of nuclear proto-oncogenes before entry into meiotic prophase of spermatogenesis. Science 1989;245:740–3.

62. O'Brien DA. Isolation, separation and short-term culture of spermatogenic cells. Methods Toxicol 1993;3(A):246–64.

63. Alcivar AA, Hake LE, Hardy MP, Hecht NB. Increased level of junB and c-*jun* mRNAs in male germ cells following testicular cell dissociation. J Biol Chem 1990;265:20160–5.

64. Gerton GL, Millette CF. Stage-specific synthesis and fucosylation of plasma membrane proteins by mouse pachytene spermatocytes and round spermatids in culture. Biol Reprod 1986;35:1025–35.

65. Tsuruta JK, O'Brien DA. Sertoli cell conditioned medium, mannose 6-phosphate-bearing glycoproteins and IGF-II are able to alter gene expression in spermatogenic cells. Mol Biol Cell 1993;4:28a.

66. Tsuruta JK, O'Brien DA. Elevated steady-state levels of c-*fos* mRNA in isolated spermatogenic cells after treatment with fetal bovine serum or phorbol ester. Mol Biol Cell 1992;3:102a.

67. Tsuruta JK, O'Brien DA. Ligands for the IGF-II/cation-independent mannose 6-phosphate receptor modulate gene expression in spermatogonia, pachytene spermatocytes and round spermatids. Mol Biol Cell 1994;5: 221a.

68. Becker-Andre M. Absolute levels of mRNA by polymerase chain reaction-aided transcript titration assay. Methods Enzymol 1993;218:420–45.

69. Sakano K, Enjoh T, Numata F, Fujiwara H, Marumoto Y, Higashihashi N, Sato Y, Perdue JF, Fujita-Yamaguchi Y. The design, expression, and characterization of human insulin-like growth factor II (IGF-II) mutants specific for either the IGF-II/cation-independent mannose 6-phosphate receptor or IGF-I receptor. J Biol Chem 1991;266:20626–35.

Part III

Macromolecules and Organelles Unique to Germ Cells

10

Testis-Specific Gene Transcription

KOUROSH SALEHI-ASHTIANI AND ERWIN GOLDBERG

The classic studies of Monesi (1, 2) in the 1960s revealed an intricate pattern of RNA synthesis during spermatogenesis, characterized by transient transcriptional activity. During the early stages of meiotic prophase, a relatively low rate of [^{3}H]uridine incorporation was detected; however, RNA synthesis increases at the mid-pachytene stage followed by diminution during the meiotic divisions. RNA synthesis once again increases in the round and elongating spermatids (up to step 8), followed by a decline in later stages where nuclear condensation occurs.

Since the discovery of *lactate dehydrogenase* (LDH)-C$_4$, many additional testis-specific gene products have been described. Table 10.1 lists a number of such genes that encode either testis-specific isoforms or structural gene products unique to the testis. In terms of expression, two broad patterns may be recognized: (i) genes whose *messenger RNA* (mRNA) expression begins prior to the first meiotic prophase, and (ii) genes that are transcribed postmeiotically. Examples of the first category include *Ldhc*, *PGK-2* (at the mRNA level), cytochrome c$_t$, and histone isoforms (see Table 10.1 for references). Expression of transition proteins, protamines, and testis-specific calpastatin occurs postmeiotically (see Table 10.1 for references).

In addition to the testis-specific genes listed in Table 10.1, a number of somatic structural genes are expressed in the testis with altered transcript structures, often showing temporal regulation during spermatogenesis (Table 10.2). Among these, alternative forms of somatic cytochrome c (3), GATA-1 (4), *pro-opiomelanocortin* (POMC) (5), pro-enkephalin (6), and a number of proto-oncogenes with altered mRNA structure can be named (7). These altered transcripts, which generally contain the same protein coding sequences, may differ in mRNA stability or translational efficiency (7). In the case of cytochrome c and GATA-1, alternative testis-specific promoters are implicated in generation of the testis-specific transcripts (3, 4).

TABLE. 10.1. A list of genes that are expressed in a testis-specific manner.

Gene/clone	Description/function	Reference
Ldhc	Lactate dehydrogenase	(35–37)
PGK-2	Phosphoglycerate kinase	(38–41)
Pdhα-2	E1α subunit of pyruvate dehydrogenase	(18)
C_t	Cytochrome c	(42–44)
Y-19	Testis-specific isoform of calpastatin	(45)
M-α-3, -7	α-tubulin isoforms	(46)
H1t	Histone isoform	(47)
H2b	Histone isoform	(48)
TP1/TP2	Transition proteins	(49, 50)
MP1/MP2	Protamines	(51)
Zfa	Zinc finger protein	(17)
Tpx-1	Sperm maturation	(52, 53)
Sby	Spermatogonia proliferation	(54)
Testis ACE	Angiotensin-converting enzyme	(55)
tsHMG	Putative regulation of haploid gene expression	(56)

Genomic Organization

A number of genes belonging to the *t*-complex region of mouse show testis-specific or testis-enhanced expression (8). Examples include *Tctex* genes (9), a CpG rich clone (designated as 117c3) (10), and transmission ratio distortion candidate genes (11). The *t*-complex is a naturally occurring variant of the murine chromosome 17 where a double inversion has occurred. The *t*-complex is approximately 15 cMorgan in size, spanning a region near the centromere to a point between the major histocompatibil-

TABLE 10.2. A list of genes with altered testis-specific transcripts.

Gene	Description/function	Reference
c-*abl*	Proto-oncogene	(57)
c-*mos*	Proto-oncogene	(58)
cytochrome c	Somatic isoform	(3)
GATA-1	Transcription factor	(4)
POMC	Neuropeptide	(5)
Pro-enkephalin	Neuropeptide	(6)
TGFβ-1	Growth factor	(59)

ity complex and the *Pgk-2* locus (12). Due to the inversions present in the *t*-complex, genes in this region form a haplotype with a very low frequency of recombination. Although the mutant *t*-complex causes sterility when homozygous, it is found at the high frequency of 40% in the population. The genes of this haplotype are believed to be important for spermatogenesis or sperm differentiation, as sperm from heterozygous males show a preferential fertilization of the eggs by sperm carrying the *t*-haplotype (13, 14).

Regardless of the functions of these genes, the fact that a number of testis-enhanced or testis-specific genes are clustered on a region of a chromosome is noteworthy.[1] While this grouping of genes may be coincidental, further characterization of these genes may reveal whether this grouping is reflective of an evolutionary strategy for generation of genes with common expression patterns.

Aside from the chromosomal location of *Pgk-2*, it is interesting to note that this gene has characteristics of a processed gene, or an expressed retroposon. While *Pgk-1* is a ubiquitously expressed gene containing 10 introns, *Pgk-2* has no introns and contains remnants of a poly(A) tail (15). The *Pgk-2* gene appears to have evolved from an aberrant transcript of *Pgk-1*, as it contains sequences corresponding to those of regulatory elements of *Pgk-1* (16). Finally, *Pgk-2* is flanked by inverted repeats (16), an arrangement that is a hallmark of transposition events. In addition to *Pgk-2*, two other testis-specific genes have been characterized as expressed retroposons. *Zfa*, a candidate testis determinant gene (17), and *Pdha-2*, a testis-specific isoform of E1α subunit of pyruvate dehydrogenase (18), both lack introns, in contrast to their somatic counterparts. Other functional mammalian retroposons (excluding the genuine transposable elements) include the rat proinsulin I (19) and N-*myc2* of the woodchuck (20). The latter shows a brain-specific expression pattern. Thus, N-*myc2* is analogous to *Pgk-2* in that both retroposons show a more restricted expression pattern as compared with their ancestral counterparts. As more functional retroposons become characterized, a trend for testis- or tissue-specific expression may become apparent for functional retroposons.

Translational Regulation

Translational regulation is a common mechanism for control of many genes during oocyte maturation and early development (22, 23). Similarly, a number of testis-specific transcripts show translational regulation during spermatogenesis. In *Drosophila*, members of a family of seven genes that

---

[1] In addition to these genes, a cluster of testis-specific genes has also been discovered in *Drosophila* (21).

encode structural proteins of the sperm tail are found to be translationally downregulated (24). This translational downregulation is mediated through a conserved 12-base motif in the 5' *untranslated region* (UTR) of these transcripts, which also appears to control changes in the poly(A) tail of the mRNA (25). In mice, examples of translationally regulated messenger RNAs include transition proteins (26, 27), Pgk-2 (28), and protamines (29). In the case of transition protein 1 and protamine 1, the transcripts are first detected in the round spermatids; however, these mRNAs are not translated for a period of 3–7 days (27). When a chimeric transcript of human growth hormone and the 3' untranslated region of protamine 1 are expressed in transgenic mice, a "protamine-like" translational regulation is observed (30). In the protamine 2 mRNA, two *cis*-acting elements (designated as Y and H elements) have been identified to interact with *trans*-acting factors. An 18-kd protein is found to interact with one of the elements (31). Purified preparations of the 18 kd protein are able to block translation of transcripts containing the 3' UTR of protamine 2 in reticulocyte lysate (32). The ability of this factor to bind and repress translation of protamine 2 appears to depend on its phosphorylation state (32). In addition, two proteins homologous to the *Xenopus* oocyte RNA/DNA binding proteins have been identified in the mouse testis (33). These proteins are not present in the immature mouse testis, brain, or liver, and appear to function in storing translationally inactive mRNAs (33).

The necessity for the presence of translational regulation of testis-specific transcripts may be the consequence of limitations set upon the differentiating spermatids by deactivation of chromatin in late spermiogenesis due to condensation of the haploid genome. Genes that are to be expressed during or after chromatin condensation need to be transcribed and maintained in a translationally inactive form prior to the differentiation stage in which the translation product is needed (34). However, this rationale does not account for the occurrence of translational regulation in *Pgk-2*. Translation of this transcript begins prior to chromatin condensation (28).

Conclusion

Development of a spermatozoan requires that a complex array of morphological changes take place in a coordinated manner. Expression of a remarkably large number of testis-specific isozymes, isoforms, unique structural genes, and genes with alternative testis-specific mRNA structure have been found (for examples, see Tables 10.1 and 10.2) in association with the spermatogenic process. The requirement for specialized gene products required to generate the spermatozoan reflects the extent to which cellular differentiation must occur. The highly coordinated nature of molecular events during spermatogenesis has provided an ideal framework for molecular analysis of structure-function relationship and of regulatory mechanisms that govern tissue-specific gene expression. As model systems, a number of representative genes have been studied in terms of their regulated expression and comparisons with their somatic counterparts. Aside from the expected regulation at the transcriptional level, several general themes have emerged with respect to spermatogenic gene expression. These include occurrence of translational regulation, clustering of genes, occurrence of alternative testis-specific transcripts, and the role of epigenetic information (i.e., DNA methylation) in regulation of testis-specific gene expression. Together, these show the multiplicity as well as convergence of regulatory mechanisms involved in testis-specific gene expression. Elucidation of these mechanisms not only has led to a better understanding of spermatogenesis but also has facilitated the study of gene function and regulation in general.

A next step toward completing our precise understanding of the molecular aspects of spermatogenesis is the analysis of the functional significance of testis-specific macromolecules. The metabolic roles played by LDH-C$_4$ and cytochrome c$_t$ are not clearly defined. There are structural differences between both of these proteins and their somatic counterparts. The function of protamine in sperm DNA condensation is well documented. The difference between testis and somatic isoforms of AgX, a cytoskeletal component of the sperm outer dense fibers, remains to be established.

References

1. Monesi V. Ribonucleic acid synthesis during mitosis and meiosis in the mouse testis. J Cell Biol 1964;22:521–32.
2. Monesi V. Synthetic activities during spermatogenesis in the mouse: RNA and protein. Exp Cell Res 1965;39:197–224.
3. Hake LE, Hecht NB. Utilization of an alternative transcription initiation site of somatic cytochrome c in the mouse produces a testis-specific cytochrome c mRNA. J Biol Chem 1993;268:4788–97.
4. Ito E, Toki T, Ishihara H, Ohtani H, Gu L, Yokoyama M, Engel JD, Yamamoto M. Erythroid transcription factor GATA-1 is abundantly transcribed in mouse testis. Nature 1993;362:466–8.
5. Gizang-Ginsberg E, Wolgemuth DJ. Expression of the pro-opiomelanocortin gene is developmentally regulated and affected by germ cells in the male mouse reproductive system. Proc Natl Acad Sci USA 1987;84:1600–4.
6. Kilpatrick DL, Millette CF. Expression of pro-enkephalin messenger RNA by mouse spermatogenic cells. Proc Natl Acad Sci USA 1986;83:5015–8.
7. Propst F, Rosenberg MP, Vande Woude GF. Proto-oncogene expression in germ cell development. Trends Genet 1988;4:183–7.
8. Yeom YI, Abe K, Bennett D, Artzt K. Testis/embryo-expressed genes are clustered in the mouse H-2K region. Proc Natl Acad Sci USA 1992;89:773–7.
9. Ha H, Howard CA, Yeom YI, Abe K, Uehara H, Artzt K, Bennett D. Several testis-expressed genes in the mouse t-complex have expression differences between wild-type and t-mutant mice. Dev Genet 1991;12:318–32.

10. Rappold GA, Stubbs L, Labeit S, Crkvenjakov RB, Lehrach H. Identification of a testis-specific gene from the mouse t-complex next to a CpG-rich island. EMBO J 1987;6:1975–80.

11. Willison KR, Hynes G, Davies P, Goldsborough A, Lewis VA. Expression of three *t*-complex genes, *Tcp-1*, *D17Leh117c3*, and *D17Leh66*, in purified murine spermatogenic cell populations. Genet Res 1990;56:193–201.

12. Silver L. Mouse *t*-haplotypes. Annu Rev Genet 1985;19:179–208.

13. Lyon MF. Transmission ratio distortion in mouse *t*-haplotype is due to multiple distorter genes acting on a responder locus. Cell 1984;37:621–8.

14. Lyon MF. Male sterility of the mouse t-complex is due to homozygosity of the distorter genes. Cell 1986;44:357–63.

15. McCarrey JR, Thomas K. Human testis-specific PGK gene lacks introns and possesses characteristics of a processed gene. Nature 1987;326:501–5.

16. McCarrey JR. Nucleotide sequence of the promoter region of a tissue-specific human retroposon: comparison with its housekeeping progenitor. Gene 1987;61:291–8.

17. Ashworth A, Skene B, Swift S, Lovell-Badge R. *Zfa* is an expressed retrotransposon derived from an alternative transcript of the *Zfx* gene. EMBO J 1990;9:1529–34.

18. Fitzgerald J, Hutchison WM, Dahl HH. Isolation and characterization of the mouse pyruvate dehydrogenase E1 alpha genes. Biochim Biophys Acta 1991;1131:83–90.

19. Soares MB, Schon E, Henderson A, Karathanasis SK, Cate R, Zeitlin S, Chirwin J, Efstratiadis A. RNA-mediated gene duplication: the rat pre-proinsulin I gene is a functional retroposon. Mol Cell Biol 1985;5:2090–103.

20. Fourel G, Transy C, Tennant BC, Buendia MA. Expression of the woodchuck N-*myc*2 retroposon in brain and in liver tumors is driven by a cryptic N-*myc* promoter. Mol Cell Biol 1992;12:5336–44.

21. Kuhn R, Kuhn C, Borsch D, Glatzer KH, Schafer U, Schafer M. A cluster of four genes selectively expressed in the male germ line of *Drosophila melanogaster*. Mech Dev 1991;35:143–51.

22. Richter JD, Paris J, McGrew LL. Maternal mRNA expression in early development: regulation at the 3′ end. Enzyme 1990;44:129–46.

23. Richter JD. Translational control during early development. Bioessays 1991; 13:179–83.

24. Schafer M, Kuhn R, Bosse F, Schafer U. A conserved element in the leader mediates post-meiotic translation as well as cytoplasmic polyadenylation of *Drosophila* spermatocyte mRNA. EMBO J 1990;9:4519–25.

25. Kempe E, Muhs B, Schafer M. Gene regulation in *Drosophila* spermatogenesis: analysis of protein binding at the translational control element TCE. Dev Genet 1992;14:449–59.

26. Heidaran MA, Showman RM, Kistler WS. A cytochemical study of the transcriptional and translational regulation of nuclear transition protein 1 (TP1), a major chromosomal protein of mammalian spermatids. J Cell Sci 1988; 106:1427–33.

27. Morales CR, Kwon YK, Hecht NB. Cytoplasmic localization during storage and translation of the mRNAs of transition protein 1 and protamine 1, two translationally regulated transcripts of the mammalian testis. J Cell Sci 1991;100:119–31.

28. Gold B, Fujimoto H, Kramer JM, Erickson RP, Hecht NB. Haploid accumulation and translational control of phosphoglycerate kinase-2 messenger RNA during mouse spermatogenesis. Dev Biol 1983;98:392–9.
29. Kleene KC, Distel RJ, Hecht NB. Translational regulation and deadenylation of a protamine mRNA during spermatogenesis in mouse. Dev Biol 1984;105:71–9.
30. Braun RE, Peschon JJ, Behringer RR, Brinster RL, Palmiter RD. Protamine 3′-untranslated sequences regulate temporal translational control and subcellular localization of growth hormone in spermatids of transgenic mice. Genes Dev 1989;3:793–802.
31. Kwon YK, Hecht NB. Cytoplasmic protein binding to highly conserved sequences in the 3′ untranslated region of mouse protamine 2 mRNA, a translationally regulated transcript of male germ cells. Proc Natl Acad Sci USA 1991;88:3584–8.
32. Kwon YK, Hecht NB. Binding of a phosphoprotein to the 3′ untranslated region of the mouse protamine 2 mRNA temporally represses its translation. Mol Cell Biol 1993;13:6547–57.
33. Kwon YK, Murray MT, Hecht NB. Proteins homologous to the *Xenopus* germ cell-specific RNA-binding proteins p54/p56 are temporally expressed in mouse male germ cells. Dev Biol 1993;158:90–100.
34. Hecht NB. Gene expression during male germ cell development. In: Desjardins C, Ewing LL, eds. Cell and molecular biology of the testis. Oxford, England: Oxford University Press, 1993:400–32.
35. Blanco A, Zinkham WH. Lactate dehydrogenases in human testes. Science 1963;139:601–2.
36. Goldberg E. Lactate and malic dehydrogenases in human spermatozoa. Science 1963;139:602–3.
37. Alcivar AA, Trasler JM, Hake LE, Salehi-Ashtiani K, Goldberg E, Hecht NB. DNA methylation and expression of the genes coding for lactate dehydrogenase A and C during rodent spermatogenesis. Biol Reprod 1991;44:527–35.
38. Vandeberg JL, Cooper DW, Close PJ. Testis specific phosphoglycerate kinase B in mouse. J Exp Zool 1976;198:231–40.
39. Vandeberg JL, Lee CY, Goldberg E. Immunohistochemical localization of phosphoglycerate kinase isozymes in mouse testis. J Exp Zool 1981;217:435–41.
40. Bluthmann H, Cicurel L, Kuntz GW, Haedenkamp G, Illmensee K. Immuno-histochemical localization of mouse testis-specific phosphoglycerate kinase (PGK-2) by monoclonal antibodies. EMBO J 1982;1:479–84.
41. Tilghman SM. DNA methylation: a phoenix rises. Proc Natl Acad Sci USA 1993;90:8761–2.
42. Goldberg E, Sberna D, Wheat TE, Urbanski GJ, Margoliash E. Cytochrome c: immunofluorescent localization of the testis specific form. Science 1997;196:1010–2.
43. Virbasius JV, Scarpulla RC. Structure of rodent genes encoding the testis-specific cytochrome c. J Biol Chem 1988;263:6791–6.
44. Hess RA, Miller LA, Kirby JD, Margoliash E, Goldberg E. Immunoelectron microscope localization of testicular and somatic cytochrome c in the seminiferous epithelium of the rat. Biol Reprod 1993;48:1299–308.
45. Liang Z-G, O'Hern PA, Yavetz B, Yavetz H, Goldberg E. Human testis cDNA identified by sera from infertile patients: a molecular biology approach to immunocontraceptive development. Reprod Fertil 1994;6:297–305.

46. Villasante A, Wang D, Dobner P, Dolph P, Lewis SA, Cowan NJ. Six mouse α-tubulin mRNAs encode five distinct isotypes: testis specific expression of two sister genes. Mol Cell Biol 1986;6:2409–19.

47. Grimes SR, Wolfe SA, Anderson JV, Stein GS, Stein JL. Structural and functional analysis of the rat testis-specific histone H1t gene. J Cell Biochem 1990;44:1–17.

48. Moss SB, Challoner PB, Groudine M. Expression of a novel histone 2B during mouse spermatogenesis. Dev Biol 1989;133:83–92.

49. Kleene KC, Flynn JF. Characterization of a cDNA clone encoding a basic protein, TP2, involved in chromatin condensation during spermatogenesis in the mouse. J Biol Chem 1987;262:17272–7.

50. Kleene KC, Bozorgzadeh A, Flynn JF, Yelick PC, Hecht NB. Nucleotide sequence of a cDNA encoding mouse transition protein 1. Biochim Biophys Acta 1988;950:215–20.

51. Howard T, Balogh R, Overbeek P, Bernstein KE. Sperm-specific expression of angiotensin-converting enzyme (ACE) is mediated by a 91-base-pair promoter containing a CRE-like element. Mol Cell Biol 1993;13:18–27.

52. Johnson PA, Peschon JJ, Yelick PC, Palmiter RD, Hecht NB. Sequence homologies in the mouse protamine 1 and 2 genes. Biochem Biophys Acta 1988;950:45–53.

53. Kasahara M, Gutknecht J, Brew K, Spurr N, Goodfellow PN. Cloning and mapping of a testis-specific gene with sequence similarity to a sperm-coating glycoprotein gene. Genomics 1989;5:527–34.

54. Mizuki N, Sarapata DE, Garcia-Sanz JA, Kasahara M. The mouse male germ cell-specific gene Tpx-1: molecular structure, mode of expression in spermatogenesis, and sequence similarity to two non-mammalian genes. Mammalian Genome 1992;3:274–80.

55. Mitchell MJ, Woods DR, Tucker PK, Opp JS, Bishop CE. Homology of a candidate spermatogenic gene from the mouse Y chromosome to the ubiquitin-activating enzyme E1. Nature 1991;354:483–6.

56. Boissonneault G, Lau YF. A testis-specific gene encoding a nuclear high-mobility-group box protein located in elongating spermatids. Mol Cell Biol 1993;13:4323–30.

57. Ponzetto C, Wolgemuth DJ. Haploid expression of a unique c-abl transcript in the mouse male germ line. Mol Cell Biol 1985;5:1791–4.

58. Goldman DS, Kisseling AA, Millette CF, Cooper GM. Expression of c-mos RNA in germ cells of male and female mice. Proc Natl Acad Sci USA 1987;84:4509–13.

59. Watrin F, Scotto L, Assoian RK, Wolgemuth DJ. Cell lineage specificity of expression of the murine transforming growth factor β3 and transforming growth factor β1 genes. Cell Growth Diff 1991;2:77–83.

11

Molecular and Cellular Biology of Novel Cytoskeletal Proteins in Spermatozoa

Richard J. Oko and Carlos R. Morales

Most of the integral components of the mature mammalian spermatozoon are made up of cytoskeletal proteins that are synthesized and assembled during the haploid phase of spermatogenesis. With the exception of various isoforms of tubulin composing the microtubules of the sperm tail (1, 2) and filamentous (3–5) and nonfilamentous (6, 7) forms of actin localized in diverse regions of the sperm head and tail of various species, the majority of sperm cytoskeletal proteins appear to have no protein or structural counterparts in somatic cells. Specialized cytoskeletal elements found in the sperm tail are the *outer dense fibers* (ODF), the *fibrous sheath* (FS), the submitochondrial reticulum (8), the annulus, and the striated collar and capitulum of the neck piece [reviewed by Oko and Clermont (9)]. In the sperm head are found the *perinuclear theca* (PT), the *outer periacrosomal layer* (OPL), and the basal plate [reviewed by Oko (10)]. The isolation or extraction of many of these sperm elements is made possible by their differential resistance to protein solubilizing agents (11–21). Compositional studies have revealed that most of these elements are made up of a heterogeneous mixture of proteins of various concentrations (11–21). Recently *complementary DNAs* (cDNAs) have been used to identify the amino acid sequence of the most prominent protein constituent found in the PT [i.e., a 15-kd polypeptide (22)], the ODF [i.e., a 27-kd polypeptide (23–25)], and the FS [i.e., a 73-kd polypeptide (26, 27)]. The sequences of these three proteins have proven to be novel, unrelated to each other, and expressed only during spermatogenesis.

This chapter presents our results on the identification and characterization of the prominent proteins of the PT, ODF, and FS; describes the ultrastructural characteristics of the respective cytoskeletal elements; outlines the differential extraction procedures used to isolate these elements; introduces our combined biochemical and immunocytochemical approach of identifying the prominent proteins of each element; compares our amino

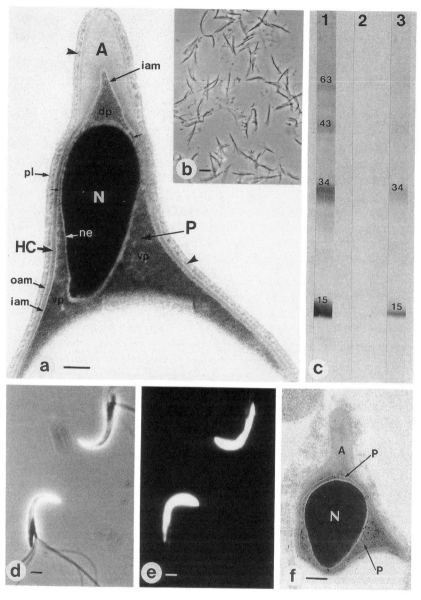

FIGURE 11.1. (a) Electron micrograph of a cross section through the apical part of the rat sperm head. In murid rodents displaying a falciform-shaped sperm head the perinuclear theca occupies a proportionally large area of the head between the nucleus (N) and the acrosome (A). This subacrosomal layer of material, often referred to as the perforatorium (P), is sandwiched between the inner acrosomal membrane (iam) and the nuclear envelope (ne). In this representative cross section, the perforatorium can be divided into a dorsal prong (dp) and two ventral prongs (vp), which are interconnected by narrow bridges (arrows). In addition to this

acid or nucleic acid sequences obtained for the major rat PT, ODF, and FS proteins (i.e., the 15-, 27- and 73-kd polypeptides, respectively) with relevant published sequences; shows the immunocytochemical results on the intracellular localization and assembly of these proteins during spermatogenesis; and compares their transcriptional and translational expressions. At least for one of these proteins, sequence and intracellular localization analysis has provided insight into its functional role. It is apparent, however, that all three of these specialized cytoskeletal proteins display unique modes of assembly and developmental regulation during spermatogenesis.

The Perinuclear Theca

Structure

The *perinuclear theca* (PT) is a rigid capsule that covers the sperm nucleus, except in the basal region of the nucleus where the tail implants into it. It has been subdivided into two regions: the subacrosomal layer (Figs. 11.1a and 11.2c), which is sandwiched between the nuclear envelope and the inner acrosomal membrane, and the postacrosomal sheath, which continues caudally between the nuclear envelope and the plasmalemma (Fig. 11.2c). In addition, there is another layer, termed the outer periacrosomal layer, which is continuous with the PT and has compositional similarities to it (21,

◄───

subacrosomal layer, a thinner layer of cytoplasmic material, referred to as the outer periacrosomal layer (arrowheads), is found sandwiched between the outer acrosomal membrane (oam) and the plasmalemma (pl). In the region overlying the acrosomic head cap (HC) the outer periacrosomal layer has similarities in composition to the perforatorium (28). Scale bar = 0.1 μm. (*b*) Phase-contrast micrograph of gradient-separated rat perforatoria. Note the characteristic three-prong structure. Scale bar = 5 μm. (*c*) Western blot of gradient-separated rat perforatoria. Perforatorial polypeptides were transferred from a linear gradient SDS polyacrylamide gel. Polypeptides are designated by molecular mass number ×10³. Lane *1*, colloidal gold stain of transferred perforatorial polypeptides. The 15-kd polypeptide is prominent. Lane 2, preimmune serum control. Lane 3, perforatorial polypeptides immunostained with affinity-purified antibody against the 15-kd perforatorial polypeptide (anti-PERF 15 antibody). Reprinted with permission from Oko and Morales (22). (*d,e*) Phase-contrast fluorescent and fluorescent micrographs, respectively, of the same field of membrane- and acrosome-denuded rat spermatozoa reacted with anti-PERF 15 antibody. The fluorescent label delineates the apical half of the sperm nuclei, the region underlying the sperm acrosome. Scale bar = 5 μm. (*f*) Electron microscope cross section through the apical part of a Lowicryl-embedded rat sperm head immunogold labeled with anti-PERF 15 antibody. The labeling is specific to the perforatorium (P), located between the membranes of the sperm acrosome (A) and nucleus (N). Scale bar = 0.2 μm.

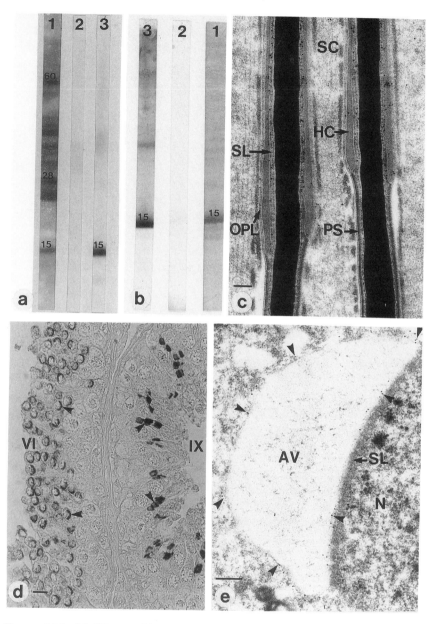

FIGURE 11.2. (*a*) Western blot of NaOH extracted bull perinuclear theca (PT) polypeptides transferred from a linear gradient SDS polyacrylamide gel. Polypeptides are designated by molecular mass number ×10³. Lane *1*, Coomassie blue dye–stained transferred bull PT polypeptides. Lane *2*, preimmune serum control. Lane *3*, bull PT polypeptides immunostained with anti-PERF 15 antibody. Note that only the 15-kd polypeptide is immunoreactive. (*b*) Western blot of NaOH extracted rat PT polypeptides transferred from a linear gradient SDS polyacrylamide gel. Lane *1*,

28). This layer of cytoplasmic material is sandwiched between the outer acrosomal membrane and plasmalemma (Figs. 11.1a and 11.2c).

Isolation

In the rat, the subacrosomal layer or perforatorium is extensively thickened (Fig. 11.1a), readily allowing for its isolation and compositional analysis (10, 17). In the bull, as in other species having spatulate-shaped sperm heads, compositional analysis of the PT is dependent on selectively extracting it from other sperm-head components (21).

The first step in the isolation and extraction protocols is to separate the sperm heads and tails by sonication and subfractionate them on a sucrose gradient. To isolate the perforatoria from rat or mouse spermatozoa, sperm heads are incubated for approximately 30 min in 0.5 to 1 N NaOH. This treatment solubilizes the membranes and acrosome and partially detaches the perforatorium from the condensed nucleus. Complete detachment is then assured by subjecting the head suspension to shear forces. The detached perforatoria are then isolated (Fig. 11.1b) from the condensed nuclei on a discontinuous sucrose gradient.

Coomassie blue dye–stained transferred rat PT polypeptides. Even under the conditions of NaOH extraction of the entire rat PT, as opposed to direct isolation of the perforatorium (see Fig. 11.1b,c), the 15-kd polypeptide remains the most prominent band. Lane 2, preimmune serum control. Lane 3, rat PT polypeptides immunostained with immune serum raised and affinity-purified against the 15-kd bull PT polypeptide seen in a. Note that the strongest reaction is with the 15-kd rat PT polypeptide. (c) EM sagittal section through portions of elongated bull spermatids immunogold labeled with the anti-15-kd bull PT antibody. This antibody, which is specific to the 15-kd bull polypeptide on Western blots (21), only labels the subacrosomal region (SL) of the PT, reminiscent of the results obtained with the anti-PERF 15 antibody in rat spermatozoa (see Fig. 11.1d–f). No gold label is found over the postacrosomal sheath (PS). SC, Sertoli cytoplasm; HC, acrosomic head cap; OPL, outer periacrosomal layer. Scale bar = 0.2 μm. (d) LM section through portions of two seminiferous tubules in stages VI and IX of the cycle of the bull seminiferous epithelium immunoperoxidase stained with the anti-15-kd bull PT antibody. The immunoperoxidase reaction product (arrowheads) is associated only with the developing acrosome of the round and elongating spermatids. Scale bar = 10 μm. (e) EM section through a portion of a step 3–4 spermatid showing the acrosomic vesicle (AV) attached to the nucleus (N). The immunogold label (arrowheads), obtained with the anti-15-kd bull PT antibody, outlines the periphery of the entire acrosomic vesicle and is in close association with the acrosomal membrane. The label also resides in the subacrosomal region (SL) between the acrosomic vesicle and nucleus. Scale bar = 0.2 μm.

To extract the entire PT from most mammalian species, including rat and mice, isolated sperm heads are exposed to three successive extraction steps consisting of incubations in 0.2% triton X-100, 1 N NaCl, and 100 mM NaOH. The first and second extraction steps solubilize the sperm-head membranes and acrosome, leaving essentially the PT covering the nucleus. The second extraction step in NaCl is not obligatory in some sperm species (e.g., human, rat, and mouse), as it has no effect on the final protein profile obtained by the NaOH extraction step. The final alkaline extraction step solubilizes the PT shell and at the same time retains the nucleus in its condensed state. Thus, by a subsequent centrifugation step, the solubilized PT proteins can be efficiently separated from the sperm nuclei.

Composition

Isolated rat perforatoria are composed of several proteins of which a 15-kd polypeptide is the most prominent (Fig. 11.1c, lane 1). This 15-kd polypeptide dominates the protein profile even when the entire rat PT is extracted (Fig. 11.2b, lane 1). The bull PT, on the other hand, is composed of several prominent polypeptides, including a 15-kd polypeptide (Fig. 11.2a, lane 1).

To confirm that the 15-kd polypeptides were indeed components of the PT in both rat and bull spermatozoa, polyclonal antibodies were raised and affinity purified against them and used as probes on Western blots of isolated or extracted PT polypeptides and on spermatozoa prepared for immunocytochemistry. On Western blots the anti-15-kd rat antibody reacted strongly with the 15-kd PT polypeptide of the rat (Fig. 11.1c, lane 3) and cross-reacted with the 15-kd PT polypeptide of the bull (Fig. 11.2a, lane 3). The anti-15-kd bull antibody reacted specifically with the 15-kd bull PT polypeptide (22) and cross-reacted with the 15-kd rat PT polypeptide (Fig. 11.2b, lane 3). The interspecies immuno–cross-reactivities found between the 15-kd polypeptides suggest a compositional similarity.

Immunocytochemical probing of rat spermatozoa with the anti-15-kd rat antibody localized the corresponding polypeptide to the subacrosomal or perforatorial region of the rat PT (Fig. 11.1d–f). Similarly the anti-15-kd bull antibody localized the corresponding polypeptide to the subacrosomal layer of the bull PT (Fig. 11.2c). Thus a consistent feature of the 15-kd PT polypeptide of each species is its localization to the subacrosomal region of the PT.

Identity of the 15-kd Rat PT Protein

Sequence analysis of a cloned cDNA encoding the major 15-kd PT polypeptide of rat spermatozoa identified a novel testicular protein with sequence similarities to a family of lipid-binding proteins (22). This PT protein, termed PERF 15 because of its localization to the perforatorium, has 132 amino acids and an estimated Mr of 15,060 (Fig. 11.3). It shares extensive sequence similarities with myelin P2 protein (29, 30), adipocyte lipid–binding protein (31), and heart fatty acid–binding protein (32). It should also be noted that PERF 15 has sequence similarities with the family of cellular retinoid-binding proteins (33). In fact, a novel, testis-specific member of the cellular lipophilic transport protein superfamily was recently identified by

```
                       1                      10
PERF 15                M  I  E  P  F  L  G  T  W  K  L  V  S
Myelin P2              S  N  K  *  *  *  *  *  *  *  *  *  *


                       20                     30
S  E  N  F  E  N  Y  V  R  E  L  G  V  E  C  E  P  R  K
*  *  *  *  D  D  *  M  K  A  *  *  *  G  L  A  T  *  *


                       40                     50
V  A  C  L  T  K  P  S  V  S  I  S  F  N  G  E  R  M  D
L  G  N  *  A  *  *  N  *  I  *  *  K  K  *  D  I  I  T


                       60                     70
I  Q  A  G  S  A  C  R  N  T  E  I  S  F  K  L  G  E  E
*  R  T  E  *  T  F  K  *  *  *  *  *  *  *  *  *  Q  *


                       80
F  E  E  T  T  A  D  N  R  K  V  K  S  L  I  T  F  E  G
*  *  *  *  *  *  *  *  *  *  T  *  *  I  *  *  L  *  R


90                     100
G  S  M  I  Q  I  Q  R  W  L  G  K  Q  T  T  I  K  R  R
*  A  L  N  *  V  *  K  *  D  *  *  E  *  *  *  *  *  K


   110                     120
I  V  D  G  R  M  V  V  E  C  T  M  N  N  V  V  S  T  R
L  *  *  *  K  *  *  *  *  *  K  *  K  G  *  *  C  *  *


   130
T  Y  E  R  V
I  *  *  K  *
```

FIGURE 11.3. Comparative best fit amino acid alignment of PERF 15 protein (22) and myelin P2 protein (29). Asterisks in myelin P2 sequence indicate identical amino acids. The PERF 15 sequence from amino acid 63 to 79, with the exception of one amino acid, is identical to the neuritogenic determinant found in myelin P2 that causes experimental autoimmune neuritis.

screening a testicular cDNA library with a certain antibody fraction raised against testicular cellular retinoic acid–binding protein (34). The sequence of this protein is identical to PERF 15.

So far, the fatty acid–binding proteins that have been examined by x-ray crystallography have shown a strikingly similar tertiary structure, irrespective of their degree of sequence similarity (35–41). They contain two layers of anti-parallel β strands enveloping a hydrophobic pocket. This binding pocket probably interacts with the carboxylate group of fatty acid or lipid ligands (42–47). Therefore it is highly likely that PERF 15 conforms to the β-pleated sheet arrangement and binds fatty acids or acidic lipids.

Of particular significance is the 60% sequence similarity found between PERF 15 and myelin P2 protein (Fig. 11.3). PERF 15 and myelin P2 are both located between membranes in the cytoplasm of respective cells. Myelin P2 is located between the cytoplasmic sides of opposing membranes in the myelin sheath of Schwann cells in the peripheral nervous system (48). It probably performs an important myelin-binding role because immunization of animals with myelin P2 leads to a T-cell–mediated peripheral nerve demyelination that mimics the acute demyelinating Landry-Guillain-Barré syndrome (49–51). In fact PERF 15 contains a stretch of amino acids from 63 to 79 (Fig. 11.3) which is nearly identical to the determinant found in myelin P2 that causes experimental autoimmune neuritis (50). Thus, based on the striking similarities in amino acid sequence and the coincident cytoplasmic locations of PERF 15 and myelin P2, it is suggested that both proteins play an important membrane-binding role in their respective cells.

Synthesis and Intracellular Localization of PERF 15

According to our immunoperoxidase results (Fig. 11.4a), PERF 15 protein first appears in mid-pachytene spermatocytes, progressively increases in concentration in late pachytene spermatocytes and round spermatids, and reaches a peak in concentration in spermatids (steps 9 to 11) undergoing the initial phase of nuclear condensation and elongation. Up until step 11 of spermiogenesis PERF 15 is present in both the cytoplasm and nucleus of these cells (52). Thereafter, in elongated spermatids (steps 12–19), the protein resides entirely in the spermatid cytoplasm. Of particular significance, as brought out by our immunogold labeling study, was the peripheral association of PERF 15 with the membrane of the forming acrosome in round spermatids (Fig. 11.4b). This acrosomal membrane association was also found by immunolabeling to be characteristic for the 15-kd PT protein of the bull (Fig. 11.2d,e) (53), which evidently shares epitopes with PERF 15 of the rat (Fig. 11.2a,b). Thus, based upon the developmental association of PERF 15 with the acrosome and its putative lipid-binding capability, we propose that this protein plays an instrumental role in attaching, spreading,

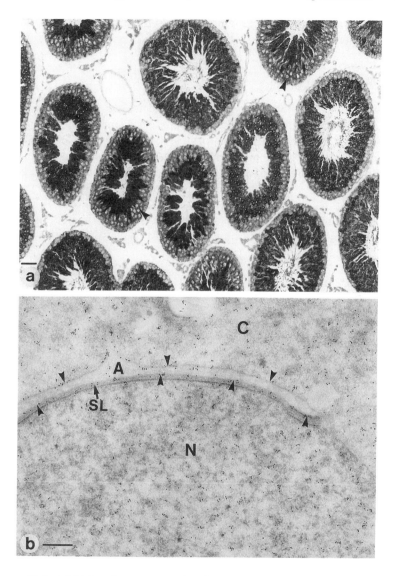

FIGURE 11.4. (*a*) Light microscope section through rat seminiferous tubules showing the pattern of immunoperoxidase staining obtained with anti-PERF 15 antibody. Regardless of the stage of the cycle of the seminiferous epithelium, immunostaining is most intense over the spermatid population of germ cells located on the inner aspect of each tubule. A weaker reaction is seen in pachytene spermatocytes (arrowheads) in later stages of the cycle. Scale bar = 20 μm. Reprinted with permission from Oko and Morales (22). (*b*) Electron microscope section of a step 7 round spermatid immunogold labeled with anti-PERF 15 antibody. In addition to labeling the cytoplasm (C) and nucleoplasm (N), the immunogold label outlines (arrowheads) the acrosome (A) and is found overlying the subacrosomal layer (SL). Scale bar = 0.2 μm.

and binding of the acrosomal membrane onto the nuclear envelope during spermiogenesis.

PERF 15 mRNA Expression

Developmental Northern blot (Fig. 11.5) and in situ hybridization (Fig. 11.6) studies showed that PERF 15 *messenger RNA* (mRNA) first begins to be transcribed in pachytene spermatocytes, reaches a peak of expression in round spermatids, and declines concomitantly with nuclear condensation and elongation of the spermatid (22). Thus it appears that the bulk of the transcript is expressed postmeiotically in round spermatids and is coordinated at this time with its translational activity. Since little of the PERF 15 mRNA remains in elongated spermatids, this transcript is most likely not subject to storage and translational regulation.

The Outer Dense Fibers

Structure

The *outer dense fibres* (ODFs) surround the axoneme in the middle piece (Fig. 11.7a) and principal piece (Fig. 11.8a) of the sperm tail. In the mid-

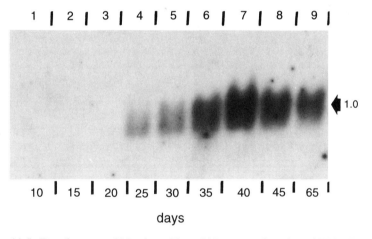

FIGURE 11.5. Developmental Northern blot of 10-µg samples of total RNA from the testis of 10- to 65-day-old rats probed with ^{32}P-labeled antisense RNA transcribed from the PERF 15 cDNA. A detectable signal first appears on a 1-kb transcript on day 25 postpartum (lane *4*), corresponding to the time in development when late pachytene spermatocytes appear. The signal continues to grow in strength through days 30, 35, and 40, which are times in development corresponding to the appearance of early round, late round, and early elongated spermatids. A reduction in signal of the 1-kb transcript occurs on day 45, corresponding to the appearance of late spermatids. The signal remains at this level into adulthood (day 65).

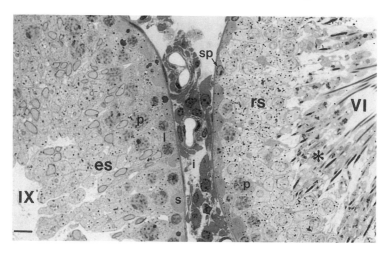

FIGURE 11.6. Radioautograph of in situ hybridized ³H-labeled PERF 15 antisense riboprobe of aldehyde fixed adult rat testis postembedded in epon. Portions of two seminiferous tubules in stages VI and IX of the cycle of the seminiferous epithelium are shown. In both tubules most of the labeling resides in the round (rs) and early-elongating (es) spermatid population of germ cells. The labeling density, however, is strongest in the round spermatids. Relatively little labeling is found in the second generation of spermatids (asterisk), and some labeling is found over pachytene spermatocytes (p). Leptotene spermatocytes (l), spermatogonia (sp), Sertoli cells (s), and interstitium (i) appear unlabeled. Scale bar = 10 μm.

piece there are nine ODFs, each one being associated with one microtubular doublet of the axoneme, while in the principal piece there are seven ODFs, because two of them are replaced in their association with the corresponding microtubular doublets by the longitudinal columns of the fibrous sheath. Each one of the ODFs has a characteristic size and shape and is composed of a massive central medulla and a thin cortex (Figs. 11.7a and 11.8a). They gradually decrease in cross-sectional profile from the proximal to the distal end of the principal piece (Fig. 11.8f). Proximally the ODFs are structurally continuous with the striated collar of the neck piece, which in turn is connected to the capitulum (9). Interestingly, both of these neck-piece components share antigenic determinants with the ODFs (16). The ODFs are common to all mammalian sperm.

Isolation

The relative insolubility of ODFs in low concentrations of ionic detergents (e.g., *sodium dodecyl sulfate* (SDS)] plus disulfide-reducing agents, as compared to other sperm-tail components, allows for their isolation (13, 14, 16, 54). Basically isolated sperm tails are extracted for 1–2 h in a buffer contain-

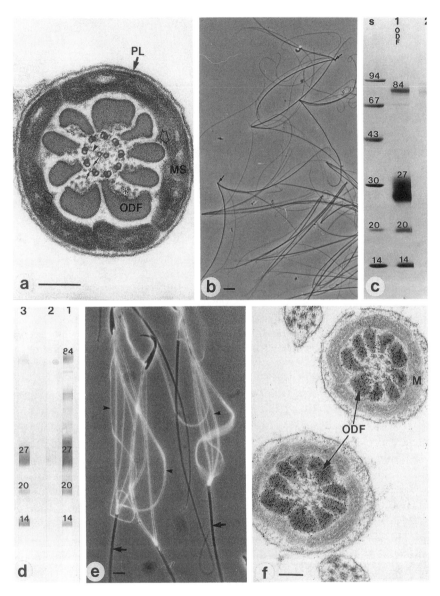

FIGURE 11.7. (*a*) Electron micrograph of a cross section through the mid-piece of the rat sperm tail. Central to the sperm tail is the axoneme made up of 9 peripheral microtubular doublets surrounding a central pair of microtubule singlets. The radial spokes (arrowhead) bridge the peripheral doublets to the central singlets. A pair of dynein arms (arrows) extend from subfiber-A of one microtubule doublet toward subfiber-B of the adjacent microtubule doublet. Each microtubule doublet is associated with an outer dense fiber (ODF) composed of a massive central medulla and a thin cortex. The ODFs display distinctive cross-sectional profiles. Satellite fibrils

ing 1% (SDS) and 2 mM *dithiothreitol* (DTT). With the exception of the ODFs and neck piece, all other tail proteins are solubilized during this time. The ODFs are then isolated (Fig. 11.7b) on a sucrose gradient.

Composition

The isolated ODFs are composed of numerous proteins (reviewed in 16), of which the 14-, 20-, 27-, and 84-kd polypeptides are the most prominent (Fig. 11.7c). The 27-kd polypeptide accounts for about 50% of the total protein of the rat ODF and contains a large amount of phosphate bound as phosphoserine (14). On carboxymethylation it has been resolved into two polypeptides (13) that have a similar amino acid content (14). However, it is possible that the molecular weight differences observed may only reflect the extent of phosphorylation at the serine residues of the 27-kd polypeptide.

To confirm that the 27-kd polypeptide was indeed a component of the ODF, immune serum was raised and affinity purified against the 27-kd

◀——————————————————————————————————

(asterisks) are found between the ODFs and, although not preserved in this section, remnants of a granular material termed the submitochondrial reticulum (open arrows) are found between the ODFs and the mitochondrial sheath (MS). This material may bind the ODFs to the mitochondria. It is apparent that the various cytoskeletal elements forming the framework of the mid-piece are interconnected. PL, plasmalemma. Scale bar = 0.2 μm. (*b*) Phase-contrast micrograph of isolated ODFs after sperm tails were extracted in SDS-DTT for 1 h. Note that the ODFs are still connected to the neck piece (arrows). This connection can be disrupted on longer treatment. Scale bar = 5 μm. (*c*) Coomassie blue–stained 8–18% linear gradient SDS-polyacrylamide gel of whole ODF fraction (lane *1*) after 1.5 h extraction. Four prominent ODF polypeptide bands having molecular masses of 84, 27, 20, and 14 kd are seen. Lane *2*, ODF gel after Western blot transfer in a solution of 25 mM Na_2HPO_2, pH 6.5. Lane *s*, molecular masses of polypeptide standards are denoted by number ×10³. (*d*) Western blot of ODF polypeptides seen in *c*. Lane *1*, ODF polypeptides immunostained with immune serum raised against the whole ODF fraction. Lane *2*, preimmune serum control. Lane *3*, ODF polypeptides immunostained with immune serum raised and affinity-purified against the major 27-kd ODF polypeptide. Note that in addition to the 27-kd band, the 20- and 14-kd bands are reactive. (*e*) Phase-contrast fluorescent micrograph of membrane-, acrosome-, and mitochondrial-sheath denuded rat spermatozoa reacted with antibody-affinity purified from the 27-kd ODF polypeptide. The fluorescent label specifically labels the splayed ODFs (arrowheads). The fibrous sheath (arrows) and sperm head are unlabeled. Scale bar = 5 μm. (*f*) EM cross sections through middle and end pieces of epon-embedded rat sperm tails immunogold labeled with antibody-affinity purified from the 27-kd ODF polypeptide. Labeling is restricted to the ODFs. M, mitochondria. Scale bar = 0.2 μm.

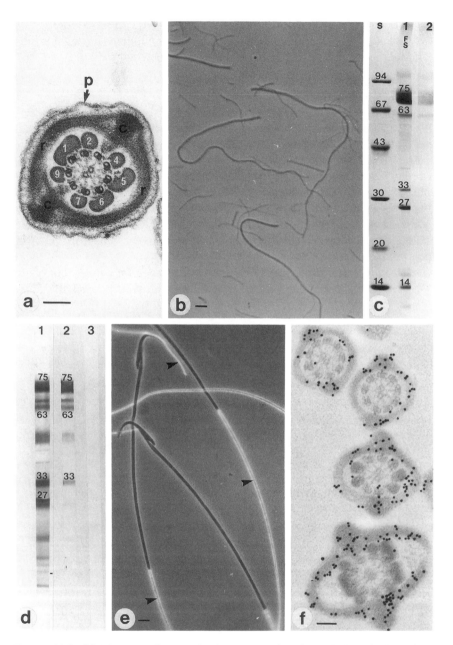

FIGURE 11.8. (*a*) Electron micrograph of a cross section through the principal piece of a rat sperm tail. The fibrous sheath surrounds the outer dense fibers and is composed of two components: the longitudinal columns (c), which run opposite microtubule doublets 3 and 8 in replacement of two corresponding outer dense fibers, and transverse ribs (r), which bridge the longitudinal columns on either side. The longitudinal columns attach to each corresponding doublet, essentially dividing

polypeptide and probed on Western blots of isolated ODF polypeptides and on fixed spermatozoa (25). On Western blots this affinity-purified antibody reacted with the 27-kd polypeptide but also cross-reacted with the 20- and 14-kd ODF polypeptides (Fig. 11.7d, lane 3). Immunocytochemical analysis revealed this antibody to be specific to the ODF of the sperm (Fig. 11.7e,f).

Identity of the 27-kd Rat ODF Protein

By immunoscreening a testicular λ-gt 11 phage cDNA library with the anti-27-kd ODF antibody, we isolated a 659 nucleotide base pair cDNA clone termed ODF 27 (25). A Genbank search showed that this cDNA had a nucleotide sequence identical to a full-length rts 5/1 cDNA isolated by Burfeind and Hoyer-Fender (24) (Fig. 11.9). Interestingly, the rts 5/1 cDNA was isolated by screening a λ-gt 11 rat testicular library with a nucleotide probe obtained from a testis-specific *Drosophila melanogaster* gene, Mst 87F, originally identified by Kuhn et al. (55). The rts 5/1 cDNA was found by Burfeind and Hoyer-Fender (24) to encode a testis-specific protein of Mr 27,000 that had amino-acid content similarities to two ODF proteins, in the 27-kd range, previously isolated by Vera et al. (14). We were able to positively identify that the rts 5/1 cDNA encoded the major 27-kd ODF

---

the principal piece into two unequally sized compartments. Outer dense fibers 1, 2, 5, 6, 7, and 9, which face the corresponding microtubule doublets, decrease in size from the proximal to the distal end of the principal piece (*f*). p, plasmalemma. Scale bar = 0.1 μm. (*b*) Phase-contrast micrograph of isolated FS after sperm tails were extracted in urea-DTT for several hours. Scale bar = 5 μm. (*c*) Coomassie blue–stained 8–10% linear gradient SDS-polyacrylamide gel of whole FS fraction (lane *1*) after 5-h extraction. Five prominent FS polypeptide bands having molecular masses of 75, 63, 33, 27, and 14-kd are seen among several other less-prominent bands. Lane 2, FS gel after Western blot transfer in a solution of 25 nM Na_2HPO_2, pH 6.5. Lane *s*, molecular standards denoted by number $\times 10^3$. (*d*) Western blot of FS polypeptides. Lane *1*, FS polypeptides stained with colloidal-gold. Lane 2, FS polypeptides immunostained with immune serum raised and affinity purified against the major 75-kd FS polypeptide. Note that in addition to the 75-kd band, 67-, 63-, 43-, and 33-kd bands are reactive. Lane 3, preimmune serum control. (*e*) Phase-contrast fluorescent micrograph of membrane-, acrosome-, and mitochondrial-sheath denuded rat spermatozoa reacted with antibody-affinity purified from the 75-kd FS polypeptide. The fluorescent label specifically labels the FS (arrowheads). Scale bar = 5 μm. (*f*) EM cross sections through principal pieces of Lowicryl-embedded rat sperm tails immunogold labeled with antibody-affinity purified from the 75-kd FS polypeptide. Labeling is restricted to the longitudinal columns and ribs of the FS. Note the gradual reduction of the ODFs as the cross sections of the principal piece diminish in size. Scale bar = 0.1μm.

```
            M   A   A   L   S   C   L   L   D   S   V   11
5/1 096 ... ATG GCC GCA CTG AGT TGT CTT TTG GAC AGT GTT
RT7 612 ... +   +   +   +   +   +   +   +   +   +   +
027

            R   R   D   I   K   K   V   D   R   E   L   R   23
    129 AGA AGG GAC ATA AAG AAG CTG GAC AGA GAA CTA AGA
    645 +   +   +   +   +   +   GTG +   +   +   +   +

            Q   L   R   C   I   D   E   I   S   S   R   C   35
    165 CAA TTG AGA TGT ATC GAC GAA ATC AGC TCC CGC TGC
    681 +   +   +   +   +   +   +   +   +   +   +   +

            L   C   D   L   Y   M   H   P   Y   C   C   C   47
    201 CTG TGT GAC TTA TAC ATG CAC CCT TAC TGC TGC TGC
    717 +   +   +   +   +   +   +   +   +   +   +   +

            D   L   H   P   Y   P   Y   C   L   C   Y   S   59
    237 GAC CTG CAC CCC TAC CCC TAC TGC CTC TGC TAC TCC
    753 +   +   +   +   +   +   +   +   +   +   +   +

            K   R   S   R   S   C   G   L   C   D   L   Y   71
    273 AAG GGA TCC CGC TCC TGT GGC CTG TGT GAC CTC TAC
    789 +   CGA +   +   +   +   +   +   +   +   +   +

            Y   P   C   C   L   C   D   Y   K   L   Y   C   83
    309 TAC CCG TGC TGC CTG TGT GAC TAC AAG CTG TAC TGC
    825 +   +   +   +   +   +   +   +   +   +   +   +
    001                                     +   +   +

            L   R   P   S   L   R   S   L   E   R   L   R   95
    345 CTC CGC CCA TCG CTC CGC AGC TTA GAG AGA CTC AGA
    861 +   +   +   +   -TC +   +   +   +   +   +   +
    010 +   +   +   +   +   +   +   +   +   +   +   +

            R   T   T   N   R   I   L   A   S   S   C   C   107
    381 AGG ACG ACA AAT AGA ATT CTG GCC TCC TCT TGC TGC
    897 +   +   +   +   +   +   +   +   +   +   +   +
    046 +   +   +   +   +   +   +   +   +   +   +   +

            S   S   N   I   L   G   S   V   N   V   C   G   119
    417 AGC AGT AAC ATT TTA GGA TCG GTG AAC GTC TGC GGC
    933 +   +   +   +   +   +   +   +   +   +   +   +
    082 +   +   +   +   +   +   +   +   +   +   +   +
```

FIGURE 11.9. Comparison and best-fit nucleotide alignment of the largest open reading frame (i.e., 735bp-245aa) of the rts 5/1 cDNA [Burfeind and Hoyer-Fender (24)] with nucleotide sequences of the RT7 gene [Van Der Hoorn et al. (23)] and our ODF27 cDNA (25). The putative amino acid sequence for the rts 5/1 cDNA is indicated and numbered for comparison. The rts 5/1 and RT7 cDNAs have common start sites, beginning at nucleotide bases 096 and 612, respectively. The partial nucleotide sequence of the 5′ end of the ODF27 cDNA begins at nucleotide base 336 of the rts 5/1 cDNA. From this base downstream to the stop codon (TAA), there is a perfect alignment of codons between these two clones, as indicated by the uninterrupted plus (+) signs. As for the RT7 cDNA, a predicted omission of one nucleotide base at position 873 of this cDNA results in a premature stop codon

```
          F    E    P    D    Q    V    K    V    R    V    K    D   131
    453  TTT  GAA  CCT  GAT  CAG  GTC  AAA  GTG  CGC  GTT  AAA  GAT
    969   +    +    +    +    +    +    +    +    +    +    +    +
    118   +    +    +    +    +    +    +    +    +    +    +    +

          G    K    V    C    V    S    A    E    R    E    N    R   143
    489  GGA  AAG  GTC  TGC  GTA  TCG  GCC  GAG  AGG  GAA  AAC  AGG
   1005   +    +    +    +   CTA   +    +    +   AG-   +    +    +
    154   +    +    +    +    +    +    +    +    +    +    +    +

          Y    D    C    L    G    S    K    K    Y    S    Y    M   155
    525  TAC  GAC  TGC  CTC  GGA  TCC  AAA  AAG  TAC  AGT  TAC  ATG
   1041   +    +    +    +    +    +    +    +    +    +    +    +
    190   +    +    +    +    +    +    +    +    +    +    +    +

          N    I    C    K    E    F    S    L    P    P    C    V   167
    561  AAC  ATC  TGC  AAA  GAG  TTC  AGT  CTG  CCG  CCG  TGC  GTG
   1077   +    +    +    +    +    +    +    +    +    +    +   -TG
    226   +    +    +    +    +    +    +    +    +    +    +    +

          D    E    K    D    V    T    Y    S    Y    G    L    G   179
    597  GAT  GAG  AAA  GAC  GTG  ACC  TAC  TCC  TAC  GGG  CTC  GGC
   1113   +    +    +    +    +    +    +    +    +    +    +    +
    262   +    +    +    +    +    +    +    +    +    +    +    +

          S    C    V    K    I    E    S    P    C    Y    P    C   191
    633  AGT  TGT  GTC  AAG  ATC  GAG  TCT  CCA  TGC  TAC  CCT  TGC
   1149   +    +    +    +    +    +    +    +    +    +    +    +
    298   +    +    +    +    +    +    +    +    +    +    +    +

          T    S    P    C    N    P    C    N    P    C    S    P   203
    669  ACG  TCT  CCC  TGC  AAC  CCC  TGC  AAC  CCC  TGC  AGC  CCC
   1185   +    +    +    +    +    +    +    +    +    +    +    +
    334   +    +    +    +    +    +    +    +    +    +    +    +

          C    S    P    C    G    P    C    G    P    C    G    P   215
    705  TGC  AGC  CCC  TGC  GGC  CCC  TGC  GGT  CCT  TGC  GGT  CCC
   1221   +    +   CC-   +    +   CC-   +    +   -CT   +    +    +
    370   +    +    +    +    +    +    +    +    +    +    +    +

          C    G    P    C    G    P    C    G    P    C    D    P   227
    741  TGT  GGC  CCC  TGT  GGT  GCC  TGC  GGC  CCC  TGC  GAC  CCT
   1257   +    +    +    +    +   CC-   +    +    +    +    +    +
    406   +    +    +    +    +    +    +    +    +    +    +    +

          C    N    P    C    Y    P    C    G    S    R    F    S   239
    777  TGC  AAC  CCC  TGC  TAT  CCC  TGT  GGA  AGC  CGA  TTC  TCC
   1293   +    +    +    +    +    +    +    +    +    +    +    +
    442   +    +    +    +    +    +    +    +    +    +    +    +

          C    R    K    M    I    L    -                          245
    813  TGT  AGG  AAG  ATG  ATC  TTG  TAA  ...   952  (An)
   1329   +    +    +    +    +    +    +    ...  1459  (An)
    478   +    +    +    +    +    +    +    ...   615  (An)
```

FIGURE 11.9. *Continued*

(TAG) nine bases downstream from the omission. Otherwise, with the exception of six other predicted nucleotide base omissions further downstream, there is a perfect alignment of the RT7 sequence with that of the rts 5/1 and ODF27 cDNAs, as indicated by the plus (+) signs. The two internal peptide sequences of the 27-kd ODF polypeptide that match the deduced amino acid sequence of the rts 5/1 cDNA are underlined. Reprinted with permission from Morales et al. (25).

polypeptide by finding two internal peptide sequences in this protein that were encoded in the 5' and 3' regions of this cDNA (Fig. 11.9). Coincidentally, one of these peptide sequences (i.e., the 3' sequence) was also identified in an internal region of the immuno–cross-reactive 20-kd ODF polypeptide shown in Figure 11.7d. Considering that there are two major transcripts of 1.5 and 1.2 kb recognized by probes to the ODF 27 cDNA (Fig. 11.10), it is likely that the smaller transcript encodes the 20-kd ODF protein while the larger transcript encodes the 27-kd ODF protein. This idea is reinforced by the results of Burfeind and Hoyer-Fender (24), who showed that a nucleotide probe specifically made to the 5' end of the rts 5/1 cDNA hybridized exclusively to the larger transcript while a probe to the entire cDNA recognized both transcripts. The possibility exists therefore that the 1.2-kb transcript (Fig. 11.10) represents an alternatively spliced product of the 1.5-kb ODF transcript. As for the immuno–cross-reactive 14-kd ODF polypeptide (Fig. 11.7d), it is likely that it is encoded by a yet unidentified gene because it possesses an amino-terminal sequence not found in the major 27-kd ODF polypeptide (25).

During the course of our investigation (25) we found that our ODF 27 cDNA and the N-terminally extended rts 5/1 cDNA had a nearly identical sequence similarity to a rat gene RT7, cloned by Van Der Hoorn et al. (23) and reported to encode a 90 amino acid protein of unknown identity (Fig. 11.9). For reasons reported in the legend of Fig. 11.9 and confirmed by Van

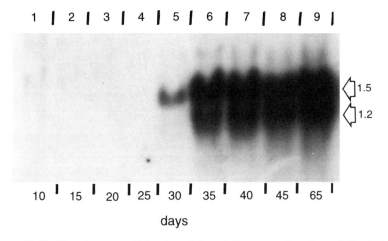

FIGURE 11.10. Developmental Northern blot of 10 µg samples of total RNA from testis of 10- to 65-day-old rats probed with [³²P]-labeled antisense RNA in vitro transcribed from ap-GEM plasmid containing the ODF 27 cDNA insert. On day 30 postpartum (lane 5), corresponding to the time in development when round spermatids first appear, a 1.5 transcript is detected. Later on day 35, two transcripts of 1.5 and 1.2 kb are detected and remain at high intensity into adulthood (day 65, lane 9).

Der Hoorn's group (56), we positively identified this gene as encoding the major 27-kd ODF protein (25).

The 27-kd ODF polypeptide contains a repetitive motif, *Cys-Gly-Pro* (CGP), at the carboxy-terminal end which is also found encoded in a family of testis-specific Mst(3) CGP genes of *Drosophila melanogaster* (57). Schäfer et al. (57) have pointed out that the best size and sequence homology between the 27-kd ODF protein and the Mst(3) CGP family is found in a gene, Mst98 Cb, which encodes a protein of 35-kd. The best homology found, however, resides in the carboxy-terminal end of both proteins and is in the order of 42%. Of particular significance is that the rat ODF proteins and the *Drosophila* Mst(3) CGP family of proteins are expressed only during the haploid phase of germ-cell development of respective testes (57, 58). Furthermore, the Mst proteins are localized to a yet unidentified region of the *Drosophila* sperm tail (55, 57). Thus, the resemblances in sequence, expression, and localization between the ODF and Mst proteins suggest an evolutionary conservation of these proteins from insects to mammals. However, the exact roles of these proteins in sperm-tail motility remain to be identified.

Synthesis and Intracellular Localization of the 27-kd ODF Protein

Based on our immunoperoxidase results (Fig. 11.11a,b), the 27-kd ODF protein is synthesized during the latter half of spermiogenesis, well after transcriptional activity in the haploid germ cell has ended (59). It is weakly concentrated in the cytoplasm of steps 9–13 spermatids undergoing the initial phase of nuclear condensation, moderately concentrated in steps 14–15 spermatids, and most concentrated in steps 16–18 spermatids. The residual ODF protein left over in the residual bodies of step 19 spermatids is phagocytosed by the Sertoli cell. During its period of synthesis, the 27-kd ODF protein accumulates in numerous granular bodies that are scattered throughout the cytoplasmic lobule of the spermatid (Figs. 11.11b and 11.12) and also assembles in a proximal to distal direction along the spermatid tail (58, 60). The observation that the maximum number and size of granular bodies are reached at the time (step 16) of maximal growth in diameter of the ODF suggests that the granular bodies may be a source of precursor proteins for the assembly of the ODF (61). If indeed the granular bodies serve as a transitory station for ODF proteins, then mechanisms must exist for protein binding and release from this unique cytoplasmic component.

ODF 27 mRNA Expression

Utilizing a probe against the ODF 27 cDNA, two potential transcripts encoding the 27-kd ODF protein were detected during rat testicular devel-

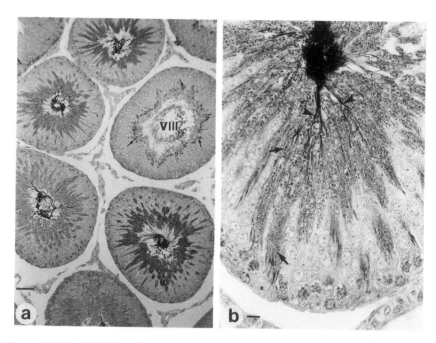

FIGURE 11.11. (a) Light microscope section through rat seminiferous tubules, representing various stages of the 14-stage cycle of the seminiferous epithelium, immunoperoxidase stained with antibody-affinity purified from the 27-kd ODF polypeptide. Note the variation in immunostaining from one stage to another. The immunostaining in reactive tubules is restricted to elongated spermatids in later steps of spermiogenesis. Residual staining is found in the residual bodies (arrowheads) of the Sertoli cell in stage VIII. Scale bar = 20 μm. (b) Higher-power light micrograph of a portion of a seminiferous tubule, at stage III of the cycle of the seminiferous epithelium, immunostained with the anti-27-kd ODF antibody. Note the intensive reaction over the sperm tails (arrowheads) and granular bodies (arrows) that are distributed numerously throughout the cytoplasm of step-16 elongated spermatids. Scale bar = 5 μm.

opment (Fig. 11.10). A 1.5-kb mRNA was first detected on day 30 postpartum, corresponding to the time when round spermatids first appear. Later, on day 35, corresponding to the time the testis is enriched in relatively more mature spermatids, an additional 1.2-kb in RNA was detected. Both mRNA species remained into adulthood. As was discussed earlier, the 1.2-kb transcript was excluded from coding for the 27-kd ODF protein on the basis that it did not contain the N-terminal end of this protein. However, because a prominent immuno–cross-reacting 20-kd ODF protein was found to contain an internal peptide sequence present in the 27-kd ODF protein, the possibility arises that the 1.2-kb transcript may encode the 20-kd ODF polypeptide and represent an alternatively spliced product of the 1.5-kb transcript.

In situ hybridization performed on adult rat testis (Fig. 11.13) confirmed our developmental Northern blot analysis (Fig. 11.10). It showed that the mRNAs encoding the ODF proteins were not yet detectable, or at very low levels, in early round spermatids. However, by steps 5–7 (late round sper-

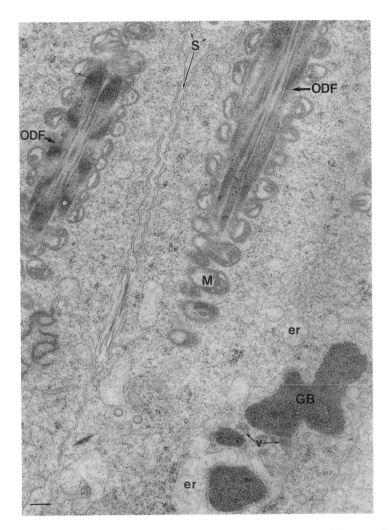

FIGURE 11.12. Electron micrograph of a section through portions of the cytoplasm of two adjacent step-16 spermatids immunogold labeled with the anti-27-kd ODF antibody. The ODFs and adjacent granular bodies (GB) are clearly immunoreactive. The immunoreactivity reaches a peak in this step of spermatid development. The cisternae of the endoplasmic reticulum (er) and vesicles with a dense content (v) are associated with the granular bodies but are unreactive. S, Sertoli cytoplasms; M, mitochondria. Scale bar = 0.2 µm.

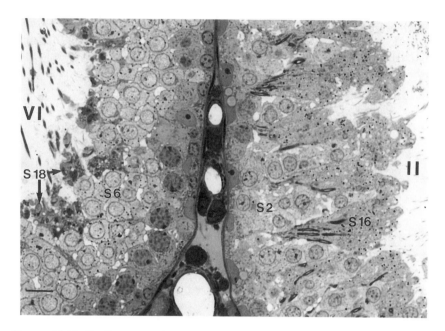

FIGURE 11.13. Radioautograph of in situ hybridized ³H-labeled ODF 27 antisense riboprobe of aldehyde-fixed adult rat testis postembedded in epon. Portions of two seminiferous tubules in stages II and VI of the cycle of the seminiferous epithelium are shown. In stage II only the elongated or step-16 spermatids (S16) are labeled; virtually no silver grains are observable over step 2 (S2) round spermatids. In stage VI labeling is apparent only in step 6 (S6) round spermatids, having at this time disappeared in step 18 (S18) elongated spermatids. No labeling is apparent in spermatocytes, spermatogonia, Sertoli cells, or interstitial cells. Scale bar = 10 μm.

matids) of spermiogenesis, the transcripts became abundant and remained at elevated levels up to step 16 spermatids, a time when maximum synthesis and assembly of ODF proteins occurs. Because the levels of the transcript are still high late into spermiogenesis, an estimated 6 days after transcription terminates, it is predicted that the synthesis of the ODF proteins is dependent on stored mRNAs that are translationally regulated.

The Fibrous Sheath

Structure

The *fibrous sheath* (FS) encases the outer dense fibers and axoneme in the principal piece of the sperm tail (Fig. 11.8a). It is composed of two structural elements: the longitudinal columns, which run opposite microtubule doublets 3 and 8 in replacement of two corresponding ODF, and numerous transverse ribs that bridge the longitudinal columns on either side (9).

Isolation

As is true for the ODF, the proteins of the FS are stabilized by disulfide bonds (62). This property, along with a relative resistance to solubilization in urea, has allowed for isolation of the FS (12, 16). Basically, isolated sperm tails are first extracted twice in a buffer containing 2% Triton X-100 and 5 mM DTT to solubilize all membrane components including the mitochondrial sheath. The pellet obtained after centrifugation is then suspended in a buffer containing 4.5–6 M urea and 25 mM DTT and incubated for 3–5 h under phase-contrast microscope observation until all cytoskeletal structures except for the FS have dissolved. The FS are then isolated (Fig. 11.8b) on a sucrose gradient.

Composition

The isolated FS is composed of numerous proteins (16) of which the 14-, 27-, 63-, and 75-kd polypeptides are the most prominent (Fig. 11.8c). The 75-kd polypeptide is by far the most dense component of the fibrous sheath and, like the major 27-kd ODF polypeptide, contains a large amount of phosphate bound as phosphoserine (63).

To confirm that the 75-kd polypeptide was a component of the FS, immune serum was raised and affinity purified against it and probed on Western blots of isolated FS polypeptides and on fixed spermatozoa. On Western blots this affinity-purified antibody reacted strongly with the 75-kd polypeptide but also cross-reacted with the 67-, 63-, 43-, and 33-kd FS polypeptides (Fig. 11.8d). Immunocytochemical analysis revealed this antibody to be specific to the ODF of the sperm (Fig. 11.8e,f).

Identity of the Major FS Protein

Recently Carrera et al. (26) cloned and sequenced the major FS polypeptide of the mouse. The sequence predicted that the mature form of this protein has a Mr of 72,890 (661 amino acids) and is synthesized as a precursor of ≈92,870 Mr (840 amino acids) in round and condensing spermatids. The length of the mature form was established from the precursor sequence by determining the N-terminal sequence of this protein isolated from mature spermatozoa. Coincidently, the N-terminal sequence (i.e., Q, S, P, S, N, P, A, T, K, S) of the mature form of the major mouse FS protein as determined by Carrera et al. (26) was found to be nearly an exact match to the N-terminally derived sequence (i.e., E, S, P, S, N, P, A, T, K, S) of the major 75-kd rat FS polypeptide as determined by us. Furthermore, the protein profile of the rat FS (Fig. 11.8c) was almost identical to the protein profile of mouse FS (not shown) obtained by the same isolation protocol. These resemblances, in addition to the strong similarity in amino acid composition found between the major FS proteins of mouse and rat (26, 27), suggest a high degree of conservation in FS proteins between these two species.

Although the major mouse FS protein was determined to be a novel cytoskeletal protein expressed only during spermiogenesis, it was found to have regional domains similar in sequence to the A-kinase anchoring proteins that are responsible for anchoring protein kinase A to the cytoskeleton (26). This activity was confirmed by ligand blotting assay and led Carrera et al. (26) to conclude that this FS protein may act as a scaffolding protein for the subcellular localization of regulatory proteins in the flagellum.

Most recently, Fulcher et al. (27) cloned and characterized an Fsc1 cDNA encoding a mouse sperm FS component. Their sequence confirmed the identity of the major mouse FS protein sequenced by Carrera et al. (26) but in addition extended the sequence of the precursor protein by 147 nucleotide bases at the 5' end. In doing so they extended the largest open reading frame predicted by Carrera et al. (26) by 27 nucleotide bases.

Synthesis and Intracellular Localization of the Major FS Protein

Based on our immunoperoxidase results (Fig. 11.14a,b), the 75-kd rat FS protein is synthesized during the latter half of spermiogenesis, well after transcriptional activity in the developing spermatid has ended. It is weakly concentrated in the cytoplasm of steps 9–12 spermatids, moderately concentrated in steps 13–14 spermatids, and most concentrated in steps 15–17 spermatids. In the cytoplasm of steps 18–19 spermatids the concentration of the 75-kd FS protein diminishes and by spermiation residual protein left over is packaged into the cytoplasmic droplet (58). In contrast to the focal distribution of ODF proteins in granular bodies, the FS proteins are diffusely distributed throughout the cytoplasm (Figs. 11.14b and 11.15) (58, 60). During its period of synthesis, the 75-kd FS polypeptide assembles in a distal to proximal direction along the tail (Fig. 11.15) characteristic of all the fibrous sheath proteins (58).

The assembly of the FS is preceded by FS anlagen, which is closely associated with the plasmalemma of the spermatid tail and assembles along the tail in a distal to proximal direction (Fig. 11.15) (reviewed in 9). This anlagen, which appears in the distal part of the spermatid tail as early as

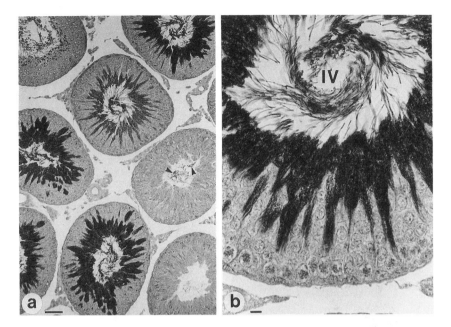

FIGURE 11.14. (a) Light microscope section through rat seminiferous tubules, representing various stages of the seminiferous epithelium, immunoperoxidase stained with antibody-affinity purified from the 75-kd FS polypeptide. The immunostaining in reactive tubules is restricted to elongated spermatids in later steps of spermiogenesis. Note that the reaction product is first deposited at the distal ends of the sperm tails (arrowheads), signifying the distal to proximal assembly of FS proteins along the sperm tail. Scale bar = 20 µm. (b) Higher power light micrograph of a portion of a seminiferous tubule, at stage IV of the cycle immunostained with the anti-75-kd FS antibody. The reaction product is evenly distributed throughout the cytoplasm of the elongated spermatids and along the principal pieces of the tails suspended in the tubular lumen. Scale bar = 5 µm.

step 2 of spermiogenesis, is not immunoreactive to FS antibodies. However, it appears as if the FS proteins, which begin to be assembled in step 11, utilize this precursor material as scaffolding for their assembly (Fig. 11.15).

mRNA Expression of the Major FS Protein

Based on developmental Northern blot and in situ hybridization studies of Fulcher et al. (27), the mRNA encoding the major mouse FS polypeptide is first transcribed in round spermatids (steps 1–6), is abundant in steps 7–12 spermatids, and declines in steps 13–15 spermatids. This time frame agrees with the late period of synthesis and assembly shown for the major rat FS

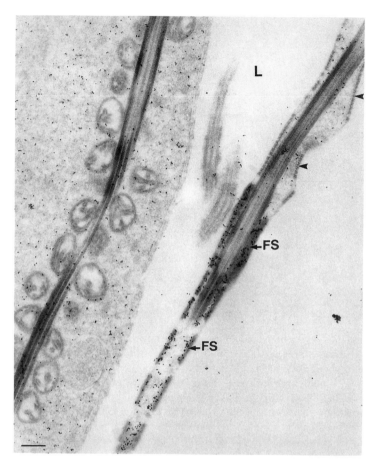

FIGURE 11.15. Electron microscope section through two different longitudinal portions of rat spermatid tails, in step 16 of spermiogenesis (stage II of the cycle of the seminiferous epithelium), immunogold labeled with the anti-75-kd FS antibody. In the more distal portion of the sperm tail, on the left, the gold label is randomly distributed throughout the abundant cytoplasm, while in the proximal portion of the sperm tail, which is suspended in the tubular lumen (L), the gold label accumulates over the FS, which is being assembled in a distal to proximal direction. The plasma associated anlagen (arrowheads), which is deposited before the appearance of the FS and may serve to trigger its formation, is clearly not immunoreactive. Note that some labeling is found along the microtubular axoneme, which may serve to transport the FS proteins distally to their site of assembly. Scale bar = 0.2 μm.

protein during spermiogenesis (see section above) and indicates that the FS mRNAs are translationally regulated.

Conclusion

Although some useful insights into the functional role of the major protein constituents of the PT, ODF, and FS have been discerned from their sequence and developmental characteristics, as reviewed in this chapter, it is envisioned that several research directives are necessary before the true significance of these specialized cytoskeletal proteins in sperm development and fertilization is understood. First, because each of these specialized cytoskeletal elements (i.e., PT, ODF, FS) is composed of multiple proteins, future research should emphasize the biochemical and structural interrelationships between protein constituents of each element and subjacent structures and membranes. Obviously the first step toward this goal will require the sequencing of at least the more prominent proteins of each cytoskeletal element. Second, because of the testicular specificity of these specialized cytoskeletal proteins, it is probable that useful functional information will be derived from genetic assays, designed to "knock out" or alter the genes encoding these proteins. Finally, the genes encoding these specialized cytoskeletal proteins could also serve as models to study the mechanisms involved in the testis-specific regulation of transcription and translation.

Acknowledgments. This work was supported by grants from the Medical Research Council of Canada and the National Sciences and Engineering Council of Canada.

References

1. Hermo L, Oko R, Hecht NB. Differential post-transcriptional modifications of microtubules in cells of the seminiferous epithelium of the rat: a light and electron microscope immunocytochemical study. Anat Rec 1991;229:31–50.
2. Distel RJ, Kleen KC, Hecht NB. Haploid expression of a mouse testis α tubulin gene. Science 1984;224:68–70.
3. Flaherty SP, Winfrey VP, Olson GE. Localization of actin in human, bull, rabbit, and hamster sperm by immunoelectron microscopy. Anat Rec 1988;221:599–610.
4. Olson GE, Winfrey VP, Flaherty SP. Cytoskeletal assemblies of mammalian spermatozoa. Ann NY Acad Sci 1987;513:222–46.
5. Oko R, Hermo L, Hecht NB. Distribution of actin isoforms within cells of the seminiferous epithelium of the rat testis: evidence for a contractile form of actin in spermatids. Anat Rec 1991;232:63–81.

6. Breed WG, Leigh CM. Distribution of filamentous actin in and around spermatids and in spermatozoa of Australian conilurine rodents. Mol Reprod Dev 1991;30:369–84.

7. Flaherty SP, Breed WG, Sarafis V. Localization of actin in the sperm head of the plains mouse, Pseudomys australis. J Exp Zool 1983;225:497–500.

8. Wierda A, Zheng L, Bartees JP. Cytoskeletal link between sperm mitochondrial sheath and outer dense fibres. Mol Biol Cell 1994;5:97a (abstract 563).

9. Oko R, Clermont Y. Mammalian spermatozoa; structure and assembly of the tail. In: Gagnon C, ed. Controls of sperm motility; biological and clinical aspects. Boca Raton, FL: CRC Press, 1990:3–27.

10. Oko R. Developmental expression and possible role of perinuclear theca proteins of mammalian spermatozoa. Reprod Fertil Dev 1995;7:777–97.

11. Olson GE, Hamilton DW, Fawcett DW. Isolation and characterization of the perforatorium of rat spermatozoa. J Reprod Fertil 1976;47:1–9.

12. Olson GE, Hamilton DW, Fawcett DW. Isolation and characterization of the fibrous sheath of rat epididymal spermatozoa. Biol Reprod 1976;14:517–30.

13. Olson GE, Sammons DW. Structural chemistry of outer dense fibres of rat sperm. Biol Reprod 1980;22:319–32.

14. Vera JC, Brito M, Zavic T, Burzio LO. Polypeptide composition of rat sperm outer dense fibres. J Biol Chem 1977;259:5970–77.

15. Longo FJ, Krohne G, Franke WW. Basic proteins of the perinuclear theca of mammalian spermatozoa and spermatids: a novel class of cytoskeletal elements. J Cell Biol 1987;105:1105–20.

16. Oko R. Comparative analysis of proteins from fibrous sheath and outer dense fibres of rat spermatozoa. Biol Reprod 1988;39:169–82.

17. Oko R, Clermont Y. Isolation, structure and protein composition of the perforatorium of rat spermatozoa. Biol Reprod 1988;39;673–87.

18. Fenderson BA, Toshimori K, Muller CH, Lane TF, Eddy EM. Identification of a protein in the fibrous sheath of the sperm flagellum. Biol Reprod 1988;38:345–57.

19. Brito M, Figueroa J, Maldonado EU, Vera JC, Burzio LO. The major component of rat sperm fibrous sheath is a phosphoprotein. Gamete Res 1989;22:205–18.

20. Eddy EM, O'Brien DA, Fenderson BA, Welch JE. Intermediate filament-like proteins in the fibrous sheath of the mouse sperm flagellum. Ann NY Acad Sci 1991;637;224–39.

21. Oko R, Maravei D. Protein composition of the perinuclear theca of bull spermatozoa. Biol Reprod 1994;50:1000–14.

22. Oko R, Morales CR. A novel testicular protein, with sequence similarities to a family of lipid binding proteins, is a major component of the rat sperm perinuclear theca. Dev Biol 1994;166:235–45.

23. Van Der Hoorn FA, Tarnasky HA, Nordeen SK. A new rat gene RT7 is specifically expressed during spermatogenesis. Dev Biol 1990;142:147–54.

24. Burfeind P, Hoyer-Fender S. Sequence and developmental expression of a mRNA encoding a putative protein of rat sperm outer dense fibres. Dev Biol 1991;148:195–204.

25. Morales CR, Oko R, Clermont Y. Molecular cloning and developmental expression of an mRNA encoding the 27 kDa outer dense fiber protein of rat spermatozoa. Mol Reprod Dev 1994;37:229–40.

26. Carrera A, Gerton GL, Moss SB. The major fibrous sheath polypeptide of mouse sperm: structural and functional similarities to the A-kinase anchoring proteins. Dev Biol 1994;165:272–84.

27. Fulcher KD, Mori C, Welch JE, O'Brien DA, Klapper DG, Eddy EM. Characterization of Fsc1 cDNA for a mouse sperm fibrous sheath component. Biol Reprod 1995;52:41–9.

28. Oko R, Moussakova L, Clermont Y. Regional differences in composition of the perforatorium and outer periacrosomal layer of the rat spermatozoon as revealed by immunocytochemistry. Am J Anat 1990;188:64–73.

29. Narayanan U, Barbosa E, Reed R, Tennekoon G. Characterization of a cloned cDNA encoding rabbit myelin P2 protein. J Biol Chem 1988;263:8332–7.

30. Narayanan U, Kaestner KH, Tennekoon GI. Structure of the mouse myelin P2 protein gene. J Neurochem 1991;57:75–80.

31. Bernlohr DA, Angus CE, Lane MD, Bolanowski MA, Kelly TJ. Expression of specific mRNAs during adipose differentiation: identification of an mRNA encoding a homologue of myelin P2 protein. Proc Natl Acad Sci USA 1984;81:5468–72.

32. Sacchettini JC, Said B, Schulz H, Gordon JI. Rat heart fatty acid-binding protein is highly homologous to the murine adipocyte 422 protein and the P2 protein of peripheral nerve myelin. J Biol Chem 1968;261:8218–23.

33. Ong DE, Newcomer ME, Chytil F. Cellular retinoid-binding proteins. In: Sporn MB, Poberts AB, Goodman DS, eds. The retinoids: biology, chemistry and medicine, 2nd ed. New York: Raven Press, 1994:283–317.

34. Schmitt MC, Jamison RS, Orgebin-Crist M-C, Ong DE. A novel, testis-specific member of the cellular lipophilic transport protein superfamily, deduced from a complementary deoxyribonucleic acid clone. Biol Reprod 1994;51:239–45.

35. Martenson RE. A general model of the P2 protein of peripheral nervous system myelin based on secondary structure predictions, tertiary folding principles and experimental observations. J Neurochem 1983;40:951–68.

36. Newcomer ME, Jones TA, Aquist J, Sundelin J, Ericksson U, Rask L, Peterson PA. The three-dimensional structure of retinol-binding protein. EMBO J 1984;3:1451–4.

37. Jones TA, Bergfors T, Sedzik J, Unge T. The three-dimensional structure of the P2 myelin protein. EMBO J 1988;7:1597–604.

38. Sacchettini JC, Gordon JI, Banaszuk LJ. The structure of crystalline *Escherichia coli* derived rat intestinal fatty acid-binding protein at 2.5-Å resolution. J Biol Chem 1988;263:5815–9.

39. Xu Z, Bernlohr DA, Banaszak LJ. Crystal structure of recombinant murine adipocyte lipid-binding protein. Biochemistry 1992;31:3484–92.

40. Xu Z, Bernlohr DA, Banaszak LJ. The adipocyte lipid-binding protein at 1.6 Å resolution: crystal structures of the apoprotein with bound saturated and unsaturated fatty acids. J Biol Chem 1993;268:7874–84.

41. Cowan SW, Newcomer ME, Jones TA. Crystallographic studies on a family of cellular lipophilic transport proteins. J Mol Biol 1993;230:1225–46.

42. Sha RS, Kane CD, Xu Z, Banaszak LJ, Bernlohr DA. Modulation of ligand binding affinity of the adipocyte lipid binding protein by selective mutation: analyses in vitro and in vivo. J Biol Chem 1993;268:7885–92.

43. Zhang J, Liu Z-P, Jones TA, Gierasch LM, Sambrook JF. Mutating the charged residues in the binding pocket of cellular retinoic acid-binding protein simulta-

neously reduces its binding affinity to retinoic acid and increases its thermostability. Proteins 1992;13:87–99.

44. Buelt MK, Bernlohr DA. Modification of the adipocyte lipid binding protein by sulfhydryl reagents and analysis of the fatty acid binding domain. Biochemistry 1990;29:7408–13.

45. Uyemura K, Yoshimura K, Suzuki M, Kitamura K. Lipid binding activities of the P2 protein in peripheral nerve myelin. Neurochem Res 1984;9:1509–14.

46. Boggs JM, Clement IR, Moscarello MA, Eylar HE, Hushim G. Antibody precipitation of lipid vesicles containing myelin proteins: dependence on lipid composition. J Immunol 1981;126:1207–11.

47. Chapman BE, James GE, Moore WJ. Conformations of P2 protein of peripheral nerve myelin by nuclear magnetic resonance spectroscopy. J Neurochem 1981;36:2032–6.

48. Trapp BD, Dubois-Dalcq M, Quarles RH. Ultrastructural localization of P2 protein in actively myelinating rat Schwann cells. J Neurochem 1984;43:944–8.

49. Kadlubowski M, Hughes AC, Gregson NA. Experimental allergic neuritis in the Lewis rat: characterization of the activity of peripheral myelin and its major basic protein, P2. Brain Res 1980;184:439–54.

50. Shin HC, McFarlane EF, Pollard JD, Watson EGS. Induction of experimental allergic neuritis with synthetic peptides from myelin P2 protein. Neurosci Lett 1989;102:309–12.

51. Rostami A, Gregorian SK. Peptide 53-78 of myelin P2 protein is a T cell epitope for the induction of experimental autoimmune neuritis. Cell Immunol 1991; 132:433–41.

52. Oko R, Clermont Y. Origin and distribution of perforatorial proteins during spermatogenesis of the rat: an immunocytochemical study. Anat Rec 1991;230:489–501.

53. Oko R, Maravei D. Distribution and possible role of perinuclear theca proteins during bovine spermiogenesis. Micro Res Tech 1995;32:520–32.

54. Calvin HI. Isolation and subfractionation of mammalian sperm heads and tails. In: Prescott DM, ed. Methods in cell biology. New York: Academic Press, 1976;13:85–104.

55. Kuhn R, Schäfer U, Schäfer M. Cis-acting regions sufficient for spermatocyte-specific transcriptional and spermatid-specific translational control of the Drosophila melanogaster gene Mst(3) gl-9. EMBO J 1988;7:447–54.

56. Higgy NA, Pastoor T, Renz C, Tarnasky HA, Van Der Hoorn FA. Testis-specific RT7 protein localizes to the sperm tail and associates with itself. Biol Reprod 1994;50:1357–66.

57. Schäfer M, Börsch D, Hülster A, Schäfer U. Expression of a gene duplication encoding conserved sperm tail proteins is translationally regulated in Drosophila melanogaster. Mol Cell Biol 1993;13:1708–18.

58. Oko R, Clermont Y. Light microscopic immunocytochemical study of fibrous sheath and outer dense fiber formation in the rat spermatid. Anat Rec 1989;225:46–55.

59. Monesi V. Synthetic activity during spermatogenesis in the mouse. RNA and protein synthesis. Exp Cell Res 1965;39:197–224.

60. Clermont Y, Oko R, Hermo L. Immunocytochemical study of fibrous sheath and outer dense fiber formation in the rat spermatid. Anat Rec 1990;225:46–55.

61. Oko R, Clermont Y. Biogenesis of specialized cytoskeletal elements of rat spermatozoa. Ann NY Acad Sci USA 1991;637:203–23.
62. Calvin HI, Bedford JM. Formation of disulfide bonds in the nucleus and accessory structures of mammalian spermatozoa during maturation in the epididymis. J Reprod Fertil 1971;Suppl 13:65–75.
63. Brito M, Figueroa J, Maldonado EU, Vera JC, Burzio LO. The major component of rat sperm fibrous sheath is a phosphoprotein. Gamete Res 1989;22:205–18.

12

Promoter Analysis of Male Germ-Cell–Specific Genes: Nuclear Transition Protein-1 and Histone H1t

MALATHI K. KISTLER, JOHN G. BARTELL, EDWARD A. SHIPWASH, WENDY R. HATFIELD, SHARON E. CLARE, MICHAEL J. DEWEY, AND W. STEPHEN KISTLER

Spermatogenesis demonstrates a regulated program of genetic expression driving a complex progression of cellular differentiation. A current challenge is to understand the factors responsible for the many examples of differential gene expression documented during spermatogenesis (1, 2). An aspect of male germ-cell differentiation that is fairly well described at the molecular level involves changes in DNA packaging by basic chromosomal proteins. Histones are responsible for the fundamental packaging unit of chromatin, the nucleosome, and early male germ cells contain the standard somatic forms of histones. However, beginning in late spermatogonia, novel histone variants that are unique to the male germ line start to appear. These include the core histone variants TH2A, TH2B, and TH3, as well as the linker histone variant H1t. The variants replace some, though not all, of their somatic-type counterparts, so that by the last third of meiotic prophase the spermatocyte nucleus is substantially enriched for testis-specific histones. This chromatin state persists into round spermatids until the spermatid nuclei elongate and condense (3, 4).

Midway through spermiogenesis (development of haploid cells), spermatid nuclei suddenly take on the characteristic morphology of the sperm head accompanied by condensation of the chromatin. Generally in parallel with these events a second change in chromosomal proteins occurs in which the majority of histones are eliminated from the nucleus, and a novel set of smaller proteins, known as nuclear transition proteins, takes their place. Two of the major transition proteins, TP1 and TP2, are widely distributed among mammals (5, 6), while some species contain additional members of this group (3, 7). The principal transition proteins are retained in the nucleus relatively briefly and are then replaced by protamines during the third major chromatin structural transition. In most mammals a single type of protamine (protamine 1) occurs in the nuclei of late spermatids and spermatozoa, but in some mammals, including mice and humans, a second type of protamine (protamine 2) occurs as well (8). Protamine 2 has the interesting feature of being made in the form of a larger precursor that is proteolytically processed in several steps to yield the final form of the protein. Because the processing is relatively slow, some spermatid-specific protein bands identified on electrophoretic gels have been initially characterized as transition proteins and later recognized to be protamine 2 precursors (9).

Isolation of recombinant clones for histone H1t and transition protein TP1 (10, 11) permitted an analysis of each *messenger RNA* (mRNA) during spermatogenesis by in situ hybridization. H1t mRNA is present beginning in late pachytene spermatocytes of about stage VII until the end of the first meiotic prophase in stage XIII (12). TP1 mRNA can first be detected in late round spermatids of stage VI and persists through the condensing spermatids of steps XIII–XIV before disappearing rapidly in step I (13, 14). Thus, the two genes offer opportunities to study transcriptional regulation at two points in spermatogenesis offset by nearly one complete cycle of the seminiferous tubule, since H1t transcription occurs in pachytene spermatocytes and TP1 transcription occurs in haploid round spermatids.

TP1 Promoter Contains a Functional CRE

The mRNAs for transition proteins and protamines first accumulate in late round spermatids, although the mRNAs are translationally repressed and do not become active for several days (15–17). Oliva and Dixon (8) noticed that the promoters of protamine 1 genes from several species, as well as the mouse TP1 gene, contain perfect or near perfect *adenosine 3':5'-cyclic monophosphate (cAMP) response elements* (CRE). The CRE consists of the 8-bp palindromic sequence 5'-TGACGTCA-3'; it is a binding site for a family of nuclear transcription factors that are responsive to phosphorylation by *protein kinase A* (PKA). The prototype for the CRE binding proteins is CREB, a transcription factor that dimerizes via a C-terminal leucine zipper located next to a basic DNA binding domain. CREB binds to strong CRE sites whether or not it is phosphorylated, but its two glutamine-rich domains are not strong transcriptional activators unless a single serine residue (at position 133 in CREB) is phosphorylated. Since PKA can phosphorylate this residue, a route is established for extracellular signals that activate adenyl cyclase to affect nuclear gene expression (18, 19). Recently a mouse line that lacks CREB has been produced by targeted homologous recombination, and the only defect described for these animals so far relates to long-term memory (20, 21). Mice that do not express CREB are fertile, so CREB does not play an indispensable function during spermatogenesis.

Other proteins related to CREB have been cloned [CRE-BP1 (22), ATFs (23)] and ATF-1 also depends upon phosphorylation for transactivation (24). The status of these factors has not been explored well in the testis. The newest member of the class of CRE binding proteins is CREM. The CREM gene is unique within the family because it gives rise to both CRE-activating and CRE-inhibiting proteins depending on tissue-specific splicing patterns (25). While both forms contain the leucine zipper and DNA-binding domains, those lacking the glutamine-rich transactivating domains of CREB (CREMα, CREMβ, CREMγ) act as repressors by binding nonproductively to CREs or by forming inactive heterodimers with CREB. In contrast, CREMτ and related forms retain the glutamine-rich transactivating domains. During spermatogenesis a remarkable change in CREM expression occurs. Only the inhibitory forms of CREM occur in the immature testis. With the development of pachytene spermatocytes, and under the stimulation of *follicle-stimulating hormone* (FSH), high levels of CREMτ mRNA appear, although translation of this mRNA is apparently repressed until the formation of haploid cells, in which CREMτ itself gradually increases, reaching a peak in late round spermatids (26–28). CREMτ mRNA levels are much higher than levels of CREB in spermatids, suggesting that even in normal animals where CREB is present, CREMτ is the predominant CRE transactivator in the cells. Furthermore, it has been shown that protein kinase A is the major kinase capable of phosphorylating CREMτ in round spermatids on the critical serine residue controlling activation (28).

We have cloned both the rat and human TP1 genes and confirmed the observation of Oliva and Dixon (8) on the presence of CRE-like DNA sequences in the TP1 promoter. While the rat CRE is a perfect palindrome, the human CRE differs at two positions from the consensus (Fig. 12.1). Reports indicate that the 8-bp CRE may not always convey cAMP induction, either because of poorly understood influences on activity by surrounding sequences (29–31) or because other proteins bound at nearby sites interfere with the occupancy of the CRE (32). We undertook an investigation to establish whether binding activity for the TP1 CRE exists in testis nuclear extracts, and, if so, whether it would recognize both the rat and human CRE sequences and could be shown to be CREMτ. We also wanted to determine whether the TP1 CRE could convey activation by PKA to a linked reporter gene.

We labeled fragments containing about 100 bp of either human or rat TP1 promoters and examined their behavior by *electrophoretic mobility shift assay* (EMSA), using nuclear extracts from 40- to 45-day-old rat testes (Fig. 12.2). Both promoter fragments gave rise to a pattern of shifted bands due to formation of apparent protein complexes (lanes 4 and 8). Competition experiments using an oligonucleotide with a GC box (SP1 binding

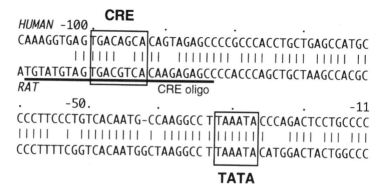

FIGURE 12.1. Sequence of TP1 promoter region upstream from TATA box. Rat sequence is from Heidaran et al. (11); human sequence taken from a genomic clone made from lymphocyte DNA (Stratagene, La Jolla, CA) and isolated by screening with a 2-kb RsaI fragment encompassing the rat gene. The CRE and TATA boxes are indicated, and the region used for the TP1 CRE oligonucleotide is underlined. Numbering is relative to the transcriptional start site.

site) eliminated the uppermost, relatively faint shifted band for the human promoter fragment (lane 1), but had less obvious effect with the rat fragment (lane 5). This oligo had no effect on the strongest shifted bands. In contrast, competition with an oligo containing the somatostatin CRE eliminated all of the strong shifted bands (lanes 2, 3, 6, and 7), while having no effect on the uppermost faint band. Thus the testis nuclear extract contained a strong binding activity for the CRE of both promoter fragments.

Testis nuclear extracts give a strong DNaseI footprint over both the GC box and the CRE region of the rat TP1 promoter (33), confirming binding activity for the CRE palindrome. To demonstrate that the TP1 CRE is competent at transcriptional induction, either the (−137/−36) rat promoter fragment or an oligonucleotide containing the TP1 CRE and flanking sequences (Fig. 12.1) was placed upstream of the thymidine kinase promoter in the *chloramphenicol acetyl transferase* (CAT) expression plasmid pBLCAT5 (34). These constructs were introduced into JEG-3 choriocarcinoma cells by the calcium phosphate technique for transient expression assays. To activate the CRE, parallel sets of cells were cotransfected with an expression vector for the catalytic subunit of PKA. In a typical experiment (Fig. 12.3), pRTP1(−137/−36)CAT was induced 10-fold. Similarly, the 26-bp sequence encompassing the rat TP1 CRE was induced nearly 6-fold by cotransfection with the PKA expression vector. To show that the CRE was responsible for the observed induction, we made a mutated version of the second plasmid (pRTP1CREmutCAT) in which the upstream half of the CRE was deleted. As expected, this construct showed much reduced induction by PKA (2-fold) in JEG-3 cells. These results established that the TP1 CRE is fully capable of conveying transcriptional induction to a fused heterologous promoter.

Evidence that CREMτ is the major CRE binding protein in our testis nuclear extracts was obtained using a CREM-specific antiserum. This antiserum specifically modified the mobility of the TP1 CRE protein complex detected by EMSA (33). In addition, a bacterially expressed form of CREMτ gave a footprint over the TP1 CRE identical to that obtained with testis extracts (33). These experiments support the conclusion that CREMτ is the predominant binding protein for the TP1 CRE.

If the promoters for several genes, such as TP1, that are expressed in round spermatids can be activated by PKA (8, 28, 33), it remains to be

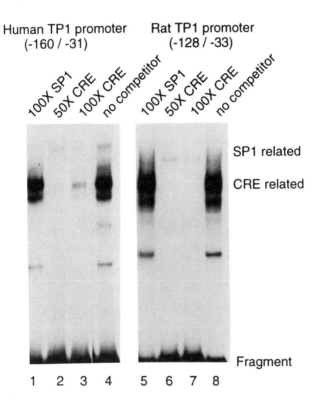

FIGURE 12.2. *Electrophoretic mobility shift assay* (EMSA) of promoter fragments of human and rat TP1 genes. The human fragment was the AluI to StuI (−160/−31) fragment cloned into the SmaI site of pUC18 and excised with EcoRI and HindIII. The rat fragment was the RsaI to StuI fragment (−128/−33) cloned and excised the same way. Testis nuclear extracts were prepared from 40-day-old rats as described (35, 36), and EMSA was performed as described (33). The top strand of the ds oligonucleotide with the somatostatin CRE was 5′-CCCGGG-TGACGTCACGGGGA-3′ and the top strand of the ds oligonucleotide with an SP1 motif was 5′-TGAGGCCCCGCCCCGTGCA-3′.

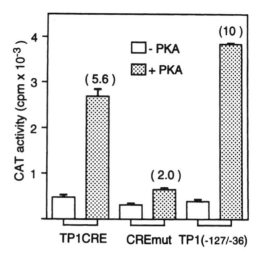

FIGURE 12.3. TP1 CRE mediates *protein kinase A* (PKA) induction of a linked gene following transient trransfection into JEG-3 cells. The TP1 promoter region (RsaI to StuI), or an oligonucleotide encompassing the TP1 CRE, or the same oligonucleotide in which the upstream half of the CRE was deleted, were fused to pBLCAT5 (34). Transfections were done with or without cotransfection with an expression plasmid for the catalytic subunit of PKA. Transfection conditions and the CAT assay have been described (33). Reprinted with permission from Kistler et al. (33).

worked out just which signaling pathways are involved. While both FSH and *luteinizing hormone* (LH), the classic gonadotrophins that control spermatogenesis, act via stimulation of adenylate cyclase, the targets for these hormones are Sertoli cells and Leydig cells, respectively. The cAMP signaling pathway in germ cells has peculiar features, including novel subunits of PKA (37), novel forms of cAMP phosphodiesterase (38), and a cytoplasmic form of adenylate cyclase (39). Recently, *pituitary adenylate cyclase–activating polypeptide* (PACAP) and its receptor have been identified in germ cells in a stage-dependent manner (40), suggesting a possible paracrine or autocrine role for this factor in germ-cell development. The ability to disrupt aspects of the cAMP pathway specifically in germ cells might well shed light on its role in promoting gene expression involved in spermatid development. The work described above makes transition protein 1 a strong candidate for regulation by cAMP in spermatids.

Investigation of the H1t Promoter in Transgenic Mice

There are two general patterns of histone expression. Most histones (replication variants) are synthesized in synchrony with DNA replication during S phase, while a minor set (replacement variants) are synthesized in nondividing cells and may eventually replace a significant fraction of the replication variants. The 3′ ends of the mRNAs for replication-dependent variants are not polyadenylated, but rather end just downstream of a characteristic stem-loop sequence. Replacement variants typically have polyadenylated mRNAs, although some histone genes give rise to both stem-loop terminated as well as polyadenylated mRNAs. The marked increases in replication variant mRNA during S phase and decrease after S phase is known to result from changes in transcription, changes in efficiency of 3′ processing, and changes in mRNA stability (41–43).

Five, closely related standard H1 variants (H1a–e) are found in mammalian somatic cells as well as the more distantly related H1°. While not all standard H1's have been investigated individually, the known genes share the features of replication-dependent variants. H1t transcription and synthesis in the rat is limited to mid-late pachytene spermatocytes (14, 44, 45). As the last period of replicative DNA synthesis occurs in preleptotene spermatocytes, H1t expression occurs not only in a tissue-specific manner, but also in a different phase of the cell cycle than that of replication variants. All in all, this contrast between H1t expression and that of the standard somatic H1's makes understanding H1t regulation an interesting challenge.

Comparison of the 5′ flanking region of the rat H1t gene with the comparable region of H1d, a standard somatic variant, indicated that both genes shared four regions of sequence homology [originally identified for H1 histones in general by Coles and Wells (46)]. These homologies include an H1-specific element (AACACA), a GC box (GGGCGG), a CCAAT motif, and a TATA box (Fig. 12.4). More recently, Grimes and coworkers identified a palindromic sequence (CCTAGG) found just upstream of the CAAT box, which is present in the promoter regions of H1t from a number of species (47, 48) (Fig. 12.4). H1t mRNA shares the stemloop 3′ end typical of replication variants and is found in the nonpolyadenylated fraction (10).

Until recently there have been no germ-cell lines from the testis that might be expected to express H1t. However, the H1t promoter was active in mouse L cells, a somatic-cell line, and Kremer and Kistler (49) examined the ability of various lengths of the H1t 5′ flanking region to drive expression of the CAT gene in both transiently and stably transfected cells. These studies indicated a potentiating role for sequences between −174 and −693 and an inhibitory role for sequences between −693 and −2kb (49). However, this system could not shed any light on the behavior of the gene in its normal environment. We therefore turned to transgenic mice to investigate the boundaries of the DNA region responsible for spermatocyte-specific expression.

The mouse and rat H1t genes can be separately identified on Northern and Southern blots due to differences in the 5′ nontranslated regions. The H1t proteins from the two species can also be resolved from one another by

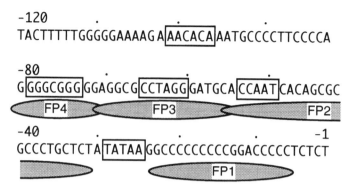

FIGURE 12.4. Sequence of the promoter region of rat H1t. Nucleotide homologies are indicated, as well as footprint regions on the H1t promoter displayed in Figure 12.9.

sodium dodecyl sulfate (SDS) gel electrophoresis. We therefore chose a 7-kb genomic fragment for initial transgenic studies containing the rat H1t gene, as well as 2.4 kb of upstream and 3.8 kb of downstream DNA. Three other constructs were made by deleting upstream or downstream sequences (Fig. 12.5). In all, 15 transgene-carrying founder animals were identified in this study, including at least two for each construct. Most founder animals were bred to provide lines that passed the transgene from generation to generation in Mendelian fashion.

Both lines bearing the largest genomic fragment (TG1) displayed high-level testis-specific expression as shown by Northern blot (Fig. 12.6), S1

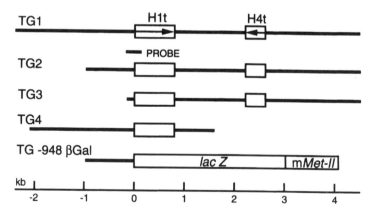

FIGURE 12.5. Diagram of constructs used in transgenic experiments. Location of a PstI-PstI fragment that serves as a rat-specific probe on northern blots is indicated. The fusion construct to *E. coli* β-galactosidase was based on placI, which includes an intron and poly(A) site from the mouse metallothionein II gene (kindly provided by R. Palmiter).

FIGURE 12.6. Northern blot
showing testis-specific
expression of rat H1t
transgene in lines derived
from the indicated founder
animals. Staining with
ethidium bromide
demonstrated equal
loading of undegraded
RNA for the various
organs. The [^{32}P]-labeled
probe fragment is
indicated in Figure 12.5.

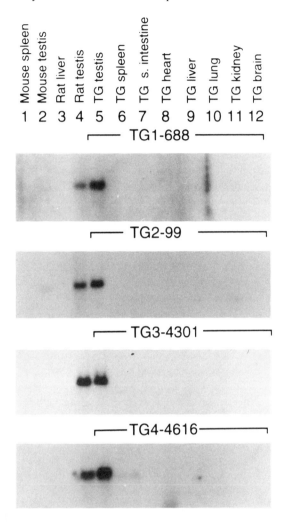

nuclease protection assays, and SDS gel electrophoresis (results not shown). At least one example of each of the other three constructs also displayed a high level of testis-specific expression (Fig. 12.6) although expression levels varied significantly among different lines, with downstream deletions (TG4) showing the greatest variability. The results from these animals indicate that the minimal sequences necessary for testis-specific expression reside between -141 and $+1578$ relative to the transcriptional start site.

From the transgenic experiments presented above, it is not possible to say whether the H1t structural gene plays a necessary role in testis-specific expression. To investigate this issue we produced transgenic mice from constructs containing 141 or 1 kb of H1t upstream sequence fused to the coding sequence for *Escherichia coli* β-galactosidase (Fig. 12.5). Two transgenic lines were established for each construct. Expression of the transgene was monitored by staining testes for β-galactosidase activity using the chromagenic substrate X-gal. One of two lines bearing the longer promoter construct expressed β-galactosidase activity in the testes (Fig. 12.7) and not above background in a number of other tissues examined. Positively stained cells were either spermatocytes or round spermatids, matching exactly the normal pattern of H1t expression. For each of several expressing animals examined histologically, an apparently random subpopulation of spermatocytes and round spermatids were positive while many cells of the same developmental stage remained unstained. We have no explanation for this phenomenon. However, the expression level of the transgene in this line is extremely low, as we have not detected β-galactosidase mRNA on Northern blots or by S1 nuclease assays of total testis RNA. None of the lines established from the short promoter construct showed a positive reaction for β-galactosidase in their testes or in other organs tested.

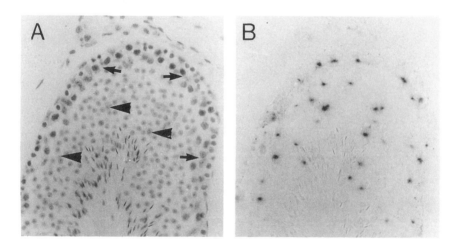

FIGURE 12.7. Demonstration of spermatocyte/spermatid expression of lacZ fusion gene in transgenic mouse testis. Testes were fixed briefly in buffered 4% paraformaldehyde and then exposed to the chromagenic substrate 5-bromo-4-chloro-3-indolyl-β-D-galactoside (X-gal) for 3 days at room temperature. They were then postfixed in paraformaldehyde for 1–2 days and processed for routine paraffin embedding and sectioning. Sections were stained with nuclear fast red. When photographed through a light green filter (*A*), the blue reaction product was difficult to detect. When the same field was photographed through a deep red filter (*B*), the reaction product was markedly intensified while the red-stained nuclei were rendered nearly invisible. Arrows (*A*) indicate positive spermatocytes. Arrowheads (*A*) indicate positive round spermatids. The tubule is at approximately stage VII.

To summarize our conclusions from the transgenic studies, 1 kb of upstream sequence is sufficient to drive spermatocyte-specific expression of a fusion gene, although at low level in the single line examined. The results for the short (141 bp) promoter fusion construct are inconclusive since we have not yet examined sufficient founder lines to conclude that expression does not occur. With the natural gene, as little as 141 bp of upstream sequence can drive testis-specific expression. Sequences further upstream or downstream of the gene may contribute to the level of expression as the most reproducibile high-level expression was found when the natural gene was flanked by at least 2 kb of its genomic surroundings.

In Vitro Studies of the Rat H1t Promoter

We have examined the ability of H1t upstream sequences to promote in vitro transcription using nuclear extracts prepared from rat testes and livers by the procedure of Gorski et al. (35). As a template, various lengths of upstream sequences were fused to the "G-less" cassette of Sawadogo and Roeder (50). In testis extracts, transcription directed by these constructs showed little dependence on sequences between −141 and −900, and transcription somewhat enhanced using the shorter construct (Fig. 12.8). A deletion to −84, which eliminates the H1 consensus element, showed no decrease in in vitro transcription. However, deletion of the promoter to −64 and −43 led to marked reduction in activity. These deletions removed the GC box region and CAAT box region, respectively. Transcription directed by the H1t promoter was also strong in liver extracts (unpublished observations), so in this regard the in vitro system did not reflect the tissue specificity of H1t.

Footprinting is a valuable technique for identifying regions of a promoter that bind prevalent nuclear proteins. DNaseI footprints of the rat H1t promoter region from both testis and liver extracts were similar (Fig. 12.9) although not identical. A marked footprint (FP1) was detected just downstream of the TATA element. Upstream of the TATA box, a long footprint (FP II) extended across the CAAT box and encompassed the H1t palindrome, CCTAGG (FP III). No footprint was seen over the GC box region on the lower strand of DNA due to the absence of DNaseI cut sites in this region. However, a footprint over this region was seen on the complementary strand (FP4) (unpublished observations). No footprint was seen over the H1-specific sequence AAACACA. The footprint obtained with liver nuclear proteins was similar, but the FP III region (H1t palindrome) did not extend as far in the 3′ direction and displayed a marked hypersensitive site within FP III (Fig. 12.9). These results are in general agreement with those from in vitro transcription. The H1 box region did not have a significant role in transcription or in binding nuclear proteins. In contrast, the region of the promoter from the GC box to the transcriptional start site was vital for in

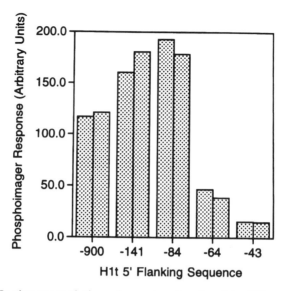

FIGURE 12.8. In vitro transcription using various lengths of the H1t upstream region fused to the G-less casette. The H1t 5'-flanking region from +6 was fused to p(C_2AT) (50), and various upstream truncations were made using restriction sites. In vitro transcription was performed as described by Gorski et al. (35) using extracts prepared from 23-day-old animals to maximize the contribution of late spermatocytes. Reaction products were separated through a denaturing polyacrylamide gel and radioactivity in the full-length transcript determined with a Molecular Dynamics phosphoimager. Duplicate results for each template are shown.

vitro transcription and displayed several clear binding sites for nuclear proteins.

To identify particular proteins that interact with footprint regions of the H1t promoter, we prepared oligonucleotides encompassing each region. Using EMSA analysis, we found that oligonucleotides for FP I and FP IV form specific complexes with nuclear proteins that are competed by a consensus oligonucleotide for transcription factor SP1 (unpublished observations). The identities of the factor(s) in testis nuclear extracts that bind to these oligonucleotides is uncertain, however, as the concentration of SP1 in immature testis is relatively low (51), and a variety of other factors can also bind to GC box-like sequences (52, 53).

H1 promoters for both standard somatic variants and H1t share a CAAT box region with an extended region of conserved nucleotides, particularly toward the 5' direction. A novel heteromeric binding protein for the H1 CAAT region has been isolated by two laboratories (54, 55), and one of the subunits has been cloned and designated H1TF2A (56). An oligonucleotide for the H1t CAAT box region (FP II) detects a prevalent protein in testis nuclear extracts, and an antiserum to bacterially expressed human H1TF2A

FIGURE 12.9. DNaseI footprint assay of the rat H1t promoter in testis and liver nuclear extracts. Extracts were prepared from 23-day-old rats as described (35, 36). The target was a BstEII to RsaI fragment cloned into the SmaI site of pUC18. It was labeled at the 3'-end of the lower strand with α[³²P]dATP and Klenow DNA polymerase. The labeled fragment (1–2 ng) was incubated with 90–100 μg of nuclear protein prior to treatment with DNaseI and resolution of the cleavage products on a denaturing gel.

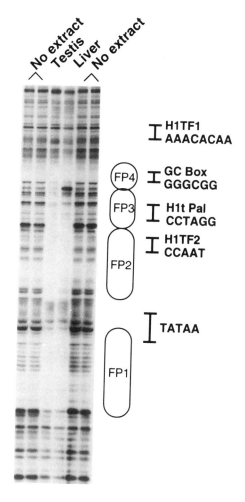

binds specifically to the testis nuclear protein that interacts with the H1t FP II oligonucleotide (judged from a supershifted band on an EMSA gel, unpublished observations). Based on this immunological identity, we conclude that H1TF2 is prevalent in testis extracts and binds specifically to the H1t CAAT box. As deletions through this area have a profound effect on in vitro transcription, we conclude that H1TF2 is an important trans-activator for H1t.

The remaining footprint covers the H1t-specific palindrome CCTAGG. Grimes and colleagues identified a testis-specific binding factor for an oligonucleotide containing this sequence (47, 48). We have confirmed a testis-specific binding activity for an oligonucleotide encompassing FP III (Fig. 12.10, band B), which is competed successfully by the same oligonucleotide but not by a series of unrelated oligonucleotides. However, this oligonucleotide also forms several additional shifted bands, of slower mobility (Fig. 12.10, band A), that are found both in the testis and also in liver and HeLa cell nuclear extracts. These additional bands have not been reported previously and are of interest because liver extracts also form a partial footprint over region III.

Oligonucleotides are useful reagents for probing the role of specific sequences in promoting in vitro transcription. Adding an excess of an oligo-

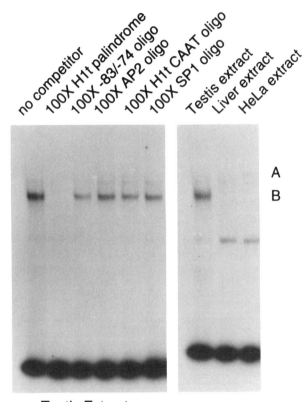

Testis Extract

FIGURE 12.10. Electrophoretic mobility shift assay of binding activity for an oligonucleotide containing the H1t-specific squence CCTAGG. The upper strand of the oligo was 5′- GATCGAGGCGCCTAGGGATGCAG-3′, and the lower strand was 5′-GATCCTGCATCCCTAGGCGCCTC-3′. It was labeled by filling in with Klenow DNA polymerase using α[³²P]dATP. Shifted complex B was competed by the same oligonucleotide used as probe (H1t palindrome) but not by a variety of other oligonucleotides. This complex was not found in liver or in HeLa cell extracts. In contrast, complexes denoted A were present in extracts from all tested sources. The lowest shifted band seen in the last three lanes on the right was not reproducible and may reflect proteolytically degraded proteins.

nucleotide to an in vitro transcription reaction can remove a particular factor from the template and thereby reveal its relative importance. Addition of oligonucleotides to in vitro transcription reactions has shown that an SP1 consensus (GC box) and an H1t CAAT box will markedly depress in vitro transcription from the H1t promoter but not from an adenoviral major late promoter control template. However, oligonucleotides for the H1 box (AACACA) or the H1t palindrome (CCTAGG) had no specific effect on the in vitro transcription from the H1t promoter (unpublished observations).

Conclusions

Tissue-specific gene expression is recognized to result from a complex interplay of widely expressed and tissue-specific transcription factors on promoter and enhancer regions of a gene of interest. We have shown that the TP1 promoter contains a functional response element for transcriptional regulation by protein kinase A. We have also shown that correct tissue-specific expression of the H1t gene can be directed by as little as 141 bp of upstream sequence. Within that region in vitro analysis supports the function of both the GC box element and the binding site for H1-specific transcription factor H1TF2. Occurrence of a testis-specific binding factor for the H1t-specific promoter element CCTAGG was confirmed, although an effect of this factor was not demonstrated by in vitro transcription reactions. These results provide some important information on the DNA sequences and binding factors that promote transcription of these genes, but much work still remains to be done to understand their developmental control.

Acknowledgment. The work reported here was supported in part by grant HD10793 from the National Institutes of Health.

References

1. Hecht NB. Gene expression during male germ cell development. In: Desjardins C, Ewing, LL, eds. Cell and molecular biology of the testis. New York: Oxford University Press, 1993:400–32.
2. Eddy EM, Welch JE, O'Brien, DA. Gene expression during spermatogenesis. In: de Kretser D, ed. Molecular biology of the male reproductive system. San Diego: Academic Press, 1993:181–232.
3. Meistrich ML. Histone and basic nuclear protein transitions in mammalian spermatogenesis. In: Hnilica LS, Stein GS, Stein JL, eds. Histones and other basic nuclear proteins. Boca Raton, FL: CRC Press, 1989:165–82.

4. Kistler WS. Structures of testis-specific histones, spermatid transition proteins and their genes in mammals. In: Hnilica LS, Stein GS, Stein JL, eds. Histones and other basic nuclear proteins. Boca Raton, FL: CRC Press, 1989:331–45.

5. Kistler WS, Geroch ME, Williams-Ashman HG. Specific basic proteins from mammalian testes, isolation and properties of small basic proteins from rat testes and epididymal spermatozoa. J Biol Chem 1973;248:4532–43.

6. Alfonso PJ, Kistler WS. Immunohistochemical localization of spermatid nuclear transition protein 2 in the testes of rats and mice. Biol Reprod 1993;48:522–9.

7. Lanneau M, Loir M. An electrophoretic investigation of mammalian spermatid-specific nuclear proteins. J Reprod Fertil 1982;65:163–70.

8. Oliva R, Dixon GH. Vertebrate protamine genes and the histone-to-protamine replacement reaction. Prog Nucleic Acid Res Mol Biol 1990;40:25–94.

9. Green GR, Balhorn R, Poccia DL, Hecht NB. Synthesis and processing of mammalian protamines and transition proteins. Mol Reprod Dev 1994;37:255–63.

10. Cole KD, Kandala JC, Kistler WS. Isolation of the gene for the testis-specific H1 histone variant H1t. J Biol Chem 1986;261:7178–83.

11. Heidaran MA, Kozak CA, Kistler WS. Nucleotide sequence of the Stp-1 gene coding for rat spermatid nuclear transition protein 1 (TP1): homology with protamine P1 and assignment of the mouse Stp-1 gene to chromosome 1. Gene 1989;75:39–46.

12. Heidaran MA, Showman RM, Kistler WS. A cytochemical study of the transcriptional and translational regulation of nuclear transition protein 1 (TP1), a major chromosomal protein of mammalian spermatids. J Cell Biol 1988; 106:1427–33.

13. Mali P, Kaipia A, Kangasniemi M, Toppari J, Sandberg M, Hecht NB, Parvinen M. Stage-specific expression of nucleoprotein mRNAs during rat and mouse spermiogenesis. Reprod Fertil Dev 1989;1:369–82.

14. Kremer EJ, Kistler WS. Localization of mRNA for testis-specific histone H1t by in situ hybridization. Exp Cell Res 1991;197:330–2.

15. Kleene KC, Distel RJ, Necht NB. Translational regulation and deadenylation of a protamine mRNA during spermiogenesis in the mouse. Dev Biol 1984; 105:71–9.

16. Heidaran MA, Kistler WS. Transcriptional and translational control of the message for transition protein 1, a major chromosomal protein of mammalian spermatids. J Biol Chem 1987;262:13309–15.

17. Kleene KC. Poly(A) shortening accompanies the activation of translation of five mRNAs during spermiogenesis in the mouse. Development 1989;106:367–73.

18. Habener JF. Cyclic AMP response element binding proteins: a cornucopia of transcription factors. Mol Endocrinol 1990;4:1087–94.

19. Montminy MR, Gonzalez GA, Yamamoto KK. Characteristics of the cAMP response unit. Recent Prog Horm Res 1990;46:219–29.

20. Hummler E, Cole TJ, Blendy JA, Ganss R, Aguzzi A, Schmid W, Beermann F, Schutz G. Targeted mutation of the cAMP response element binding protein (CREB) gene: compensation within the CREB/ATF family of transcription factors. Proc Natl Acad Sci USA 1994;91:5647–51.

21. Bourtchuladze R, Frenguelli B, Blendy J, Cioffi D, Schutz G, Silva AJ. Deficient long-term memory in mice with a targeted mutation of the cAMP-responsive element-binding protein. EMBO J 1994;79:59–68.

22. Maekawa T, Skura H, Kanes-Ishii C, Sudo T, Yoshimura T, Fujisawa J, Yoshida M, Ishii S. Leucine zipper structure of the protein CRE-BP1 binding to the cyclic AMP response element in brain. EMBO J 1989;8:2023–90.

23. Hai T, Liu F, Coukos WJ, Green MR. Transcription ATF cDNA clones: an extensive family of leucine zipper proteins able to selectively form DNA-binding heterodimers. Genes Dev 1989;3:2083–90.

24. Rehfuss RP, Walton KM, Loriaux MM, Goodman RH. The cAMP-regulated enhancer-binding protein ATF-1 activates transcription in response to cAMP-dependent protein kinase A. J Biol Chem 1991;266:18431–4.

25. de Groot RP, Sassone-Corsi P. Hormonal control of gene expression: multiplicity and versatility of cyclic adenosine 3′,5′-monophosphate-responsive nuclear regulators. Mol Endocrinol 1993;7:145–53.

26. Foulkes NS, Mellstrom B, Benusiglio E, Sassone-Corsi P. Developmental switch of CREM function during spermatogenesis: from antagonist to transcriptional activator. Nature 1992;355:80–4.

27. Foulkes NS, Schlotter F, Pevet P, Sassone-Corsi P. Pituitary hormone FSH directs the CREM functional switch during spermatogenesis. Nature 1993; 362:264–7.

28. Delmas V, van der Hoorn F, Mellstrom B, Jegou B, Sassone-Corsi P. Induction of CREM activator proteins in spermatids: down-stream targets and implications for haploid germ cell differentiation. Mol Endocrinol 1993;7:1502–14.

29. Montminy MR, Sevarino KA, Wagner JA, Mandel G, Goodman RH. Identification of a cyclic AMP responsive element within the rat somatostatin gene. Proc Natl Acad Sci USA 1986;83:6682–6.

30. Deutsch PJ, Hoeffler JP, Jameson L, Habener JL. Cyclic AMP and phorbol ester-stimulated transcription mediated by similar DNA elements that bind distinct proteins. Proc Natl Acad Sci USA 1988;85:7922–6.

31. Deutsch PJ, Hoeffler JP, Jameson L, Lin JC, Habener JF. Structural determinants for transcriptional activation by cAMP-responsive DNA elements. J Biol Chem 1988;263:18466–72.

32. Miller CP, Lin JC, Habener JF. Transcription of the rat glucagon gene by the cyclic AMP response element-binding protein CREB is modulated by adjacent CREB-associated proteins. Mol Cell Biol 1993;13:7080–90.

33. Kistler MK, Sassone-Corsi P, Kistler WS. Identification of a functional cyclic adenosine 3′,5′-monophosphate response element in the 5′-flanking region of the gene for transition protein 1 (TP1), a basic chromosomal protein of mammalian spermatids. Biol Reprod 1994;51:1322–9.

34. Boshart M, Kluppel M, Schmidt A, Schütz G, Luckow B. Reporter constructs with low background activity utilizing the cat gene. Gene 1992;110:129–30.

35. Gorski K, Carnerro M, Schibler U. Tissue specific in vitro transcription from the mouse albumin promoter. Cell 1986;47:767–76.

36. Lichtsteiner S, Wuarin J, Schibler U. The interplay of DNA-binding proteins on the promoter of the mouse albumin gene. Cell 1987;51:963–73.

37. Oyen O, Myklebust F, Scott JD, Cadd GG, McKnight GS, Hansson V, Jahnsen T. Subunits of cyclic adenosine 3′,5′-monophosphate dependent protein kinase show differential and distinct expression patterns during germ cell differentia-

tion: alternative polyadenylation in germ cells gives rise to unique smaller-sized mRNA species. Biol Reprod 1990;43:46–54.

38. Welch JE, Swinnen JV, O'Brien DA, Eddy EM, Conti M. Unique adenosine 3′, 5′ cyclic monophosphate phosphodiesterase messenger ribonucleic acids in rat spermatogenic cells: evidence for differential gene expression during spermatogenesis. Biol Reprod 1992;46:1027–33.

39. Onoda JM, Braun T, Wrenn SM Jr. Characterization of the purine-reactive site of the rat testis cytosolic adenylate cyclase. Biochem Pharmacol 1987; 36:1907–12.

40. Kononen J, Paavola M, Penttila T-L, Parvinen M, Pelto-Huikko M. Stage-specific expression of pituitary adenylate cyclase-activating polypeptide (PACAP) mRNA in the rat seminiferous tubules. Endocrinology 1994;135: 2291–4.

41. Heintz N. The regulation of histone gene expression during the cell cycle. Biochim Biophys Acta 1991;1088:327–39.

42. Harris ME, Bohni R, Schneiderman MH, Ramamurthy L, Schümperli D, Marzluff WF. Regulation of histone mRNA in the unperturbed cell cycle: evidence suggesting control at two posttranscriptional steps. Mol Cell Biol 1991;11:2416–24.

43. Stein GS, Stein JL, van Wijnen AJ, Lian JB. Regulation of histone gene expression. Curr Opin Cell Biol. 1992;4:166–73.

44. Brock WA, Trostle PK, Meistrich ML. Meiotic synthesis of testis histones in the rat. Proc Natl Acad Sci USA 1980;77:371–5.

45. Meistrich ML, Bucci LR, Trostle-Weige PK, Brock WR. Histone variants in rat spermatogonia and primary spermatocytes. Dev Biol 1985;112:230–40.

46. Coles LS, Wells JRE. An H1 histone gene-specific 5′ element and evolution of H1 and H5 genes. Nucleic Acids Res 1985;13:585–94.

47. Grimes SR, Wolfe SA, Koppel DA. Tissue-specific binding of testis nuclear proteins to a sequence element within the promoter of the testis-specific histone H1t gene. Arch Biochem Biophys 1992;296:402–9.

48. Wolfe SA, Grimes SR. Histone H1t: a tissue-specific model used to study transcriptional control and nuclear function during cellular differentiation. J Cell Biochem 1993;53:156–60.

49. Kremer EJ, Kistler WS. Analysis of the promoter for the gene encoding the testis-specific histone H1t in a somatic cell line: evidence for cell-cycle regulation and modulation by distant upstream sequences. Gene 1992;110: 167–73.

50. Sawadogo M, Roeder RG. Factors involved in specific transcription by human RNA polymerase II: analysis by a rapid and quantitative in vitro assay. Proc Natl Acad Sci USA 1985;81:308–12.

51. Saffer JD, Jackson SP, Annarella MB. Developmental expression of Sp1 in the mouse. Mol Cell Biol 1991;11:2189–99.

52. Imataka H, Sogawa K, Yasumoto K, Kikuchi Y, Sasano K, Kobayashi A, et al. Two regulatory proteins that bind to the basic transcription element (BTE), a GC box sequence in the promoter region of the rat P-450 1A1 gene. EMBO J 1992;11:3663–71.

53. St-Arnaud R, Moir JM. Wnt-1-inducing factor-1: a novel G/C box-binding transcription factor regulating the expression of wnt-1 during neuroectodermal differentiation. Mol Cel Biol 1993;13:1590–8.

54. van Wijnen AJ, Massung RF, Stein J, Stein G. Human H1 histone gene promoter CCAAT-box binding protein HiNF-B is a mosaic factor. Biochemistry 1988:27:6534–41.
55. Gallinari P, LaBella F, Heintz N. Characterization and purification of H1TF2, a novel CCAAT-binding protein that interacts with a histone H1 subtype specific consensus element. Mol Cell Biol 1989:9:1566–75.
56. Martinelli R, Heintz N. H1TF2: the large subunit of a heterodimeric, glutamine rich CCAAT-binding transcription factor involved in histone H1 cell cycle regulation. Mol Cell Biol 1994:14:8322–32.

Part IV

Hormone Action and Transport Mechanisms

13

Androgen Receptor Distribution in the Testis

C.A. Suarez-Quian, B.O. Oke, W. Vornberger, G. Prins, S. Xiao, and N.A. Musto

Germ cells contain *androgen receptor* (AR). Germ cells do not contain androgen receptor. These diametrically opposed views are at the center of a long-running dispute regarding the cell site of androgen action within the testis (reviewed in 1, 2). In this chapter we examine AR distribution in the rat and mouse testis using an affinity-purified rabbit polyclonal antibody made to a 21 amino acid peptide of the amino terminus of the rat AR (3–5). Results reveal the presence of AR in testicular somatic cells, as well as in elongated spermatids.

Procedure

Antibody

PG-21 is an affinity-purified, rabbit polyclonal antibody made to a synthetic peptide corresponding to the first 21 amino acids of the amino terminus of the rat AR. Its use as a valid immunological probe for the rat AR has been established (3–5).

Tissue Fixation, Embedding, and Immunocytochemistry

The procedure for immunocytochemistry was described in detail previously (6). We employed Bouin's fixed testes that were embedded in polyester wax and immunostained using Zymed (San Francisco, CA) Histostain-SP kits. Reaction product was generated using DAB-Black from Zymed. The only modification we employed from the previously described staining protocol was microwaving sections prior to immunostaining. After rehydrating polyester wax sections attached to glass slides, slides were placed in 0.1 M citrate buffer, pH 6.0, and microwaved for 30 min using a 600 W oven. Care was taken that the buffer did not boil over the container leaving the sections to dry. After microwaving, sections were allowed to come to room temperature and were then immunostained as described (6). Counterstaining with hematoxylin was done for only 1–2 sec.

The primary antibody to AR was used at a concentration of 2 µg/mL. Controls included preadsorption of the primary antibody with 10-fold excess of the antigenic peptide, or with an unrelated peptide of the AR, and then using the preadsorbed antibody as the probe. In addition, we employed immunofluorescence instead of biotin-streptavidin immunoperoxidase to examine AR immunoreactivity. The procedure employed resembled that described above, except that the secondary antibody was replaced with rhodamine-conjugated goat anti-rabbit antibody (Cappel) at a 1:80 dilution.

Tissue Fractions and Western Immunoblotting

Nuclear and cytosol fractions from rat prostates, epididymis, testes, and elongated spermatids were prepared as described (7).

An enriched, elongated spermatid fraction was prepared as described by Grove and Vogl (8). Adult rat testes were decapsulated, placed in ice-cold PBS, pH 7.3, containing 5 mM *ethylenediaminetetraacetic acid* (EDTA), and minced for 20 min using fine scissors. At this point a fraction of the minced testis was collected, doused, and separated into nuclear and cytosolic fractions; these fractions were used for immunoblotting. The elongated spermatid fractions were then prepared from the remaining minced testis. The minced testes were continuously aspirated for 15 min using a 10-mL pipette and the resulting tissue suspension was centrifuged at 600 g for 5 min in a clinical centrifuge, pelleting intact tubules and leaving sheared germ cells in the supernatant. The supernatant was collected and the pellet was resuspended and centrifuged again to increase germ-cell yield. The two supernatants were pooled, pelleted at 3,200 g at 4°C for 5 min, then washed, resuspended, and pelleted three times in 0.25 M sucrose. The final pellet was then treated as described above for prostate to generate nuclear and cytosolic fractions from the enriched elongated spermatids.

The enrichment of elongated spermatids was assessed by preparing cytospins of the final cell pellet (prior to separating nuclei from cytosol) onto glass slides and examining the spun cell by phase microscopy. Approximately 80% of all cells exhibited features of elongated spermatids, i.e., elongated nuclei and condensed chromatin. The contaminating cells appeared to be pachytene spermatocytes or round spermatids. In addition, the attached cells were immunostained for AR to verify the presence of a robust immunoperoxidase product in the spun cells. The cytospins were prepared using a Shandon Cytospin 2 for pelleting cells at 1,000 rpm for 10 min. In these preparations all of the cells appeared positive for AR.

However, it was not possible to distinguish cell boundaries in the cytospins. Indeed, it is likely that some of the cells appeared positively stained for AR due to overlapping of the elongated spermatid cytoplasm. Protein concentrations of all preparations were measured by the procedure of Bradford (9) using bovine serum albumin as a standard.

Next, 50 μg of prostate and epididymis nuclear and cytosolic proteins and 250 μg of both nuclear and cytosolic proteins from the testis and the enriched, elongated spermatid fraction were dissolved in Laemli buffer (10) and separated by 7.5% polyacrylamide gel electrophoresis using a Biorad Mini-Protean II Dual Slab Cell chamber system and then transferred to nitrocellulose. The procedure used for immunoblotting was essentially that of Johnson et al. (11). Affinity-purified anti-AR was used at a concentration of 1.5 μg/mL and alkaline-phosphatase goat anti-rabbit 2nd IgG (Polyscience, Inc.) was used at a 1:400 dilution.

Nucleic Acid In Situ Hybridization

The *chromosomal RNA* (cRNA) probe was synthesized from the NruI-HindIII fragment of rat AR cDNA provided by Dr C. Chang (Madison, WI). This rat AR *complementary DNA* (cDNA) fragment was subcloned into SmaI-HindIII-digested pBluescript II SK(+) (Stratagene, San Diego, CA). The plasmid was purified by a Qiagen Maxiprep kit (Chatsworth, CA). The insert, along with its vector, was digested with AlwN I to yield a 236-bp template for the antisense probe synthesis. Digestion with AlwN I also yielded a 180-bp template, which did not contain the corresponding sense sequence for the antisense probe, but did contain a sequence of the AR cDNA and served as a control. The antisense and sense probes were transcribed in vitro using the templates and T7 or T3 polymerases (Promega Corporation, Madison, WI), respectively. The probes were labeled by incorporating ^{35}S-CTP (>1,000 Ci/mmol; Amersham Corporation, Arlington, IL) in the transcription reaction. The labeled probes were purified twice by ethanol precipitation and used for in situ hybridization.

Preparation of testes sections for in situ hybridization was performed as described above for immunocytochemistry. In situ hybridization was carried out as described by Angerer and Angerer (12) with the following modifications. The sections were first dewaxed and hydrated using descending grades of ethanol (100%, 95%, 70%, 50%) for 10 min each, including 1% lithium carbonate in 70% ethanol to remove residual picric acid. The sections were then treated with 300 mM glycine for 10 min and washed in distilled water twice. Proteinase K digestion was carried out for 15 min in 1 mM Tris-HCl, pH 7.4, 50 mM EDTA, pH 8.0, containing 1 μg/mL of proteinase K (Ambion, Austin, TX). The slides were then washed for 10 min with distilled water, 0.1 M triethanolamine-HCl, pH 8.0, containing

0.25% acetic anhydride, 2X SSC for 10min, and dehydrated in ascending grades of ethanol (50%, 70%, 90%, 95%, and 100%). Prehybridization was carried out at room temperature for 2h in a buffer containing 50% formamide, 0.3M NaCl, 20mM Tris-HCl pH 8.0, 1mM EDTA, 1X Denhardt's solution, 500µg/mL yeast tRNA, 10% dextran sulfate, and 100mM *dithiothreitol* (DTT). Hybridization was carried out overnight at 48°C with either the antisense or the sense probes (1×10^6 cpm) in 30µL of the above buffer. Posthybridization washes included a wash in a large volume of hybridization buffer at 60°C for 10min and a high stringency wash with 0.1X SSC at 50°C for 15min. RNAse treatment (20µg/ mL RNAse A in 0.5M NaCl, 10mM Tris-HCl, 1mM EDTA, pH 8.0) for 30min was also included in the wash regimen. The slides were then dehydrated, dipped in Kodak NTB-2 emulsion diluted 50% with 600mM ammonium acetate, and exposed in a desiccated light-tight box at 4°C for 2 weeks.

Cell Culture and Transfection Studies

The cell lines COS-7 and LnCap were cultured in *Dulbecco modified Eagle medium* (DMEM) supplemented with 10IU µg/mL of streptomycin and 5% *fetal bovine serum* (FBS) and grown on glass coverslips. All cultures were maintained at 37°C with 5% CO_2. Cells were transfected with plasmid DNA using lipofectamine reagent. In brief, 4–10µl of lipofectamine and 1–2µg of plasmid were diluted separately with 100µl of Opti-MEM I reduced-serum medium. The two solutions were then mixed gently and incubated for 30min to form DNA-liposome complexes. The complexes were diluted with 0.8mL DMEM medium (antibiotic and serum free) and the sub-confluent cells were washed once with DMEM medium and exposed to complexes for 5h under standard culture conditions. Cells were fed their normal growth medium for 48h after transfection. For COS-7 cells, FBS was replaced with charcoal stripped serum and the cells were grown either in the presence of 10^6M testosterone or in its absence. At the end of the culture, cells were processed for immunocytochemistry as described.

Results

AR Distribution in Adult Rat and Mouse Testis

Immunocytochemical localization of AR in testis was achieved using biotin streptavidin immunoperoxidase staining, employing diaminobenzidine as the chromogen. In this protocol positive results at the sites of antigen-antibody interaction are identified by the deposition of a dark brown reaction product. Because the AR was expected to localize to the nuclei, counterstaining of tissues with hematoxylin was performed for only 1–2 sec. Previous AR immunocytochemistry studies from our laboratory employed aminoethyl carbazole as the chromogen, followed by brief counterstaining with hematoxylin. In this method, the chromogen renders a red deposit at sites of antigen distribution and the surrounding tissues, not containing a positive reaction, are distinguished by the blue counterstaining of hematoxylin. The reader is referred to our previous publication (7) for a comparison in which similar results were first published.

Survey observations of AR distribution in the adult rat testis at low magnification revealed positive deposition of reaction product in the nuclei of Sertoli cells at stages IV–VIII of the cycle of the seminiferous epithelium, in the cytoplasm of elongated spermatids, in the nuclei of peritubular myoid cells, in the nuclei of smooth muscle cells forming the walls of blood vessels and in some Leydig cells of the interstitium (Fig. 13.1A). In addition, the intensity of AR staining in Sertoli cell nuclei varied as a function of the cycle of the seminiferous epithelium. Specifically, reaction product in Sertoli cell nuclei was first detected at stage IV and then it increased markedly up to stage VIII, the stage at which the intensity reached its maximum (Fig. 13.2A,B). In contrast, all peritubular myoid cells detected, at all stages of the cycle, were AR positive and no variation in staining intensity was discerned.

Within the interstitial compartment of the rat, the principal staining intensity detected was in smooth muscle cells forming the walls of blood vessels (Fig. 13.2C). In contrast, endothelial cells found in the inner layer of blood vessels were AR negative. Although Leydig cells were clearly AR positive as well, staining intensity varied and was never as great as in the smooth muscle cells or in the most intense Sertoli cells.

Similar observations were made in the adult mouse testis. Sertoli cell AR staining varied as a function of the cycle, as did elongated spermatid cytoplasmic staining, and all peritubular myoid cells and smooth muscle cells of blood vessels were AR positive. A marked contrast existed between the AR staining intensity somatic cells of rat and mouse; in the mouse all Leydig cells detected were AR positive and the intensity of the staining was as great, if not greater, than the most intense Sertoli cells at stage VIII (Fig. 13.3).

AR staining of elongated spermatids was examined to determine at which time in their differentiation AR first appeared. In step 11 elongated spermatids, at the stage in their development where elongation is clearly evident but nuclear condensation is not yet apparent, AR staining was present in all elongated spermatids of a particular cross section at stage XI of the cycle of the seminiferous epithelium (Fig. 13.4). With the onset of chromatin condensation at the subsequent stage, AR staining in the nuclei of elongated spermatids disappeared in a head to tail direction, concomitant with the appearance of AR staining in the cytoplasm (data not shown, but results reported in 7).

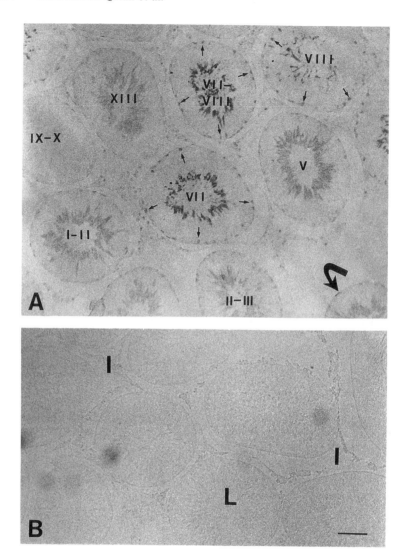

FIGURE 13.1. Androgen receptor (AR) distribution in adult rat testis. (A) A low-power profile of AR immunostained rat testis is illustrated. Roman numerals indicate different stages of the cycle of the seminiferous epithelium. Note that AR staining intensity differs between stages. Small arrows point to Sertoli cell nuclei differentially stained for AR. The curved arrow at right indicates an example of AR stained peritubular myoid cells. Although some Leydig cells staining is noted in the interstitium, staining intensity is weak. (B) Control section immunostained with preadsorbed antibody. I, interstitium. Note the absence of reaction product. Bar = 100 μm.

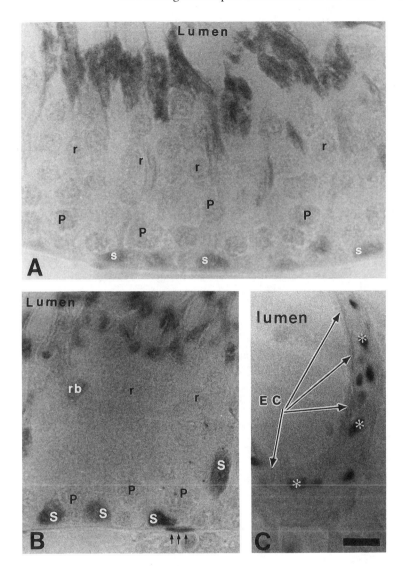

FIGURE 13.2. AR distribution in adult rat testis. (*A*) Positive AR immunostaining is clearly evident in Sertoli cell nuclei (s) and cytoplasm of elongated spermatids near the lumen of the tubule at stage VII. Pachytene spermatocytes (P) and round spermatids (r) are AR negative. (*B*) AR staining intensity is greater in Sertoli cell nuclei and residual bodies (rb) of a stage VIII tubule. AR-stained myoid cell nuclei are indicated with short arrows. (*C*) AR staining is evident in nuclei of smooth muscle cells (asterisks) of blood vessels, whereas endothelial cells (EC) are negative. Bar = 13 μm.

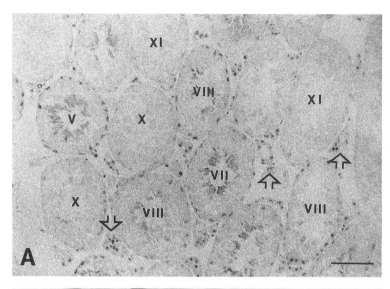

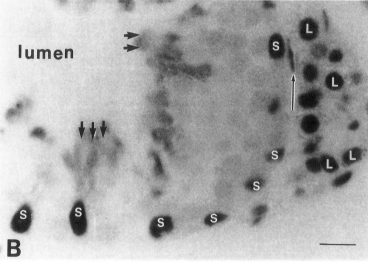

FIGURE 13.3. AR distribution in adult mouse testis. AR staining of adult mouse testis is illustrated at low power (A) and at high power in (B). As in the rat, AR staining intensity in elongated spermatids and Sertoli cell nuclei varies as a function of the cycle of the seminiferous epithelium, indicated by roman numerals. Open arrows indicate clumps of Leydig cells in interstitium that are strongly positive for AR. (B) A stage VIII tubule is demonstrated. Note that both Sertoli cell (S) and Leydig cell (L) nuclei stain intensely for AR. Cytoplasm of elongated spermatids (short arrows) is also positive. A peritubular myoid cell is indicated by the long arrow. Bar = 100 μm (A) and 13 μm (B).

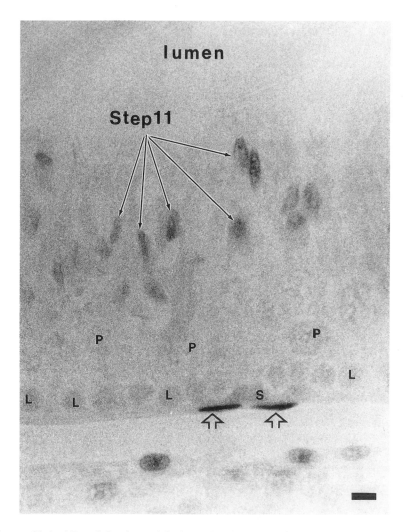

FIGURE 13.4. AR staining in nuclei of step 11 elongated spermatids. At stage XI of the cycle of the seminiferous epithelium nuclei of elongated spermatids were AR positive. Leptotene spermatocytes (L), pachytene spermatocytes (P) and Sertoli cells, however, were AR negative. As an internal control, peritubular myoid cells (open arrows) that are AR positive are shown. Bar = 10 μm.

Results of nucleic acid in situ hybridization using a rat cRNA antisense probe for AR revealed specific and robust hybridization at the periphery of the seminiferous tubules at stage IX of the cycle, whereas no specific hybridization was observed when a control probe was used (Fig. 13.5A,B). This pattern is consistent with hybridization of the labeled probe to Sertoli cells and to germ cells residing in this area of the epithelium at this stage.

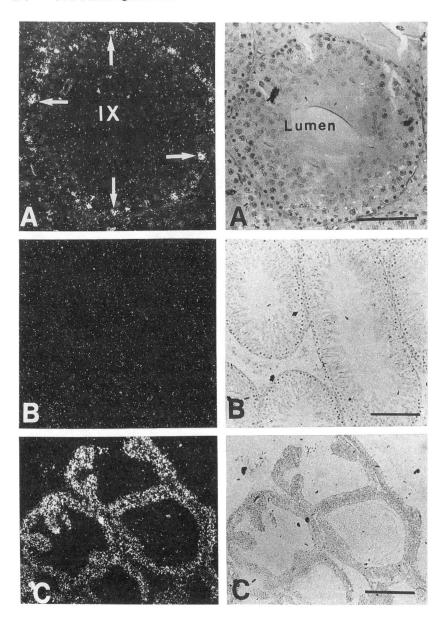

FIGURE 13.5. Nucleic acid in situ hybridization of AR. (*A*) Robust ^{35}S-cRNA hybridization to seminiferous tubules was detected at stage IX, at the periphery of the tubule, in the area occupied by Sertoli cells and leptotene spermatocytes. (*B*) Control section hybridized with sense cRNA is demonstrated. (*C*) A positive control for AR is shown; robust hybridization in seminal vesicles was observed. Bar = 100 μm (*A*) and 150 μm (*B*, *C*).

Although it was not possible to discern the specific cell types to which the labeled cRNA had hybridized, at stage IX, the basal area of the seminiferous epithelium is occupied principally by leptotene spermatocytes. Positive method controls using the same antisense probe for AR demonstrated specific hybridization to epithelial cells of seminal vesicles and caput epididymis, two cell types known to contain abundant levels of AR *messenger RNA* (mRNA).

AR Distribution in the Developing Testis (Fig. 13.6)

AR in the postnatal testis was first discerned in peritubular myoid cells at day 5 (unlike the flattened nuclei of myoid cells in the adult testis, prepubertal myoid cell nuclei are more oval in shape). Sertoli cell AR staining was not detected until day 15 after birth, when all Sertoli cell nuclei were AR positive. Initial immunocytochemical experiments of day 15 testes, in which sections were not microwaved prior to staining, did not yield positive results. Rather, in the absence of microwaving, positive AR staining of Sertoli cell nuclei was not observed until day 20. These results may indicate that 20-day-old Sertoli cells contain more AR than 15-day-old Sertoli cells. Day 25 testes exhibit similar AR distribution as day 20, but by day 30 the adult pattern of AR staining in Sertoli cell nuclei became evident. Whereas some tubules exhibit positive AR staining in Sertoli cells, other tubules lacked AR positive Sertoli cells. At day 40, the first elongated spermatid staining was discerned (data not shown).

Control Studies

The validity of immunocytochemistry results relies heavily on the quality of control studies. To this end, we conducted a series of conventional control studies using PG21 that included both positive and negative methodologies.

First, we determined that PG21 indeed recognized a protein band by Western immunoblotting at 110kd, the corresponding molecular weight of rat AR. Significantly, detection of the 110-kd band in either the nuclear or cytosolic fractions of testicular or elongated spermatid extracts coincided precisely with the immunocytochemical results (Fig. 13.7). AR was detected exclusively in the cytosolic fraction of both elongated spermatids and whole testis extracts. In contrast, the two positive control tissues examined in this study, epididymis and prostate, rendered positive 110-kd bands solely in the nuclear fractions. AR distribution in developing testes, however, up to day 30 after birth, was detected exclusively in nuclear fractions (Fig. 13.8). Here, again, the immunoblotting results coincided precisely with the immunocytochemical localization of AR. Further, no AR detection was obtained in 40-day-old testes. These results were not surprising, since, by immunocy-

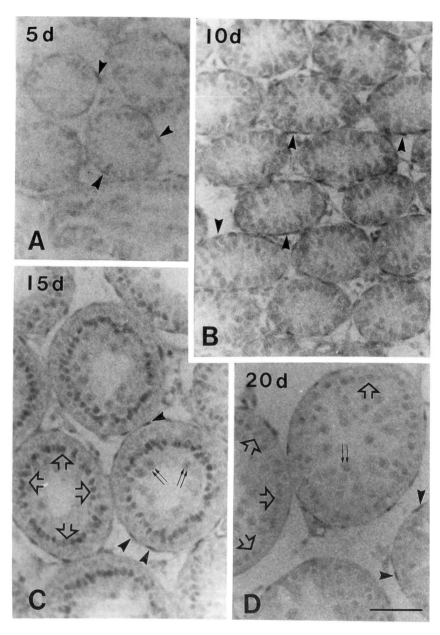

FIGURE 13.6. AR distribution in the developing rat testis. AR distribution in testes of 5-, 10-, 15-, and 20-day-old rats is illustrated. The first positive AR signal was observed in nuclei of peritubular myoid cells (arrowheads) in day 5 testis, and in all myoid cells thereafter. In contrast, AR positive Sertoli cell nuclei (open arrows) did not appear until day 15 and remained positive at day 20. Double arrows point to AR negative germ cells in the forming lumens of day 15 and 20 tubules. Their apparent darkness is an artifact of slight counterstaining with hematoxylin, which in color photographs appears blue. Bar = 50 μm.

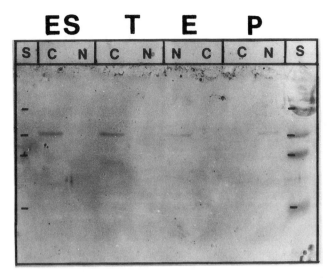

FIGURE 13.7. AR immunoblots in adult rat testis; 250 μg of protein were loaded in lanes for each nuclear (N) and cytosolic (C) fraction of elongated spermatid (ES) and whole testicular extract (T), but only 50 μg of epididymal (E) and prostate (P) fractions were loaded per lane. Standards (S) at 116, 106, 80, 40 kd are indicated. Note that the antibody immunoblots a specific band at approximately 110 kd.

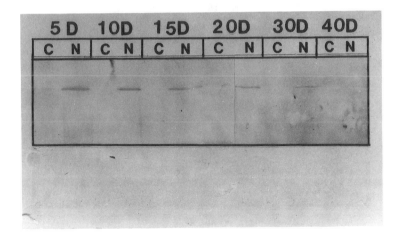

FIGURE 13.8. AR immunoblots in developing rat testis. Approximately 200 μg of protein were loaded per lane. A specific band at approximately 110 kd in the nuclear fraction of developing testes was observed until day 30. No bands were detected in day 40 testicular extracts.

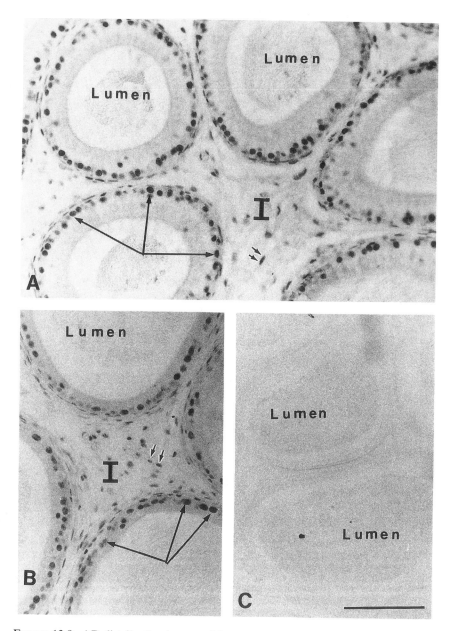

FIGURE 13.9. AR distribution in rat epididymis (positive control 1). The proximal (*A*) and distal (*B*) caput of rat epididymis were used as positive controls for AR staining. The nuclear AR distribution in cells of the epithelium (long arrows) and most cells of the interstitium (short arrows) is apparent. (*C*) Preadsorbed antibody was used as a negative control of the distal caput. Bar = 100 μm.

tochemistry, AR positive elongated spermatids were limited and Sertoli cell nuclear AR staining was also minimal.

Positive cellular and tissue control AR staining was performed to demonstrate the validity of the PG21 antibody as a specific probe for AR in the testis. The proximal and distal caput of the epididymis were processed for AR immunostaining using the same protocol used for the testis. Results revealed that AR staining was limited to the nuclei of cells forming the epithelial lining of this tube, as well as the nuclei of interstitial cells (Fig. 13.9A,B); that is, the pattern of AR staining in these positive control tissues was precisely as expected (3–5). Further, preadsorption of PG21 with the antigenic peptide eliminated all immunostaining (Fig. 13.9C). LnCAP cells, a prostatic cell line known to contain AR, were immunostained for AR. Again, all cells were AR positive and AR staining was limited to the nuclei (Fig. 13.10A). The last positive control performed was the transfection of COS-7 cells with AR to immunolocalize it in these cells grown either in the presence or absence of physiological concentrations of androgens. Untransfected COS-7 cells were AR negative (Fig. 13.10B); however, transfection with AR led to approximately 10–15% positive AR staining of the cells. In the absence of androgens AR distribution was detected maximally in the cytoplasm, whereas AR staining shifted to the nucleus upon stimulation with androgens for as little as 15 min (Fig. 13.10C,D). These observations are consistent with those made by French and colleagues in which intracellular AR partitioning between the nucleus and the cytoplasm was demonstrated to be androgen dependent (13).

Results of negative controls performed to test the validity of PG21 staining were as follows. PG21 was preadsorbed with the antigenic peptide, or another peptide of the rat AR, and the preadsorbed antibodies were then used for immunostaining. Preadsorption of PG21 with the antigenic peptide completely eliminated the staining reaction (Fig. 13.1B), whereas the unrelated peptide had no effect on staining intensity (data not shown). Next, we examined whether identical immunostaining results could be obtained by using a different reporter molecule (fluorescence) conjugated to the secondary antibody. Results demonstrated that the staining of elongated spermatids was not an artifact of the immunoperoxidase reaction, since identical staining results were achieved using immunofluorescence (Fig. 13.11).

Discussion

Immunocytochemistry is a powerful technique to demonstrate protein distribution in tissues; it is not a method to prove definitively where these proteins are not. Thus, given appropriate methodological, tissue, and reagent controls, positive immunocytochemical results are always more readily explained than negative observations. For example, among the

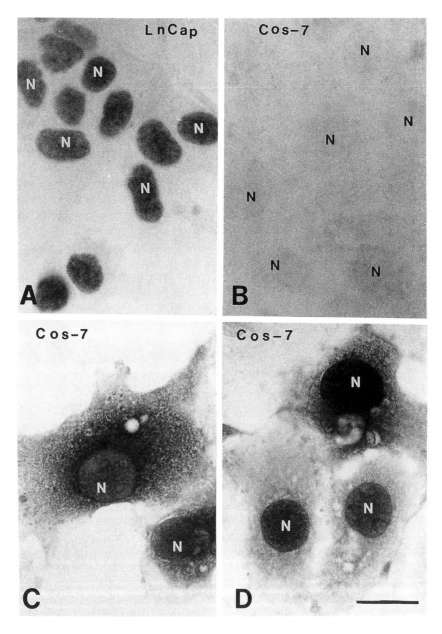

FIGURE 13.10. AR in cultured cells (positive control 2). LNCap cells (A) and COS-7 cells transfected with the full-length rat AR gene (C and D) were AR positive. In C, COS-7 cells were grown in the absence of androgens; in D they were treated with 10^{-6} M testosterone for 15 min. Note that most of the reaction product in D is found in the nucleus. In B, untransfected COS-7 cells stained for AR are shown. Examples of nuclei (N) are indicated. Bar = 20 μm.

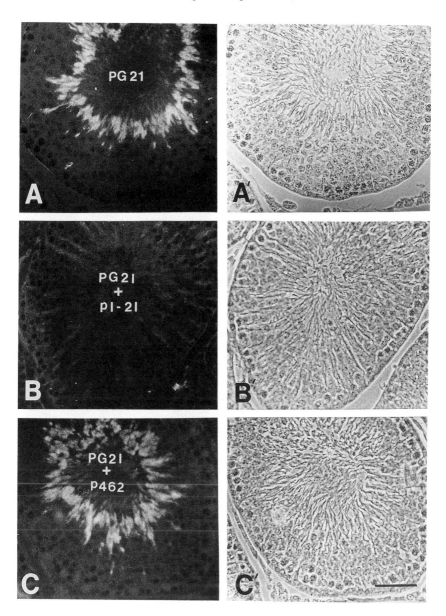

FIGURE 13.11. AR distribution in testis (positive control 3). Adult rat testis sections were immunostained for AR using fluorescein-conjugated second antibody (*A–C*) as the reporter molecule and the corresponding phase images are presented in (*A'–C'*). (*A*) Elongated spermatids near the lumen of the tubule are AR positive with the PG21 antibody. (*B*) Preadsorption with the antigenic peptide p1-21 abolishes the reaction. (*C*) Preadsorption with an unrelated peptide of AR, p462, had no effect on positive staining. Bar = 50 μm.

myriad reasons that one may fail to detect specific cellular distribution of a desired protein is that harsh fixation may mask epitopes recognized by the antibody, even though an identical fixation/staining protocol, when used in a positive control tissue, leads to immunostaining (12). Such phenomena may give rise to false-negative immunocytochemical results and may yield a biologically incorrect understanding of a particular tissue system. In contrast, positive immunostaining provides structural evidence for functionality of the protein being localized. Although it is true that false-positive results may be a problem with particular antibodies, negative control studies, performed with the PG21 antibody, significantly minimized this possibility. To this end, we report that the PG21 antibody recognizes the presence of AR in the nuclei of somatic cells of the testis, including Sertoli cells at stages IV–VIII, all peritubular myoid cells, Leydig cells and smooth muscle cells of blood vessels. In addition, we detected AR in the nuclei of step 11 elongated spermatids, as well as in the cytoplasm of step 12–19 elongated spermatids.

The immunocytochemical results presented herein, that germ cells exhibit immunoreactive AR, corroborate previous studies reporting similar observations. Table 13.1 is a summary of recent publications in which AR immunolocalization in the testis was described. This table makes it clear that there are now different antibody probes available for AR and that some of these will render positive AR staining in germ cells. It is also clear from this list that germ cell AR staining was not achieved by all investigators. Although the reasons for this disparity are not readily apparent, again, we wish to emphasize that positive AR staining results may be interpreted to indicate that germ cells contain AR, whereas negative results do not prove that AR is absent from these cells.

Although our AR immunolocalization results in somatic cells do not provide functional evidence of androgen action during spermatogenesis, they are consistent with past studies in which Sertoli, peritubular, and Leydig cells in vitro have all been shown to respond in some fashion to androgens (reviewed in 2). Thus, our results fit in well within the current understanding of androgen action in spermatogenesis. That somatic cells respond directly to androgens, however, does not preclude germ cells from also being androgen responsive.

Not everyone is in agreement that germ cells are AR positive, or, even if they are, that they respond directly to androgens. This concept evolved, or at least gained wide acceptance, after an elegant and landmark review written by Irving Fritz (1) in 1978 summarized available knowledge regarding androgen action during spermatogenesis. In this review Fritz argued that androgen action in spermatogenesis is likely to occur via somatic cells and he separated the available evidence into two types, theoretical considerations and experimental data. There were three theoretical considerations. First, the AR gene loci had been shown to reside on the X

TABLE 13.1. Immunohistochemical localization of androgen receptors.

Reference	Antibody	Results
	Rat	
Takeda et al., 1990 (14)	MAb N-term-fusion protein Rb N-term-fusion protein	Somatic cells
Sar et al., 1990 (15)	Rb52 18aa N-term to DNA binding domain RB32 N-term 9–29	Somatic cells
Vornberger et al., 1994 (7)	RB N-term 1–21	Somatic + germ cells
Bremner et al., 1994 (16)	Rb N-term 1–17	Somatic cells
	Human	
Ruizeveld de Winter et al., 1991 (17)	MAb 39.4 N-term 301–320	Somatic cells
Rajpert de Meyts and Skakkebaek, 1992 (18)	MAb 39.4 N-term 301–320 MAb N-term 1–15	Normal germ cells 44% Seminoma 40% CIS 45% Seminoma 42% CIS
Kimura et al., 1993 (19)	Rb 55-kd hAR	Spermatogonia, spermatocytes, somatic cells

MAb, monoclonal antibodies; Rb, rabbit antisera; N-term, amino terminus and numbers indicate amino acids used to raise antibody; CIS, carcinoma in situ.

chromosome, implying that after meiotic segregation of chromosome Y–bearing sperm would likely lack AR. Since no evidence existed (or exists) to suggest that X- and Y-bearing sperm have different hormonal requirements, it was reasonable to suggest that spermatogenesis could proceed without a direct androgenic stimulation of germ cells. Second, the X chromosome was believed to undergo inactivation early during spermatogenesis. Thus, even if the AR gene product could be transferred to clones of germ cells via existing cytoplasmic bridges, evidence suggested that it was not even transcribed in post-meiotic germ cells. Finally, in 1963, Ohno and colleagues (20) reported that all spermatogonia and more differentiated germ cells of the creeping vole, *Microtus oregoni*, are deficient in the X chromosome. Given that the AR gene locus is on the X chromosome, the apparent X chromosome deficiency argued against a direct androgenic effect on germ cells. The strongest argument made by Fritz against germ cells requiring a direct stimulation by androgens was based on the experimental results of Lyon et al. (21), in which they generated two chimeric mice that were *tfm*/Y-XY. These animals were able to transfer the *tfm* gene to their offspring, implying that androgens could not possibly have acted directly on the haploid germ cells since the *tfm* component of the chimeras lacked a functional AR.

Data accumulated during the last 15 years, however, provide plausible, alternative arguments to the theoretical concerns raised by Fritz that germ cells do not respond directly to androgens. First, Braun et al. (22) reported in 1989 that genetically haploid spermatids are phenotypically diploid, demonstrating that clones of germ cells, even after segregation of their chromosomes, possess the ability to transfer large macromolecules among themselves. This observation is consistent with the interpretation that even though the AR locus is on the X chromosome, germ cells have a mechanism to ensure equal transmission of the gene product to all haploid germ cells if indeed the gene is transcribed. Second, Disteche (23) recently published a review detailing that a number of X-linked genes escape X-inactivation, although the case for AR in germ cells has not been examined. Clearly, if the AR locus escapes X-inactivation, then germ cells may contain the potential to respond directly to androgenic stimulation during spermatogenesis. Alternatively, even if the AR locus is inactivated, recent studies by Handel provide compelling evidence that germ cells possess a mechanism to overcome X-inactivation (24). Working with the *hprt* gene, an X-linked gene whose function is general cell housekeeping, Handel demonstrated that robust transcription of the gene occurs in leptotene spermatocytes, possibly to ensure sufficient mRNA for later translation by haploid germ cells. In this context it is important to note that the AR in situ studies presented herein also demonstrated a robust hybridization to leptotene spermatocytes. Thus, if the AR locus undergoes X inactivation, then our results are consistent with the mechanism Handel proposed by which germ cells may bypass the inactivation. Third, although Ohno's observation of the XY dysgenesis in the creeping vole remains intriguing, to our knowledge it has neither been corroborated, nor the level of true XY dysgenesis examined. In particular, given the presence of other X chromosome gene products required for general cell survivability, it would seem unreasonable to find complete absence of the X chromosome in the diploid spermatogonia as originally described.

To date, the two *tfm*/Y-XY chimeric mice generated by Lyon et al. (21) remain the strongest argument against germ cells requiring a direct androgen stimulation. This observation, however, does not preclude either germ cells from exhibiting AR, as we demonstrate in the present study, or androgens from directly stimulating germ cells. The ability of the chimeric mice to reproduce may simply reveal that absence of AR in germ cells is not fully incompatible with fertility, but it addresses neither the quality nor quantity of viable sperm produced if AR is present in germ cells. Indeed, the presence of AR in germ cells may only have to minimally enhance the spermatogenic process to become a significant evolutionary advantage. Absence of AR function in the *tfm* sperm component of the chimeric mice may not impede fertility during an artificial, laboratory fertility test. Out-

TABLE 13.2. Androgen receptors in germ cells.

Reference	Method	Somatic cells	Germ cells
Biochemical Studies			
Galena et al., 1974 (25)	Radioreceptor assay	+	+
Sanborn et al., 1975 (26)	Nuclear exchange	+	+
Sanborn et al., 1975 (27)	Nuclear exchange	+	+
Wilson and Smith, 1975 (28)	Radioreceptor assay	+	+
Wright and Frankel, 1980 (30)	Radioimmunoassay	N.E.*	+
Tsai et al., 1977 (29)	Nuclear exchange	+	+
Tsai and Steinberger, 1982 (31)	Nuclear exchange	+	+
Frankel, 1984 (32)	Nuclear exchange	+	+
Frankel and Chapman, 1984 (33)	Nuclear exchange	+	+
Structural studies			
Sar et al., 1975 (34)	Autoradiography	+	+
Schulz et al., 1989 (35)	T immunolocalization	+	+
Molecular biology studies			
Huang et al., 1992 (36)	Northern analysis	+	+

*Not examined.

side the laboratory, however, even a minimal absence of a direct androgen effect on germ cells may have catastrophic effects for a population.

That germ cells contain AR does not depend solely on our and other's immunolocalization evidence. Table 13.2 presents an abbreviated list of studies from the past 20 years in which a variety of methods have been utilized to demonstrate the presence of AR in germ cells. Only the study by Grootegoed et al. (37), also using a binding assay for AR, reported that germ cells are AR negative. In this study, however, animal models were utilized that lacked elongated spermatids, the precise germ cell type in which we report immunoactive AR. Our observations that elongated spermatids contain AR are consistent with the various studies presented in Table 13.2, all demonstrating that germ cells are AR positive. However, it does not provide functional evidence that, even if present, AR is required for germ-cell function. Nevertheless, given our immunocytochemical findings, along with the previous 20-year history in the literature that germ cells are AR positive, we suggest that the question of whether germ cells may respond directly to androgens during spermatogenesis is not yet settled. Indeed, we like to suggest that our results indicate that further experimentation to resolve this issue is now warranted.

Acknowledgments. We would like to thank Drs. Mary Ann Handel, William Wright, Terry Brown, and Stephen Byers for critical analysis of our results during the course of this study. Their insights into androgen action during spermatogenesis significantly helped formulate our own hypothesis in this area. Financial support of this work was provided in part by NIH Grants HD-24633 to C.A.S.-Q. and N.A.M. and DK-40890 to G.P. Dr. B.O. Oke was a recipient of a Rockefeller Biotechnology Fellowship.

References

1. Fritz I. Sites of action of androgens and follicle stimulating hormone on cells of the seminiferous tubule. In: Litwack G, ed. Biochemical actions of hormones. New York: Academic Press, 1978:249–81.
2. Sharpe R. Regulation of spermatogenesis. In: Knobil E, Neill JD, eds. The physiology of reproduction, 2nd ed. New York: Raven Press, 1994:1363–434.
3. Prins GS, Birch L, Greene GL. Androgen receptor localization in different cell types of the adult rat prostate. Endocrinology 1991;129:3187–99.
4. Prins GS, Cooke PS, Birch L, Donjacour AA, Yalcinkaya TM, Siiteri PK, Cunha GR. Androgen receptor expression and 5a-reductase activity along the proximal-distal axis of the rat prostatic duct. Endocrinology 1992;130: 3066–73.
5. Prins GS, Birch L. Immunocytochemical analysis of androgen receptor along the ducts of the separate rat prostate lobes after androgen withdrawal and replacement. Endocrinology 1993;132:169–78.
6. Oke B, Suarez-Quian CA. Localization of secretory, membrane-associated and cytoskeletal proteins in rat testis using an improved immunocytochemical protocol that employs polyester wax. Biol Reprod 1993;48:621–31.
7. Vornberger W, Prins G, Musto NA, Suarez-Quian CA. Androgen receptor distribution in rat testis: new implications for androgen regulation of spermatogenesis. Endocrinology 1994;134:2307–16.
8. Grove BD, Vogl AW. Sertoli cell ectoplasmic specializations: a type of actin-associated adhesion junction? J Cell Sci 1989;93:309–23.
9. Bradford MM. A rapid and sensitive method for the quantitation of microgram quantities of protein using the principle of protein dye binding. Anal Biochem 1976;72:248–54.
10. Laemmli UK. Cleavage of structural proteins during assembly of the head of bacteriophage T4. Nature 1970;227:680–5.
11. Johnson DA, Gautsch JW, Sportsman JR, Edler JH. Improved technique utilizing nonfat dry milk for analysis of proteins and nucleic acid transferred to nitrocellulose. Gene Anal Tech 1984;1:13–18.
12. Angerer LM, Angerer RC. Localization of mRNAs by in situ hybridization. In: Setlow JK, Hollander A, eds. Genetic engineering. New York: Plenum Press, 1985:37–66.
13. Simental JA, Sar M, Lane MV, French FS, Wilson EM. Transcriptional activation and nuclear targeting signals of the human androgen receptor. J Biol Chem 1991;266:510–8.
14. Takeda H, Chodak G, Mutchnik S, Nakamoto T, Chang C. Immunohistochemical localization of androgen receptors with mono- and polyclonal antibodies to androgen receptors. J Endocrinol 1990;126:17–25.
15. Sar M, Lubahn DB, French FS, Wilson EM. Immunohistochemical localization of the androgen receptor in rat and human tissues. Endocrinology 1990; 127:3180–6.

16. Bremner WJ, Millar MR, Sharpe RM, Saunders PTK. Immunohistochemical localization of androgen receptors in the rat testis: evidence for stage-dependent expression and regulation by androgens. Endocrinology 1994;135: 1227–34.

17. Ruizeveld de Winter JA, Trapman J, Vermey M, Mulder E, Zegers ND, van der Kwast TH. Androgen receptor expression in human tissues: an immunohistochemical study. J Histochem Cytochem 1991;39:927–36.

18. Rajpert-de Meyts E, Skakkebaek NE. Immunohistochemical identification of androgen receptors in germ cell neoplasia. J Endocrinol 1992;135:R1–R4.

19. Kimura N, Mizokami A, Oonuma T, Sasano H, Nagura H. Immunocytochemical localization of androgen receptor with polyclonal antibody in paraffin-embedded human tissues. J Histochem Cytochem 1993;41:671–8.

20. Ohno S, Jainchill J, Stenius C. The creeping vole (*Microtus oregoni*) as a gonosomic mosaic. I. The OY/XY constitution of the male. Cytogenetics 1963;2:232–9.

21. Lyon MF, Glenister PH, Lamoreux ML. Normal spermatozoa from androgen-resistant germ cells of chimeric mice and the role of androgen in spermatogenesis. Nature 1975;258:620–2.

22. Braun RE, Behringer RR, Peschon JJ, Brinster RL, Palmiter RD. Genetically haploid spermatids are phenotypically diploid. Nature 1989;337:373–6.

23. Disteche C. Escape from X inactivation in human and mouse. Trends Genet 1995;11:17–22.

24. Shannon M, Handel MA. Expression of the Hprt gene during spermatogenesis: implications for sex-chromosome inactivation. Biol Reprod 1993;49:770–8.

25. Galena HJ, Pillai AK, Terner C. Progesterone and androgen receptors in non-flagellate germ cells of the rat testis. J Endocrinol 1974;63:223–37.

26. Sanborn BM, Elkington JSH, Steinberger A, Steinberger E. Androgen binding in the testis: in vitro production of androgen binding protein (ABP) by Sertoli cell cultures and measurement of nuclear bound androgen by a nuclear exchange assay. In: French FS, Hansson V, Ritzen EM, Nayfeh SN, eds. Hormonal regulation of spermatogenesis. New York: Plenum Press, 1975: 293–310.

27. Sanborn BM, Steinberger A, Meistrich ML, Steinberger E. Androgen binding sites in testis cell fractions as measured by a nuclear exchange assay. J Steroid Biochem 1975;6:1459–65.

28. Wilson EM, Smith AA. Localization of androgen receptors in rat testis: biochemical studies. In: French FS, Hansson V, Ritzen EM, Nayfeh SN, eds. Hormonal regulation of spermatogenesis. New York: Plenum Press, 1975: 281–6.

29. Tsai Y-H, Sanborn BM, Steinberger A, Steinberger E. The interaction of testicular androgen-receptor complex with rat germ cell and Sertoli cell chromatin. Biochem Biophys Res Commun 1977;75:366–72.

30. Wright WW, Frankel AI. An androgen receptor in the nuclei of late spermatids in testes of male rats. Endocrinology 1980;107:314–18.

31. Tsai Y-H, Steinberger A. Effect of sodium molybdate on the binding of androgen-receptor complexes to germ cell and Sertoli cell chromatin. J Steroid Biochem 1982;17:131–6.

32. Frankel AI. Nuclear androgen binding sites in the male rat II. Seminiferous tubules. J Steroid Biochem 1984;20:1295–300.

33. Frankel AI, Chapman JC. Nuclear androgen binding sites in the male rat—III. Late spermatids and spermatozoa in the testis, with an introduction to epididymal spermatozoa. J Steroid Biochem 1984;20:1301–11.
34. Sar M, Stumpf WE, McLean WS, Smith AA, Hansson V, Nayfeh SN, French FS. Localization of androgen target cells in the rat testis: autoradiographic studies. In: French FS, Hansson V, Ritzen EM, Nayfeh SN, eds. Hormonal regulation of spermatogenesis. New York: Plenum Press, 1975:311–19.
35. Schulz R, Paris F, Lembke P, BlumV. Testosterone immunoreactivity in the seminiferous epithelium of rat testis: effect of treatment with ethane demethanesulfonate. J Histochem Cytochem 1989;37:1667–73.
36. Huang HFS, Li MT, Qian L, Pogach LM. The presence of mRNA of androgen receptor and androgen binding protein in germ cells. 74th Annual Meeting of Endocrine Society, June 24–27, 1992, San Antonio, TX. 1992:300.
37. Grootegoed JA, Peters MJ, Mulder E, Rommerts FFG, van der Molen JJ. Absence of a nuclear androgen receptor in isolated cells of rat testis. Mol Cell Endocrinol 1977;9:159–67.

14

Testicular Androgen Receptor Protein: Distribution and Control of Expression

P.T.K. Saunders, M.R. Millar, G. Majdic, W.J. Bremner, T.T. McLaren, K.M. Grigor, and R.M. Sharpe

Androgens are essential in fetal life for development of the male phenotype (1) and in the adult for maintenance of normal spermatogenesis (2). Androgen action is mediated by a specific intracellular receptor expressed in target tissues that binds testosterone and dihydrotestosterone with high affinity (3). Ligand binding is essential for activation of the receptor, which then binds to specific targets on DNA resulting in modulation of the level of gene expression (4). Recently we have successfully used immunocytochemistry, following microwave antigen retrieval, to demonstrate that *androgen receptor* (AR) expression in adult rat *Sertoli cells* (SC) occurs predominantly at stages II–VII of the spermatogenic cycle, with highest levels at stage VII (5)—results in agreement with other investigators (6). In our study AR immunostaining was also detectable in peritubular myoid cells, arterioles, and Leydig cells, but not in germ cells (5).

The aims of the current study were to use immunohistochemistry (i) to examine the ontogeny of expression of androgen receptor in the rat fetus and neonate, (ii) to determine where AR protein is expressed in testes from normal and infertile humans and from nonhuman primates, and (iii) to examine whether manipulation of hormones or germ-cell complement in the adult rat affected stage-dependent detection of AR in Sertoli cells.

Procedure

Animals and Tissues

Adult Wistar rats (aged 75–100 days) obtained from our colony were maintained under standard animal house conditions. Fetal samples were obtained from time-mated females (presence of a vaginal plug in the morning was taken as evidence of mating during the previous 12 hours, i.e., day 0.5). Whole fetuses (days 11.5 to 17.5) and testes removed from fetuses on days 16.5 to 20.5 (delivery on day 21–23 in our colony), from neonates (days 3, 5, 7), and from immature males (days 14 to 45) were immersion fixed in Bouin's solution for 6–7 h. Testicular tissue from adult rats was obtained following perfusion fixation carried out as previously described (7). To induce selective degeneration/loss of pachytene and later spermatocytes, rats were administered *methoxyacetic acid* (MAA) (Aldrich Chemical Co. Ltd) as a single oral dose of 650 mg/kg (day 0). On the basis of our previous studies (8, 9) this dose results in the selective destruction/loss of >80% of pachytene and later spermatocytes at all stages other than early- to mid-stage VII of the spermatogenic cycle and has no other discernible effect. Thereafter, spermatogenesis proceeds normally with normal kinetics so that the initial loss of pachytene and later spermatocytes is manifest as the selective loss of round and then elongate spermatids at later time points after treatment (9). In the present studies, MAA-treated rats were killed at 3, 7, 14, 18, and 21 days after treatment. To induce complete testosterone withdrawal, rats were administered a single intraperitoneal injection of 75 mg/kg *ethane dimethane sulfonate* (EDS) in 3:1 (v/v) water:dimethyl sulfoxide and perfusion fixed 6 days later. This treatment results in destruction and removal of all of the Leydig cells within 30–36 h (10). Some EDS-treated rats were supplemented with *testosterone esters* (TE) (Sustanon, Organon Laboratories, Cambridge, England) administered subcutaneously at a dose of 25 mg every 3 days, commencing at the time of EDS treatment. This dose of TE is able to maintain virtually normal spermatogenesis and fertility for at least 10 weeks in the absence of Leydig cells (10).

Testes from four ex-breeder adult marmoset monkeys (*Callithrix jacchus*) and one stump-tailed macaque (*Macaca archtoides*) were cut into 0.5-cm segments and immersion fixed in Bouin's or 4% paraformaldehyde. Human tissue samples were obtained by wedge biopsy during routine surgical investigation for a variety of clinical conditions including infertility and immersion fixed in Bouin's as above. After fixation, all tissue samples were stored in 70% ethanol and processed into paraffin wax on an automatic tissue processor using a standard 20-h cycle (11).

Immunocytochemistry

Sections (5 μm) were cut and mounted on slides coated with 3-aminopropyl triethoxy-silane (Sigma Chemical Co. Poole, Dorset, England), dried overnight (50°C), dewaxed, rehydrated in graded ethanols, washed in water, submerged in 0.01 M citrate buffer pH 6, and microwaved on full power (650 W, 4 times 5 min). After standing for 20 min without disturbance in the microwave oven, sections were washed once (5 min) in TBS (0.05 M Tris-HCl pH 7.4, 0.85% NaCl) and blocked using normal swine serum diluted in

TBS (1:5, NSS-TBS). Anti-human AR antibody raised in rabbits against the first 17 amino acids of the AR was purchased from Novocastra (Newcastle, UK). This polyclonal antibody was diluted 1:10–1:20 in NSS-TBS (see above) and incubated on the sections overnight at 4°C under plastic coverslips. After removal of coverslips, sections were washed twice in TBS (5 min), incubated for 30 min with biotinylated swine anti rabbit immunoglobulin (Dako, High Wycome, Bucks), diluted 1:500 in NSS-TBS, then washed again in TBS (2 times 5 min). For detection of bound antibodies, sections were first incubated with alkaline phosphatase conjugated to avidin-biotin (Dako) for 30 min, then washed in TBS (2 times 5 min), followed by a final wash in Tris-Mg buffer (100 mM Tris-HCl pH 9.5, 100 mM NaCl, 50 mM $MgCl_2$). Color reaction product was developed by incubation in a solution containing 337.5 µg/mL nitro-blue tetrazolium, 175 µg/mL 5-bromo-4-chloro-3-indolyphosphate, and 1 mM levamisole in Tris-Mg buffer for 30 to 120 min (12). Sections were counterstained with hematoxylin, dehydrated in absolute alcohol, cleared in xylene, and coverslipped using Pertex mounting medium (Cell path plc).

Quantitation of AR Immunostaining

Stage-dependent changes in nuclear AR immunostaining in rat testis were quantitated as previously described (5). To determine whether AR staining of Sertoli cell nuclei in sections of normal human testis was stage dependent, sections of testis from three different patients were either stained with *hematoxylin and eosin* (H&E) or immunostained for AR. The number of stained SC nuclei in each section was determined by counting SC nuclei falling at intersections on a grid containing 121 intersections. The number of SC nuclei visualized by each staining method was then expressed as a percentage of the total area examined. If AR immunostaining in SC nuclei is stage dependent, more nuclei per unit area should be found in the H&E-stained sections than in those immunostained with AR antibody.

Results

Ontogeny of Expression of Androgen Receptor in Fetal, Neonatal, and Immature Rats

In the fetal rat, AR was detectable by immunocytochemistry on day 16.5 in the nuclei of mesenchymal cells surrounding the Wolffian duct and within the epithelium of the mesonephric tubules and their underlying mesenchyme, but was absent from the cells around the degenerating Müllerian duct (not shown). Within the fetal testis AR was first detected at day 17 p.c. and was confined to interstitial cells surrounding the seminiferous cords. An

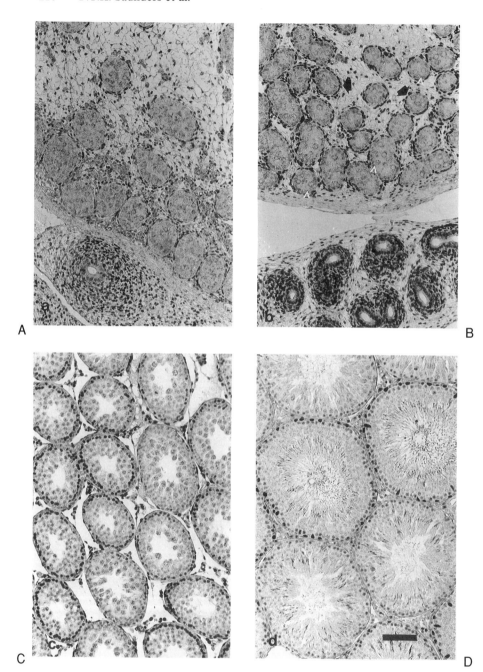

A

B

C

D

Figure 14.1. Ontogeny of androgen receptor immunostaining in the rat testis. During pregnancy (A) and early neonatal life (B) nuclear AR were prominent within the interstitial cell population of the testis, especially presumptive peritubular cells surrounding the solid seminiferous cords (arrows). Staining of Sertoli cells (SC)

example of a section of fetal rat testis and associated structures on day 19.5 of gestation is shown in Figure 14.1A. Note the prominent staining of nuclei of cells surrounding the seminiferous cords and other interstitial cells but the lack of significant staining of Sertoli cell nuclei. In the day 3 neonatal rat (Fig. 14.1B) abundant AR was present in the nuclei of peritubular cells and the nuclei of other interstitial cells. At this age, staining of SC remained weak and unconvincing. AR in SC increased significantly during the remainder of the first week of fetal life but exhibited no difference in abundance between individual seminiferous tubules (not shown). As maturation of spermatogenesis progressed and differences between the germ-cell complement of individual seminiferous tubules became established, the intensity of SC nuclear staining with the antibody increased and differences between individual tubules emerged (Fig. 14.1C, day 23) so that at day 45 the pattern of SC staining was virtually the same as in the adult. In adults (Fig. 14.1D) nuclear immunostaining of SC increased progressively in intensity from stages II–VII of the spermatogenic cycle, then declined precipitously during stage VIII to become barely detectable in stages IX–XIII. Prominent AR immunostaining was also evident in peritubular myoid cells, arterioles, and interstitial cells, but immunostaining in these cells did not vary with the stage of the cycle of the adjacent tubules (5). There was no evidence for immunostaining for AR in germ cells.

Expression of Androgen Receptors in the Human and Nonhuman Primate

In sections of testicular tissue from normal fertile humans (Fig. 14.2A) nuclear AR were present in Sertoli cells, Leydig cells, and peritubular cells but not in germ cells (Fig. 14.2B). A strong positive reaction was evident in the SC nuclei in sections of fixed testicular tissue from the common marmoset (Fig. 14.2C) and stump tailed macaque (Fig. 14.2E). In the sections of marmoset and macaque testis viewed under high-power magnification (Fig. 14.2D and F, respectively) there appeared to be no evidence of stage-dependent expression of the AR in SC.

To determine whether nuclear ARs were present in testes of individuals with abnormalities in spermatogenesis, sections of testicular tissue were stained with H&E to determine the gross morphology of the tissue (Fig. 14.3A,C,E) or subjected to AR immunostaining (Fig. 14.3B,D,F). In the

---

(arrowheads) remained very faint until after birth (*B*). As the rat matured, SC nuclear AR staining increased and differences in the abundance of AR in SC of different tubules emerged (*C*). In the adult rat, AR were present in peritubular cells and Leydig cells regardless of the stage of the tubules they surrounded. However, staining of SC nuclei was stage dependent with highest levels at stage VII. (*A*) Fetal day 19.5; (*B*) neonatal day 3; (*C*) immature day 21; (*D*) adult. Magnification ×10; black bar = 100 μm.

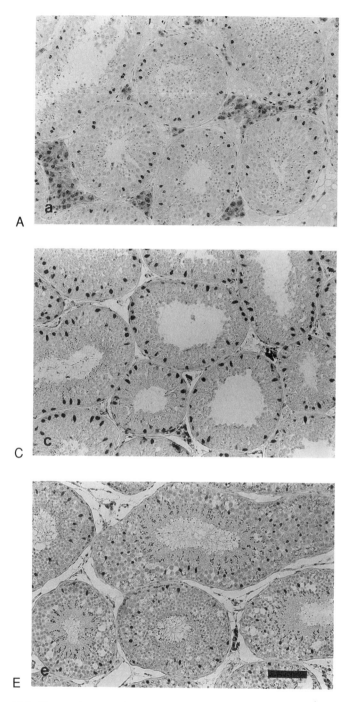

FIGURE 14.2. Expression of androgen receptors in the human and nonhuman primate testis. Panels show sections viewed under low and high power magnification of testis samples from a normal human male (*A*, *B*), common marmoset (*Callithrix jacchus*) (*C*, *D*) and stump-tailed macaque (*Macaca arctoides*) (*E*, *F*). Sertoli cell

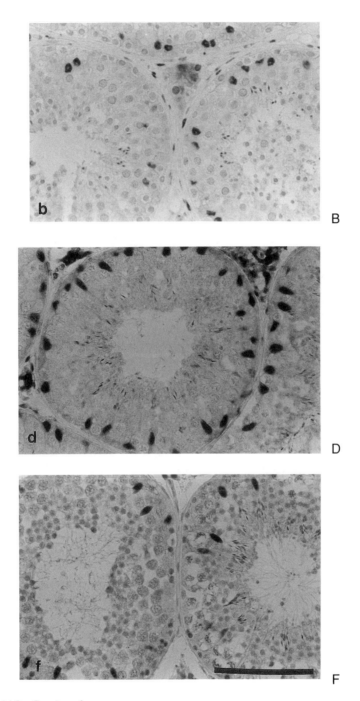

FIGURE 14.2. *Continued*
nuclei showed prominent nuclear AR immunostaining in each case. Nuclear AR
were also present in peritubular and Leydig cells but were not found in germ cells.
Magnification ×10 (*A, C, E*) and ×25 (*B, D, F*); black bar = 100 μm.

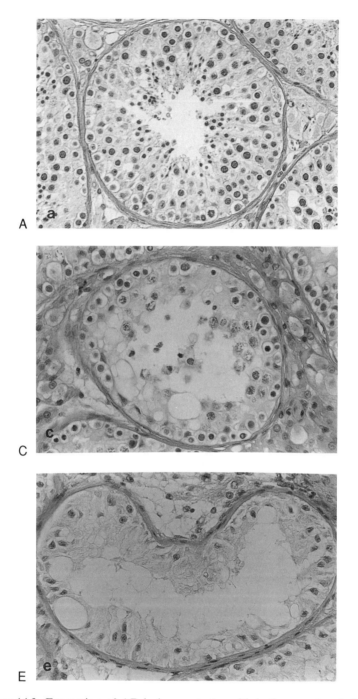

FIGURE 14.3. Expression of AR in human testes with both normal and abnormal morphology. Sections of human testis from three individuals stained either with hematoxylin and eosin (*A, C, E*) or with AR antibody (*B, D, F*). Sections *A* and *B* were from a normal fertile male, histology of sections *C* and *D* is consistent with

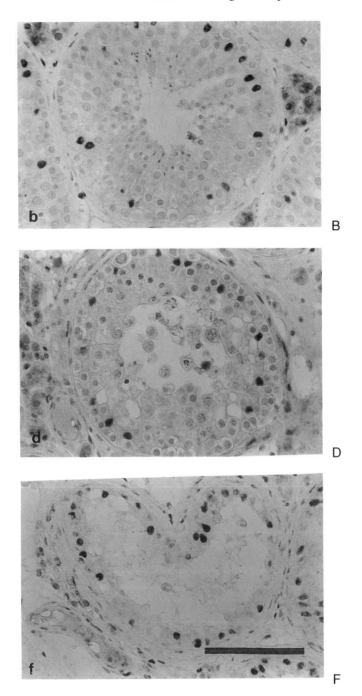

FIGURE 14.3. *Continued*
incomplete spermatogenesis (no spermatids), and sections *E* and *F* are from an
individual with Sertoli cell only syndrome. Positive staining of SC nuclei with AR
antibody was observed in all three cases.

sections stained with H&E, SC nuclei could be identified easily by their irregular shape and prominent nucleoli. Nuclear AR were present in SC, Leydig cells, and peritubular cells of patients diagnosed with incomplete spermatogenesis (Fig. 14.3D) and Sertoli cell-only syndrome (Fig. 14.3F). Surprisingly, they did not appear less strongly stained than those from normal fertile controls and there was no evidence that fewer SC nuclei were immunostained.

The pattern of AR distribution within SC of normal human testes was more difficult to determine than that in the rat or the marmoset because of the complex helical arrangement of spermatogenesis that results in the presence of several stages of the spermatogenic cycle within each cross section of a tubule. Additional analysis of sections of testicular tissue taken from three patients with an apparently normal germ-cell complement was undertaken using sections stained with H&E or using AR immunocytochemistry to determine whether all SC nuclei in the sections were stained for the AR. A histogram of the results obtained is presented in Figure 14.4. There was no difference between the numbers of SC nuclei in the sections

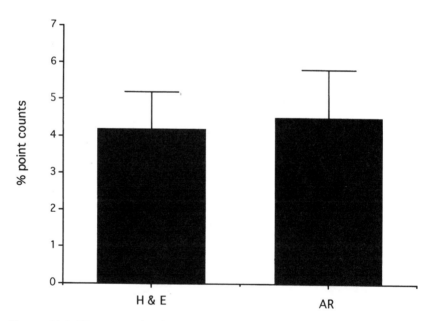

FIGURE 14.4. Histogram showing percentage of Sertoli cell nuclei in sections of normal human testis visualized by staining with hematoxylin and eosin (H&E) compared with those stained by AR antibody. Mean ± SEM for three different testicular samples with five grids per section.

visualized using H&E and those detected by AR immunostaining, suggesting that ARs are not expressed in an obvious stage-dependent fashion in the human SC.

Determination of the Pattern of Expression of AR in Testes from Adult Rats Following Androgen Withdrawal and Manipulation of Germ-Cell Complement

On sections of testis taken from rats treated 6 days previously with EDS to induce complete androgen withdrawal, no AR immunostaining was detected in any of the cell types (Fig. 14.5B) in comparison to sections of untreated (control) rat testis developed on the same slides (Fig. 14.5A upper), where the normal staining pattern was observed. Replacement of testosterone by injections, either from the time of EDS treatment or only 2 h prior to tissue recovery, resulted in restoration of a normal pattern of staining with stage-specific nuclear AR in SC but no staining of germ cells or SC cytoplasm (Fig. 14.5C). Stage-dependent staining of AR in SC was maintained when selected germ cells were absent following MAA induced depletion; an example of the pattern of staining in the testis of a rat lacking round spermatids (MAA 14 days previously) is shown in Fig. 14.5D.

Discussion

Using antigen retrieval (13) and immunocytochemistry we have been able to examine the pattern of expression of AR in rat, primate, and human testis. In the fetal rat we failed to find convincing nuclear AR in the testis before day 17.5 p.c., at which time a few cells of the interstitial cell population did appear positive. As testicular development continued with increasing differentiation of the seminiferous cords, AR staining increased but remained convincing only in cells outside the cords. The nuclei in a population of cells largely one layer thick and surrounding the seminiferous cords were stained prominently, as were some other cells within the interstitium, which also had a flat elongated nucleus. Based on their locations within the interstitial region of the testis, we would identify these AR-positive cells as being peritubular and interstitial mesenchymal cells, respectively, both of which have a fibroblastic appearance. In an interesting series of experiments in vitro, Buehr and coworkers (14) found that cells from the mesonephric region migrated into the testis and contributed to the interstitial cell population, including those in the flattened peritubular layer. In the absence of an influx of cells from the mesonephros, normal differentiation of testis cords did not occur, consistent with the synthesis of components of the extracellular matrix by peritubular cells contributing to organization of the

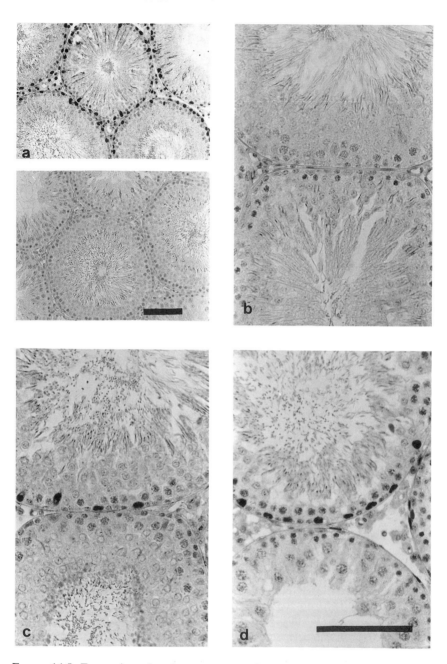

FIGURE 14.5. Expression of androgen receptor in testes from untreated (control) adult rats (*A* upper) compared with those treated with EDS 6 days before tissue recovery (testosterone withdrawal—*B*), those treated with EDS with testosterone (T) replacement (*C*), and testes lacking spermatids (MAA day 14—*D*). The lower half of *A* shows a normal adult rat section in which the anti-AR antibody had

seminiferous cords. In the context of the current findings it is interesting to speculate that the cells in the fetal testis containing AR have developed from the same cell population that expresses AR in the mesonephros. Our results would indicate that the peritubular cells are responsive to androgens during fetal life, although the influence this might have on fetal testicular development is uncertain.

Positive staining of AR protein within the cells of the seminiferous cords was unconvincing prior to day 20.5 of gestation, when nuclei of a few Sertoli cells around the periphery of the cords did appear faintly stained. In postnatal samples nuclear AR in Sertoli cells was increased, although it remained much less intense than that in the peritubular cells during the first 3 weeks of life. Peritubular cells from immature rats (postnatal days 15–25) have recently been shown to secrete activin-A (15) and to respond to androgens with increased expression of an androgen response element reporter (16). As maturation of the testis proceeded, AR immunostaining in SC became stage dependent and resembled that in the adult rat on day 45.

In adult life, immunohistochemically detectable AR in ST was confined to the nucleus of the SC, and in the adult rat, but not in the marmoset, macaque, or human, was more prominent at specific stages of the spermatogenic cycle. In the rat, nuclear staining of AR increased progressively in intensity from stages II–VII and then declined precipitously during stage VIII to become barely detectable at stages IX–XIII (5). In all species, prominent AR immunostaining was also evident in peritubular myoid cells, arterioles, and interstitial cells, and even in the rat, AR immunostaining in these cell types did not appear to vary with the stage of the cycle of adjacent tubules. The finding of stage-dependent AR in SC in the rat was consistent with other observations we have made of marked differences in androgen action on ST at different stages of the spermatogenic cycle. For example, histological changes induced by androgen withdrawal occur first at stages VII–VIII, and overall protein secretion is controlled by *testosterone* (T) specifically at stages VI–VIII (2, 17). Our results do not suggest that AR in SC of marmoset, stump tailed macaque, or human exhibits the same marked stage dependence as has been seen in the rat, and we did not find evidence that AR was present in germ cells as has been reported for the rat (6) and human (18), although in the latter study interpretation of results was hampered by poor tissue preservation. In the ram (our unpub-

---

been preabsorbed with the AR peptide used as immunogen. T withdrawal resulted in the loss of AR staining from all cell types within the testis, but the normal pattern of stage-dependent SC AR staining was maintained by exogenous administration of T. Absence of germ cells had no affect on this pattern of staining (*D*). Bar = 100 μm.

lished observations) AR in SC did appear slightly stage dependent, and the availability of AR for immunostaining appears therefore to be species dependent.

In the rat, testosterone withdrawal is known to disrupt spermatogenesis (19, 20), and we therefore tested the effects of T withdrawal, using EDS, and T replacement on the pattern of AR immunostaining in the adult rat. The amount of nuclear AR, detected immunohistochemically, varied with the time after removal of Leydig cells; 4 days after EDS faint and variable AR staining was detectable (unpublished observations), but on EDS plus 6 days no ARs were detectable in any cell type. Maintenance of spermatogenesis by replacement of T beginning at the time of EDS treatment resulted in a pattern of AR immunostaining indistinguishable from that of controls. In a preliminary experiment we also found that AR staining was partially restored in EDS plus 6-day animals given an injection of T only 2 h prior to death. In the EDS plus T–treated animals, although the pattern of staining was very similar to controls, quantitative analysis revealed that levels of staining were somewhat lower (5), possibly reflecting lower levels of *follicle-stimulating hormone* (FSH) in these animals.

In immature rats, AR immunostaining in SC developed gradually and differences between tubules emerged as the germ-cell population increased (days 14 to 35). There is evidence that where stage-dependent differences are found in the expression of genes and their protein products in SC, a major factor is the changing germ-cell complement (2). We have previously used specific germ-cell depletion by MAA to confirm that synthesis of proteins by SC can be modulated by germ cells (21, 22). However, we have so far been unable to show that depletion of selected populations of spermatocytes or round or elongating spermatids leads to any major change in AR immunolocalization in SC. Further studies are under way to discover if co-depletion of more than one class of germ cells is effective in altering the pattern of SC staining in rats. In the human, where we did not find evidence of stage specificity of SC AR immunostaining, SC nuclei were immunopositive in samples where a full germ-cell complement was either partially or totally absent.

To detect the AR protein in our sections of tissue it was necessary to pretreat the samples by microwaving in citrate buffer. In the absence of this pretreatment, which was recommended by the supplier of the antiserum, no immunostaining was detected (our unpublished observations). However, AR immunostaining in SC at stages IV–VII has been reported in a separate study (6) in which samples of tissue were embedded in polyester wax and not subjected to antigen retrieval. The immunogen used to raise the antiserum is located at the extreme N terminal end of the receptor protein in a region associated with ligand-independent transcriptional activation (23). Antigen retrieval, due to the high temperatures used, is believed to cause "unmasking" of antigenic sites; this has been particularly applicable to proteins with a nuclear location and can sometimes be mimicked by treatment of sections with proteolytic enzymes (13). ARs are known to associate with other proteins both before and after ligand binding (3). A recent study has shown that retention of receptor-bound androgen is enhanced by an interaction between the AR N-terminal and steroid-binding domains (24). In the current study we have not determined if stage-dependent AR staining in rat SC reflects simply the availability of this antigenic site on the protein only at selected stages and that the AR is present in all SC but masked. If this is the case, then the presence of AR available for immunochemical localization in all SC nuclei in the marmoset, macaque, and human might reflect a different conformation of the protein in these species compared with the rat, leaving this antigenic site exposed at all times. Experiments using antisera raised against epitopes selected from within other portions of the receptor protein (25, 26) combined with antigen retrieval might answer these questions.

References

1. George FW, Wilson JD. Sex determination and differentiation. In: Knobil E, Neill JD, eds. The physiology of reproduction, 2nd ed. New York: Raven Press, 1994:3–28.
2. Sharpe RM. Regulation of spermatogenesis. In: Knobil E, Neill JD, eds. The physiology of reproduction, 2nd ed. New York: Raven Press, 1994:1363–434.
3. Carson-Jurnica MA, Schrader WT, O'Malley BW. Steroid receptor superfamily: structure and functions. Endocr Rev 1990;11:201–19.
4. Rundlett SE, Wu S-P, Miesfeld RL. Functional characterizations of the androgen receptor confirm that the molecular basis of androgen action is transcriptional regulation. Mol Endocrinol 1990;4:708–14.
5. Bremner WJ, Millar MR, Sharpe RM, Saunders PTK. Immunohistochemical localization of androgen receptors in the rat testis: evidence for stage-dependent expression and regulation by androgens. Endocrinology 1994;135:1227–34.
6. Vornberger W, Prins G, Musto N, Suarez-Quian C. Androgen receptor distribution in rat testis: new implications for androgen regulation of spermatogenesis. Endocrinology 1994;134:2307–16.
7. Millar M, Sharpe RM, Maguire SM, Saunders PTK. Cellular localisation of messenger RNAs in rat testis; application of digoxigenin-labelled probes to embedded tissue. Cell Tissue Res 1993;273:269–77.
8. Bartlett JMS, Kerr JB, Sharpe RM. The selective removal of pachytene spermatocytes using methoxy acetic acid as an approach to the study in-vivo of paracrine interactions in the testis. J Androl 1988;9:31–40.
9. Allenby G, Foster PMD, Sharpe RM. Evaluation of changes in the secretion of immunoactive inhibin by rat seminiferous tubules in-vitro as an indicator of early toxicant action on spermatogenesis. Fundam Appl Toxicol 1991;16:710–24.
10. Sharpe RM, Maddocks S, Kerr JB. Cell-cell interactions in the control of spermatogenesis as studied using Leydig cell destruction and testosterone replacement. Am J Anat 1990;188:3–20.

11. Gordon K. Tissue processing. In: Bancroft J, Stevens A, eds. Theory and practice of histological techniques. New York: Churchill Livingstone, 1982.
12. de Jong ASH, van Kessel-van Vark M, Raap AK. Sensitivity of various visualization methods for peroxidase and alkaline phosphatase activity in immunoenzyme histochemistry. Histochemistry 1985;17:1119–30.
13. Shi S-R, Chaiwun B, Young L, Cote R, Taylor C. Antigen retrieval technique utilizing citrate buffer or urea solution for immunohistochemical demonstration of androgen receptor in formalin-fixed paraffin sections. J Histochem Cytochem 1993;41:1599–604.
14. Buehr M, Gu S, McLaren A. Mesonephric contribution to testis differentiation in the fetal mouse. Development 1993;117:273–81.
15. de Winter JP, Vanderstichele HMJ, Verhoeven G, Timmerman MA. Peritubular myoid cells from immature rat testes secrete activin A and express activin receptor type II in vitro. Endocrinology 1994;135:759–67.
16. Ku C-Y, Loose-Mitchell DS, Sanborn BM. Both Sertoli and peritubular cells respond to androgens with increased expression of an androgen response element reporter. Biol Reprod 1994;51:319–26.
17. Sharpe RM, Maddocks S, Millar M, Saunders PTK, Kerr JB, McKinnell C. Testosterone and spermatogenesis: identification of stage-dependent, androgen regulated proteins secreted by adult seminiferous tubules. J Androl 1992; 13:172–84.
18. Kimura N, Mizokami A, Oonuma T, Sasano H, Nagura H. Immunocytochemical localization of androgen receptor with polyclonal antibody in paraffin-embedded human tissues. J Histochem Cytochem 1993;41:671–8.
19. Bartlett JMS, Kerr JB, Sharpe RM. The effect of selective destruction and regeneration of rat Leydig cells on the intratesticular distribution of testosterone and morphology of the seminiferous epithelium. J Androl 1986;7:240–53.
20. Kerr JB, Millar M, Maddocks S, Sharpe RM. Stage-dependent changes in spermatogenesis and Sertoli cells in relation to the onset of spermatogenic failure following withdrawal of testosterone. Anat Rec 1993;235:547–59.
21. Maguire SM, Miller MR, Sharpe RM, Saunders PTK. Stage-dependent expression of mRNA for cyclic protein 2 during spermatogenesis is modulated by elongate spermatids. Mol Cell Endocrinol 1993;94:79–88.
22. Allenby G, Foster PMD, Sharpe RM. Evidence that secretion of immunoactive inhibin by seminiferous tubules from the adult rat testis is regulated by specific germ cell types: correlation between in vivo and in vitro studies. Endocrinology 1991;128:467–76.
23. Jenster G, van der Korput J, van Vroonhoven C, van der Kwast T, Trapman J, Brinkman A. Domains of the human androgen receptor involved in steroid binding, transcriptional activation, and subcellular localization. Mol Endocrinol 1991;5:1396–404.
24. Zhou Z-X, Lane MV, Kemppainen JA, French FS, Wilson EM. Specificity of ligand-dependent androgen stabilization: receptor domain interactions influence dissociation and receptor stability. Mol Endocrinol 1995;9:208–18.
25. Sar M, Lubahn DB, French FS, Wilson EM. Immunohistochemical localization of the androgen receptor in rat and human tissues. Endocrinology 1990; 127:3180–6.

26. Husman D, Wilson C, McPhaul M, Tilley W, Wilson J. Antipeptide antibodies to two distinct regions of the androgen receptor localise the receptor protein to the nuclei of target cells in the rat and human prostate. Endocrinology 1990;126:2359–68.

15

Role of Carrier Proteins in the Movement and Metabolism of Retinoids in the Seminiferous Tubule

DAVID E. ONG

Vitamin A is required for maintenance of the proper state of many of the differentiated epithelia of the body and for processes as diverse as morphogenesis and vision. As details about the structure and biochemistry of vitamin A have been revealed, it has become clear that a family of compounds, the retinoids, are involved in fulfilling the functions of vitamin A. Retinol is the only "required" retinoid because it can serve as a precursor to all other retinoids and provides the appropriate forms for storage and transport (reviewed in 1). It is present in the blood, bound to its carrier protein, *retinol-binding protein* (RBP), at a relatively constant level in the normally nourished animal. This serves to supply most of the organs and cells that then produce the retinoids that act as hormones, principally retinoic acid. It is clear that the hormonal effects of retinoids can be explained in many cases by the presence of nuclear receptor proteins that bind retinoids and then activate and repress the expression of specific genes (2). But for the forms of vitamin A that appear to function as hormones, we still know little of their sites of production, the regulation of that production, and what means are present to modulate their action.

While 11-*cis*-retinal is known to function as a chromophore of the visual pigments, the retinoids that may have active roles in regulating differentiation or function of various cells of the body are less well defined. Candidates include all-*trans*- and 9-*cis*-retinoic acid, didehydroretinoic acid, 14-OH,4,14 *retro* retinol, and perhaps retinol itself (3). Other candidates exist, such as 4-oxo-retinoic acid (4) and perhaps retinoids as yet undescribed (or just underappreciated). However, for most processes, the dominant role seems to be played by all-*trans*-retinoic acid.

The ability of retinoids to control gene expression can be fully appreciated in retrospect from the detailed account of the histopathology of vitamin A deficiency in the rat reported by Wolbach and Howe (5). The widespread pathological changes observed in organs were often characterized by squamous, keratinizing cells replacing the normal, columnar epithelial cells. This suggested that certain cells were directed along different pathways of differentiation by the presence or absence of retinoids. Although pathways induced in response to dietary deficiency are clearly pathological, perhaps such alternate paths might be selected under normal physiology for some cells by controlling the local presence of retinoids. The mechanisms by which supply of active retinoids to responsive cells is regulated are still largely a matter of conjecture. There is clearly no obvious central "endocrine" organ for the production of retinoic acid, for example; it is more likely that it is generated within the organ/tissue or cell where it is required, making retinoic acid an autocrine or paracrine hormone. This appears to be particularly true for the testis. Retinoic acid is apparently needed for spermatogenesis and more than 99% of the endogenous retinoic acid of the testis is produced locally (6).

While retinol is delivered to cells by RBP, four cellular retinoid-binding proteins are found within cells; they are members of a superfamily of intracellular lipid-transport proteins. These four proteins have different cellular locations. Two bind both retinol and retinal and are called *cellular retinol-binding protein* (CRBP) types I and II; two bind retinoic acid and are called *cellular retinoic acid–binding protein* (CRABP) types I and II. These proteins channel the movement and metabolism of retinoids within the cell (reviewed in 7). CRBP and CRABP are both present in the testis and epididymis (8, 9).

Requirement of Vitamin A for Spermatogenesis

The effect of vitamin A deficiency on spermatogenesis was first examined in detail by Mason (10), who described sloughing of germ cells into the lumen of the seminiferous tubule; only Sertoli cells, spermatogonia, and a small number of early spermatocytes remained in the testis of the deficient animal. The germ cells that show signs of degeneration are late spermatocytes and spermatids, found on the luminal side of the blood-testis barrier (11, 12). There is also an arrest in the cell cycle for early spermatogonia (A_1 stage), preventing both formation of later spermatogonia (A_{2-4}, I, and B) and replenishment of the A_1 population. One study suggests that the arrest occurs before the S phase (during G1, 13), while other studies are consistent with an arrest after the S phase, during G2 (14, 15). A similar arrest occurs in the preleptotene primary spermatocytes in the G2 phase, preventing progression through meiosis (14). There is no obvious degeneration of spermatogonia (11, 16). Instead of indicating use of retinoids, the lack of later-stage spermatogonia observed during deficiency may actually indicate that they do not require retinoids and have continued to progress to the spermatocyte stage, only to be arrested at that point.

Retinoic Acid Is a Required Retinoid for Spermatogenesis

When all-*trans*-retinoic acid, not normally present in the diet, is substituted for naturally occurring forms of vitamin A in the diets of laboratory animals, all organs except the testis and the eye appear to be morphologically and functionally normal. The failure of retinoic acid to support vision indicates that it cannot be reduced to retinal or retinol in vivo (17). The histological lesions produced in the testis of rats maintained on retinoic acid only (18) are indistinguishable from those described for "orthodox" vitamin A deficiency. Spermatogenesis can be reinitiated and fertility restored by returning retinol to the diet (18, 19), but increasing dietary retinoic acid (18–20), or even direct injection (21), did not prevent degeneration. For many years it was believed that retinoic acid had no function in spermatogenesis. In fact, supplying retinoic acid in place of other forms of vitamin A has allowed the study of the effects of deficiency on spermatogenesis in animals apparently uncompromised in other aspects of their physiology, except for vision, including several studies referred to above. However, van Pelt and de Rooij (22) supplemented dietary retinoic acid with additional amounts injected intraperitoneally in retinol-deprived rats and restored the stages of spermatogenesis through elongated spermatids. There were fewer elongated spermatids than round spermatids, suggesting that not all of the round spermatids survived to the next stage. Fertility was never fully restored, suggesting a further role for retinoids (or the need for a different retinoid), at the critical stage of spermiogenesis. Although van Pelt and de Rooij conclude that "retinoic acid is able to support the full development of spermatogenic cells into elongated spermatids" (22), they note that the dosage required to maintain spermatogenesis is 30 times higher than the amount of retinoic acid needed to maintain normal body growth.

This apparent elevated requirement for spermatogenesis, compared with the needs of other tissues, may simply reflect a problem in delivery due to the cellular architecture of the testis. Tight junctions between adjacent Sertoli cells create a major element of the blood-testis barrier, with the late germ cells (pachytene and beyond) sequestered in the luminal compartment of the seminiferous tubule, restricted from direct access to blood-borne nutrients or hormones. This makes them completely dependent on nutrient supply through the Sertoli cell. The apparent inability of Sertoli cells to take up retinoic acid (23) would limit the amount of retinoic acid available to those cells. The possibility that dietary retinoic acid fails to "penetrate to the site of action" had been suggested previously (18). Retinoic acid appears indeed to be one of the forms of vitamin A required for spermatogenesis, but it may need to be generated in situ. If supplied by diet or injection, large amounts might be needed to overcome the blood-testis barrier.

Other evidence also supports a role for retinoic acid in spermatogenesis. Rat testis is a rich source of CRABP (8) and some germ cells clearly contain CRABP, as shown by radioimmunoassay and in situ localizations of CRABP mRNA (24, 25). The testis also contains *messenger RNA* (mRNA) for both alpha and beta nuclear *retinoic acid receptors* (RAR)-α,β (26–28). Transgenic mice that have had the gene for RAR-α ablated show testicular degeneration indistinguishable from that of the vitamin A–deficient animal (29). Thus, it is clear that retinoic acid does function in the testis. What is not clear at this time is where the necessary retinoic acid is produced. It must come from within the testis given that less than 1% of the endogenous retinoic acid in this organ is obtained from the plasma (6). However, it is quite possible that other retinoids that cannot be derived from retinoic acid are also required for certain steps in the production of viable sperm, as will be discussed below.

Delivery of Vitamin A to the Seminiferous Epithelium

Role of the Peritubular Cell

Retinol-RBP is clearly present in the interstitial space of the testis, outside the vascular bed (30). However, the peritubular (myoid) cells may provide a significant barrier to the movement of this complex into the seminiferous tubule. Only 10–15% of peritubular cell-cell junctions appear to be open. The movement of molecules such as ferritin, horseradish peroxidase (MW = 44,000), and lanthanum into the intercellular space between the peritubular cells and the germinal epithelium is clearly restricted, penetrating the space only above the open cell junctions (31, 32). Because RBP (MW = 21,000) circulates in a 1:1 complex with another blood protein, *transthyretin* (TTR) (MW = 55,000), it may not be able to circumnavigate the peritubular cells sufficiently rapidly to meet the needs of Sertoli and germ cells. In support of this idea, RBP injected directly into the testis of the rat showed a complete failure to penetrate to the Sertoli cell or germinal epithelium (33).

The peritubular cell is known to be rich in CRBP, suggesting it might play an important role in vitamin A metabolism or processing (24, 34). The presence of CRBP is a reliable marker for cells that process considerable retinol (7). Cultured peritubular cells had previously been shown to continue to express CRBP (34), and we have found that to be true as well (35). Further, we observed that the cultured cells will internalize [³H]retinol from RBP and this internalization was competed for by the presence of unlabeled retinol-RBP (Fig. 15.1). There is considerable debate about the mechanism(s) by which cells acquire retinol from RBP (36). Some favor dissociation from RBP with simple diffusion across the cell membrane (37); others provide evidence for a specific recognition of the complex either with internalization of the complex (38) or with removal of the retinol without RBP internalization (39). Our results with peritubular cells, and with Sertoli cells, discussed below, favor the last mechanism, in which the RBP "receptor" functions as a transporter. We found no evidence for specific uptake of free retinol (35). It is possible that different cells use different mechanisms. For example, a putative RBP receptor has been isolated from the retinal pigment epithelium but it appears to be restricted to that cell type (40).

Cells rich in CRBP frequently store retinol as esters, synthesized by the enzyme *lecithin-retinol acyltransferase* (LRAT). However, less than 2% of the retinol internalized by the peritubular cell was recoverable as ester and no LRAT activity could be detected in microsomal preparations from those cells (35). This suggested that retinol might be moving out of the cell, perhaps by being secreted bound to a newly synthesized molecule of RBP. It had been assumed that RBP synthesis and release was restricted to the liver hepatocyte (41), until it was discovered that RBP mRNA could'be detected in other organs (42). Thus, retinol movement across blood-organ barriers might involve retinol-RBP release into the protected compartments by the barrier cells. An appropriate analogy is the ability of the Sertoli cell to synthesize and release transferrin to provide iron to the sequestered, late germ cells (43). To investigate this possibility, we exploited the high affinity of RBP for TTR to collect any RBP in the medium from peritubular cells cultured with radioactive amino acids. The TTR was coupled to Sepharose-4B; RBP binds to TTR in solutions of moderate ionic strength, but is released when the ionic strength is to very low levels. By this technique, metabolically labeled RBP was recovered from the culture medium of peritubular cells provided with labeled methione (Fig. 15.2); its identity was confirmed by a number of biochemical criteria, including comigration with authentic RBP on *sodium dodecyl sulfate–polyacrylamide gel electrophoresis* (SDS-PAGE) gels (Fig. 15.3). Several other cells known to synthesize RBP also synthesize and release TTR, including the hepatocyte (44) and the retinal pigment epithelial cell (45). By the reciprocal method of collecting any TTR on an RBP-Sepharose column, we examined the ability of the peritubular cell to secrete TTR. No synthesis was detected (Fig. 15.2).

This ability of the peritubular cell to obtain retinol from RBP and synthesize and release RBP suggests that retinol may move across the peritubular cell, rather than around it. The rate of entry of the TTR-RBP-retinol complex into the intercellular space between peritubular cells and Sertoli cells may be too slow or too restricted to meet the vitamin A needs of spermatogenesis. The lack of synthesis of TTR suggests that, if plasma TTR as well as TTR-RBP are somewhat restricted from entry, the RBP released

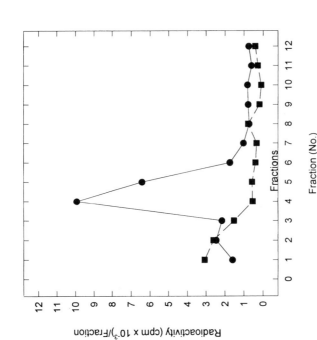

FIGURE 15.2. Synthesis of RBP and TTR by peritubular cells. Presence of [³⁵S]-labeled RBP (●) and TTR (■) in peritu-bular cell conditioned medium was examined by affinity chromato-graphy on TTR-Sepharose or RBP-Sepharose, respectively, after incubating cells with 100 μCi [³⁵S]methionine for 72h. Authentic TTR eluted from the RBP-Sepharose column at fraction 5, but no radioactivity was recovered from the medium. Authentic RBP eluted from the TTR-Sepharose column coincident with the radioactive peak shown. Reprinted with permission from Davis and Ong (35).

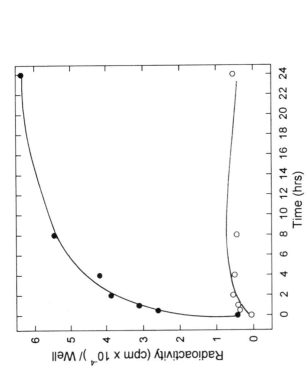

FIGURE 15.1. Uptake of [³H]retinol from the retinol-RBP complex by peritubular cells. Incorporation was monitored with time (●) when 1.0 μM [³H]retinol-RBP was incubated with peritubular cells for 0 to 24h. When 25 μM unlabeled retinol-RBP was incubated with each time course, the incorporation of radioactivity was significantly reduced (○). Reprinted with permission from Davis and Ong (35).

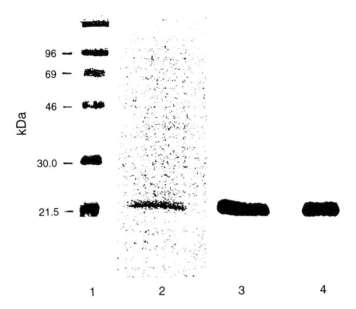

FIGURE 15.3. Examination of material isolated by TTR-affinity chromatography by SDS-PAGE. Lane 1 contains Coomassie-stained molecular weight markers. Lane 3 is the Coomassie stain of the material isolated from the TTR-affinity column. Human RBP was added to the media before isolation. Lane 4 is the Coomassie stain of human RBP alone. Lane 2 is the PhosphorImager scan of Lane 3. Lane 2 superimposes on lane 3. Reprinted with permission from Davis and Ong (35).

from the peritubular cell would be present uncomplexed with TTR, more free to diffuse within this intercellular space that contains considerable extracellular matrix. A role for the peritubular cell in providing nutrients to the interior of the tubule has not been previously noted, to our knowledge (reviewed in 46).

There is no known delivery system for retinoic acid, which is not a component of the normal diet. But if provided to animals in an artificial diet, it circulates in the blood bound to serum albumin (47). Since serum albumin is a large, highly asymmetric protein (30 by 150 Å), it may also be slow to move into and through the space behind the peritubular cells. Thus, administered retinoic acid would have to cross two cellular barriers, explaining why such high doses are required to support spermatogenesis. The possibility that the peritubular cell might also produce retinoic acid to meet the needs of the seminiferous epithelium needs to be examined.

Role of the Sertoli Cell

We had previously characterized the ability of Sertoli cells in culture to internalize retinol from RBP (48). Uptake slowed markedly when sufficient retinol was internalized to saturate the amount of CRBP present in the cell, suggesting a coupling of uptake to availability of apoCRBP. ApoCRBP has been demonstrated to be able to affect the activity of enzymes, activating a liver retinyl ester hydrolase (49), but inhibiting LRAT, the enzyme that esterifies retinol (50). Thus, CRBP can attenuate cellular metabolism of retinol, depending on its degree of saturation, and perhaps also regulate uptake. CRBP expression in Sertoli cells varies during the spermatogenic cycle in the adult (30, 51). We found that CRBP was demonstrable in Sertoli cells by immunohistochemistry in sections prepared from fetuses at the 20th gestational day, about 1 day before birth, with all tubules staining with equal intensity. Differential expression of CRBP in the Sertoli cells of adjacent tubules began to be discernible, as assessed by the intensity of immunoreactivity, by the 4th postnatal day, becoming more apparent throughout puberty (52). Thus, the variable expression of CRBP is established early, independently of the presence of late germ cells, and seems to anticipate the cyclical variation seen in the adult. This indicates that functional differences in Sertoli cells can precede the appearance of late germ cells.

Once internalized, the retinol is esterified to a considerable degree within the Sertoli cell (48, 53, 54), in contrast to the fate of retinol in the peritubular cell. That esterification is due to LRAT (54). Our initial observations of Sertoli cells isolated from adult rats indicated that they might contain higher amounts of LRAT than those isolated from 20-day-

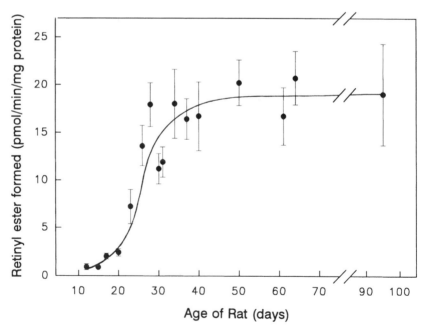

FIGURE 15.4. Developmental profile of LRAT specific activity in rat testis microsomes. Values shown are averages ± SD ($n = 3$). Reprinted with permission from Schmitt and Ong (52).

old rats (54). In a study of the endogenous retinoids of spermatozoa (55), we had observed that testicular spermatozoa contained retinyl ester (140 fmol/10^6 sperm). This opened the possibility that the Sertoli cell might be exporting esters to germ cells, similar to the export of LRAT-produced retinyl esters from absorptive cells (56). However, if Sertoli cells from the testes of mature animals were cultured to remove any contaminating germ cells, they were found to have levels of LRAT as low as that observed for cells from the 20-day-old animal (52). Since the LRAT activity in microsomes from whole testis of the mature rat is high (54), a careful developmental study of LRAT activity in whole testis and isolated cells was undertaken (52). The specific activity of microsomal LRAT from whole testis increased 10-fold between postnatal days 20 and 35, coincident with the great increase in late germ cells that occurs during the period (Fig. 15.4). This increase was due to the presence of LRAT in the round spermatids; their microsomes had a specific activity 2–3 times higher than those from whole testis and 5 times higher than pachytene microsomes, and could account for the majority of the LRAT activity of the testis. This suggested that the origin of the retinyl esters in spermatozoa was by esterification of retinol provided to the spermatids, rather than by import as the ester itself.

The source of this retinol is likely RBP retinol secreted from the Sertoli cell. Just as observed for cultured peritubular cells, the Sertoli cell synthe-

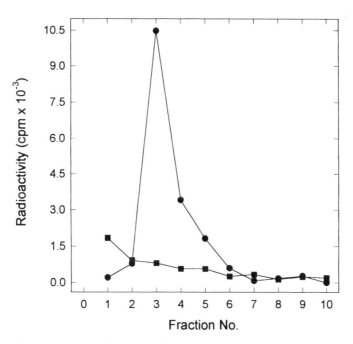

FIGURE 15.5. Synthesis of RBP and TTR by Sertoli cells. The presence of [^{35}S]-labeled RBP (●) and TTR (■) was determined as described in the legend to Figure 15.3. Only labeled-RBP was detected.

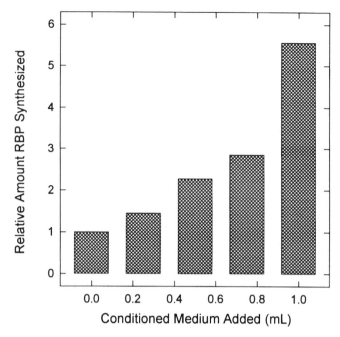

FIGURE 15.6. Stimulation of RBP synthesis and secretion by factor(s) present in the media from cultures of peritubular cells. Serum-free medium from cultures of peritubular cells was concentrated 60-fold, diafiltered with fresh medium to remove small molecules, and provided to cultures of Sertoli cells 24h prior to establishing RBP synthesis.

sizes and secretes RBP, but not TTR (Fig. 15.5). We have not yet examined if this release might be preferentially from the apical side, as it is for the pigment epithelial cell (45). Interestingly, the rate of Sertoli cell RBP synthesis could be stimulated up to 5-fold in a dose-dependent manner by concentrated, dialyzed medium collected from serum-free cultures of peritubular cells, suggesting that a secreted peritubular cell product might be involved in regulating RBP synthesis (57) (Fig. 15.6). The varying expression seen for CRBP in Sertoli cells at the different stages of the spermatogenic cycle may well reflect the amount of retinol processed by the cell. It will be of interest to determine whether RBP and CRBP expression will prove to be co-regulated in the cultured Sertoli cell by peritubular cell secretions.

Immunolocalization of CRABP in Testis

The studies described above suggest the mechanism by which retinyl esters are accumulated by the spermatozoa but do not elucidate the site of production of retinoic acid that appears to be required by A_1 spermatogonia and primary spermatocytes. To begin to address this question, we have recently reexamined the cellular location of CRABP in the testis by immunohistochemistry. Our previous study (51) that suggested CRABP was present primarily in late germ cells is now established to be incorrect, due to the presence of antibodies to a closely related member of the same superfamily (58) in the antiserum we used in that study. This novel protein has now been identified as a testis-specific protein (58, 59) and is present in considerable abundance, about 1.5% of the total soluble testicular protein (Kingma and Ong, unpublished). Its staining intensity was consequently very high and obscured staining for CRABP.

We have produced new preparations of antiCRABP *immunoglobulin G* (IgG), affinity-purified on a recombinant CRABP-Sepharose column, that do not recognize that testis-specific protein. With this preparation, we found strongest staining in spermatogonia, consistent with the results from the in situ hybridization of CRABP mRNA reported by others (25) and clearly different than the staining we had seen with our previous preparations. Most striking, and surprising, was the compartmentalization that was observed, in which CRABP staining was strongly cytoplasmic, with clear exclusion from the nucleus (Fig. 15.7).

A similar staining pattern, showing exclusion from the nucleus, has also been observed for CRABP-II in the luteal cells of the rat corpus luteum (60). This exclusion is not seen for the other, comparably sized members of the family that we have examined by immunolocalization: CRBP in Sertoli cells (52), CRBP-II in absorptive cells (61), or TLBP in late germ cells (58). We have also clearly seen CRBP in both the nuclear and cytoplasmic compartments of retinal pigment epithelial cells by immunolocalization at the EM level (62).

Given the small size of these proteins (15.5 kd, about $3 \times 3 \times 4$ nm), free access to the nucleus is expected since the nuclear pores have an opening (diameter of 7–9 nm) that permits diffusion of proteins of $<60,000$ kd into the nucleus. A protein of about 17,000 daltons equilibrates between the cytoplasm and nucleus in 2 min (63). The conclusion then is that CRABP must be physically restrained from entry into the nucleus, by association either with a soluble protein of sufficient size to block movement through the pores or with a structural element of the cell. The exclusion phenomenon is seen in what appear to be late type A and in type B spermatogonia. No cytoplasmic staining was seen in spermatocytes or spermatids; it was not possible to assess whether any A_0/A_1 spermatogonia exhibited such staining. However, in the later spermatogonia, it would appear that CRABP is preventing retinoic acid from reaching the nucleus, where the nuclear receptor proteins for retinoic acid are located. There might be not only restriction of movement into the nucleus but also acceleration of metabolism to other forms (64). It has been suggested that CRABP might protect certain cells from the effects of retinoic acid (65). This barrier function could either block the activation of expression of specific genes or serve to

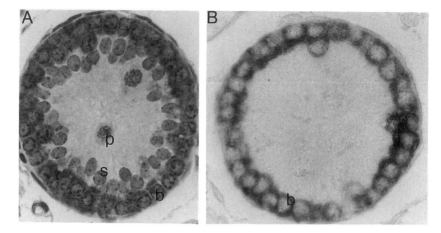

FIGURE 15.7. Immunolocalization of CRABP in pubertal rat testis. Sections (5 μm) were stained using an immunostaining kit (Serotec, Harlan) and affinity-purified anti-CRABP IgG. (*A*) Postnatal day 17 at a stage corresponding to stages I–IV of the adult testis. Note the strong staining of type B spermatogonia (b) along the basement membrane, in contrast to the more centrally located Sertoli cells (s) and early pachytene spermatocytes (p). (*B*) The exclusion of CRABP immunostaining from the nuclei of type B spermatogonia (b) is evident in this uncounterstained section of rat testis at postnatal day 17.

relieve the repression of expression of specific genes. For example, if certain genes necessary for the progression of spermatogonia are normally repressed by retinoic acid, the induction of CRABP expression (and any attendant retinoic acid-metabolizing enzymes) would then allow differentiation/function to proceed. Note that this would explain the previous observations that the later spermatogonia show no obvious degeneration in the vitamin A–deficient animal and support the suggestion put forward here that their eventual disappearance with prolonged deficiency may be due to a normal progression to the spermatocyte. Their numbers would not be replenished because of the block in the cell cycle observed for the A_1 spermatogonia in the deficient animal.

The ability to create a CRABP barrier within a cell would allow different cell types to respond differently to the local presence of retinoic acid depending on their expression of CRABP. This suggests that retinoic acid is produced by nongerminal cells of the tubule and then is generally supplied, in some manner, to the germinal epithelium. Clearly, possible production by peritubular cells and Sertoli cells must be considered and will be the focus of future work.

Summary

From the observations detailed in this discussion, the following scenario can be proposed (Fig. 15.8): retinol is first moved into the seminiferous tubule by uptake from interstitial retinol-RBP by the peritubular cell, which then releases the retinol to the interior on a new molecule of RBP. The retinol is then taken up from this complex by Sertoli cells, and perhaps by some of the germ cells not sequestered behind the Sertoli cell tight junctions. Some of the retinol is then released from the Sertoli cell on a new molecule of RBP, to supply the retinol needed for the accumulation of the retinyl ester found in sperm. Retinoic acid is synthesized from retinol within the tubule (site unknown). This retinoic acid is then provided to the A_1 spermatogonia and early spermatocytes, which are shown to require retinoic acid to progress through the cell cycle, but it is blocked from acting in the later spermatogonia that appear not to require retinoic acid, by their expression of CRABP and subsequent restriction of that protein to the cytoplasm. This may serve to accelerate the catabolism of retinoic acid by cytochrome P-450 activity, known to be present in the testis (64).

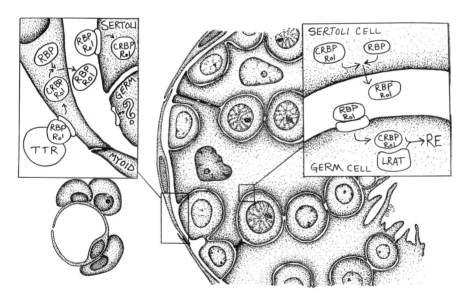

FIGURE 15.8. Model for the delivery of retinol to the cells of the seminiferous tubule. The retinol-RBP-TTR would reach the peritubular cell after escape from a testicular capillary, shown with associated interstitial cells in the lower left of the figure. Reprinted with permission from Davis and Ong (35).

Acknowledgments. This work was supported by NIH grant HD25206. The author is particularly indebted to collaborators Frank Chytil, Ph.D., Marie-Claire Orgebin-Crist, Ph.D., and Michael Skinner, Ph.D., and to students and postdoctoral fellows Jan Shingleton, Ph.D., James Davis, Ph.D., Christie Schmitt, Ph.D., Steve Pappas, Ph.D., and Steve Porter, M.D., Ph.D., from whose work this chapter was drawn.

References

1. Blomhoff R, Green MH, Green JB, Berg T, Norum KR. Vitamin A metabolism: new perspectives on absorption, transport, and storage. Physiol Rev 1991;71:951–90.
2. Mangelsdorf DJ, Umesono K, Evans RM. The retinoid receptors. In: Sporn MB, Roberts AB, Goodman DS, eds. The retinoids, 2nd ed. New York: Raven Press, 1994:319–49.
3. Blaner WS, Olson JA. Retinol and retinoic acid metabolism. In: Sporn MB, Roberts AB, Goodman DS, eds. The retinoids, 2nd ed. New York: Raven Press, 1994:229–56.
4. Pijnappel WWM, Hendriks HFJ, Folkers GE, Dekker EJ, Edelnbosch C, van der Saag PT, Durston AJ. 4-Oxo-retinoic acid is a highly active modulator of positional specification. Nature 1993;366:340–4.
5. Wolbach SB, Howe PR. Tissue changes following deprivation of fat soluble A. J Exp Med 1925;42:753–77.
6. Blaner WS, Wei S, Kurlandsky SB, Episkopou V. Retinoid transport in rodents. In: Livrea MA, Vidali G, eds. Retinoids: from basic science to clinical applications. Basel: Birkhauser Verlag, 1994:53–78.
7. Ong DE, Newcomer ME, Chytil F. Cellular retinoid-binding proteins. In: Sporn MB, Roberts AB, Goodman DS, eds. The retinoids, 2nd ed. New York: Raven Press, 1994:283–318.
8. Ong DE, Chytil F. CRABP from rat testis. Purification and characterization. J Biol Chem 1978;253:4551–4.
9. Ong DE, Crow JA, Chytil F. Radioimmunochemical determination of cellular retinol- and cellular retinoic acid-binding proteins in cytosols of rat tissues. J Biol Chem 1982;257:13385–9.
10. Mason KE. Differences in testis injury after vitamin A deficiency, vitamin E deficiency, and inanition. Am J Anat 1933;52:153–239.
11. Mitranond V, Sobhon P, Tosukhowong P, Chindaduangrat W. Cytological changes in the testes of vitamin A-deficient rats. Quantitation of germinal cells in the seminiferous tubules. Acta Anat 1979;103:159–68.
12. Griswold MD, Bishop PD, Kim KH, Ren P, Siiteri KE, Morales C. Function of vitamin A in normal and synchronized seminiferous tubules. Ann NY Acad Sci 1989;564:154–72.
13. van Pelt AM, de Rooij DG. The origin of the synchronization of the seminiferous epithelium in vitamin A-deficient rats after vitamin A replacement. Biol Reprod 1990;42:677–82.
14. Ismail N, Morales C, Clermont Y. Role of spermatogonia in the stage-synchronization of the seminiferous epithelium in vitamin-A-deficient rats. Am J Anat 1990;188:57–63.

15. Wang Z, Kim KH. Vitamin A-deficient testis germ cells are arrested at the end of S phase of the cell cycle: a molecular study of the origin of synchronous spermatogenesis in regenerated seminiferous tubules. Biol Reprod 1993;48: 1157–65.

16. Sobhon P, Mitranond V, Tosukhowong P, Chindaduangrat W. Cytological changes in the testes of vitamin A-deficient rats II: ultrastructural study of the seminiferous tubule. Acta Anat 1979;103:169–83.

17. Dowling JE, Wald G. The biological function of vitamin A acid. Proc Natl Acad Sci USA 1960;46:587–608.

18. Thompson JN, Howell JMcC, Pitt GAJ. Vitamin A and reproduction in rats. Proc R Soc Biol Sci 1964;159:510–35.

19. Howell JM, Thompson JN, Pitt GAJ. Histology of lesions produced in the reproductive tract of animals fed a diet deficient in vitamin A alcohol but containing vitamin A acid: the male rat. J Reprod Fertil 1963;5:159–67.

20. Thompson JN, Pitt GAJ. Vitamin A acid and hypervitaminosis A. Nature 1960;188:672–3.

21. Ahluwalia B, Bieri JG. Local stimulatory effect of vitamin A on spermatogenesis in rat. J Nutr 1971;101:141–51.

22. van Pelt AM, de Rooij DG. Retinoic acid is able to reinitiate spermatogenesis in vitamin A-deficient rats and high replicate doses support the full development of spermatogenic cells. Endocrinology 1991;128:697–704.

23. Ahluwalia B, Gambhir K, Sekhon H. Distribution of labeled retinyl acetate and retinoic acid in rat and human testes. A possible site of incorporation in rat testes. J Nutr 1975;105:467–75.

24. Blaner WS, Galdieri M, Goodman DS. Distribution and levels of cellular retinol- and cellular retinoic acid binding protein in various types of rat testes cells. Biol Reprod 1987;36:130–7.

25. Rajan N, Kidd GL, Talmage DA, Blaner WS, Suhara A, Goodman DS. Cellular retinoic acid-binding protein messenger RNA: levels in rat tissues and localization in rat testis. J Lipid Res 1991;32:1195–204.

26. Rees JL, Daly AK, Redfern CPF. Differential expression of the α and β retinoic acid receptors in tissues of the rat. Biochem J 1989;259:917–9.

27. Kim KH, Griswold MD. The regulation of retinoic acid receptor mRNA levels during spermatogenesis. Mol Endocrinol 1990;4:1679–88.

28. Eskild W, Ree AH, Levy FO, Jahnsen T, Hansson V. Cellular localization of mRNAs for retinoic acid receptor-alpha, cellular retinol-binding protein, and cellular retinoic acid-binding protein in rat testis: evidence for germ cell-specific mRNAs. Biol Reprod 1991;44:55–61.

29. Lufkin T, Lohnes D, Mark M, Dierich A, Gorry P, Gaub M-P, LeMeur M, Chambon P. High postnatal lethality and testis degeneration in retinoic acid receptor α mutant mice. Proc Natl Acad Sci USA 1993;90:7225–9.

30. Kato M, Sung WK, Kato K, Goodman DS. Immunohistochemical studies on the localization of cellular retinol-binding protein in rat testis and epididymis. Biol Reprod 1985;32:173–89.

31. Fawcett DW, Leak LV, Heidger PM. Electron microscopic observations on the structural elements of the blood-testis barrier. J Reprod Fertil (Suppl 10) 1970:105–22.

32. Dym M, Fawcett DW. The blood testis barrier in the rat and the physiological compartmentalization of the seminiferous epithelium. Biol Reprod 1970;3:308–26.

33. McGuire BW, Orgebin-Crist MC, Chytil F. Localization of retinol-binding protein in rat testis. Endocrinology 1981;108:658–67.
34. Huggenvik J, Griswold MD. Retinol binding protein in rat testicular cells. J Reprod Fertil 1981;61:403–8.
35. Davis JT, Ong DE. Retinol processing by the peritubular cell from rat testis. Biol Reprod 1994;52:356–64.
36. Soprano DR, Blaner WS. Plasma retinol binding protein. In: Sporn MB, Roberts AB, Goodman DS, eds. The retinoids, 2nd ed. New York: Raven Press, 1994:255–82.
37. Noy N, Blaner WS. Interactions of retinol with binding proteins: studies with rat cellular retinol-binding protein and with rat retinol-binding protein. Biochemistry 1991;30:6380–6.
38. Malaba L, Kindberg GM, Norum KR, Berg T, Blomhoff R. Receptor-mediated endocytosis of RBP by liver parenchymal cells: interference by radioactive iodination. Biochem J 1993;291:187–91.
39. Bok D, Heller J. Transport of retinol from the blood to the retina: an autoradiographic study of the pigment epithelial cell surface receptor plasma retinol-binding protein. Exp Eye Res 1976;22:395–402.
40. Bavik CO, Busch C, Eriksson U. Characterization of a plasma retinol-binding protein membrane receptor expressed in the retinol pigment epithelium. J Biol Chem 1992;267:23035–42.
41. Goodman DS. Plasma retinol-binding protein. In: Sporn MB, Roberts AB, Goodman DS, eds. The retinoids, vol. 2. New York: Academic Press, 1984: 42–89.
42. Soprano DR, Soprano KJ, Goodman DS. Retinol-binding protein messenger RNA levels in the liver and in extrahepatic tissues of the rat. J Lipid Res 1986;27:166–71.
43. Skinner MK, Griswold MD. Secretion of testicular transferrin by cultured Sertoli cells is regulated by hormones and retinoids. Biol Reprod 1982;27:211–21.
44. Fielding P, Fex G. Cellular origin of prealbumin in the rat. Biochem Biophys Acta 1982;716:446–9.
45. Ong DE, Davis JT, O'Day WT, Bok D. Synthesis and secretion of retinol-binding protein and transthyretin by cultured retinol pigment epithelium. Biochemistry 1994;33:1835–42.
46. Skinner MK. Cell-cell interactions in the testis. Endocr Rev 1991;12:45–77.
47. Smith JE, Milch PO, Muto Y, Goodman DS. The plasma transport and metabolism of retinoic acid in the rat. Biochem J 1973;132:821–7.
48. Shingleton JL, Skinner MK, Ong DE. Characteristics of retinol accumulation from serum retinol-binding protein by cultured Sertoli cells. Biochemistry 1989;28:9641–7.
49. Boerman MHEM, Napoli JL. Cholate-independent retinyl ester hydrolase: stimulation by apo-cellular retinol-binding protein. J Biol Chem 1991; 266:22273–8.
50. Herr FM, Ong DE. Differential interaction of lecithin-retinol acyltransferase with cellular retinol binding-proteins. Biochemistry 1992;31:6748–55.
51. Porter SB, Ong DE, Chytil F, Orgebin-Crist M-C. Localization of cellular retinol-binding protein and cellular retinoic acid-binding protein in the rat testis and epididymis. J Androl 1985;6:197–212.

52. Schmitt MC, Ong DE. Expression of cellular retinol-binding protein and lecithin retinol acyltransferase in developing rat testis. Biol Reprod 1993;49:972–9.
53. Bishop PD, Griswold MD. Uptake and metabolism of retinol in cultured Sertoli cells: evidence of a kinetic model. Biochemistry 1987;26:7511–7.
54. Shingleton JL, Skinner MK, Ong DE. Retinol esterification in Sertoli cells by LRAT. Biochemistry 1989;28:9647–53.
55. Pappas SR, Newcomer ME, Ong DE. Endogenous retinoids in rat epididymal tissue and rat and human spermatozoa. Biol Reprod 1993;48:235–47.
56. Quick TC, Ong DE. Vitamin A metabolism in the human intestinal Caco-2 cell line. Biochemistry 1990;29:11116–23.
57. Davis JT, Ong DE. Synthesis and secretion of retinol-binding protein by cultured Sertoli cells. Biol Reprod 1992;47:528–33.
58. Schmitt MC, Jamison RS, Orgebin-Crist M-C, Ong DE. A novel, testis-specific member of the cellular lipophilic transport protein superfamily, deduced from a cDNA clone. Biol Reprod 1994;51:239–45.
59. Oko R, Morales CR. A novel testicular protein, with sequence similarities to a family of lipid binding proteins, is a major component of the rat sperm perinuclear theca. Dev Biol 1994;166:235–45.
60. Bucco RA, Melner MH, Gordon DS, Leers-Sucheta S, Ong DE. Inducible expression of cellular retinoic acid-binding protein II in rat ovary: gonadotropin regulation during luteal development. Endocrinology 1995;136:2730–40.
61. Ong DE, Lucas PC, Kakkad B, Quick TC. Ontogeny of two vitamin A-metabolizing enzymes and two retinol-binding proteins present in the small intestine of the rat. J Lipid Res 1991;32:1521–7.
62. Bok D, Ong DE, Chytil F. Immunocytochemical localization of cellular retinol binding protein in the rat retina. Invest Ophthalmol Vis Sci 1984;25:877–83.
63. Lang I, Scholz M, Peters R. Molecular mobility and nucleocytoplasmic flux in hepatoma cells. J Cell Biol 1986;102:1183–90.
64. Fiorella PD, Napoli JL. Microsomal retinoic acid metabolism. J Biol Chem 1994;269:10538–44.
65. Ruberte E, Dolle P, Chambon P, Morriss-Kay G. Retinoic acid receptors and cellular retinoid binding proteins. Differential pattern of transcription during early morphogenesis in mouse embryos. Development 1991;111:45–60.

16

Transport Mechanisms for Endocrine and Paracrine Factors in the Testis

RICHARD M. SHARPE, MICHAEL R. MILLAR, SIMON MADDOCKS, AND JACQUI CLEGG

As in every organ in the body, mechanisms for the delivery and distribution of nutrients, hormones, and other messengers operate within the testis. In contrast to other organs (excepting the brain), the testis has a much greater dependence on these transport systems because of its unusual anatomy. The fact that the bulk of the testis is composed of the avascular seminiferous tubules, which have a very high energy/nutritional demand because of the proliferating germ cells, means that extravascular transport systems have to be highly developed if normal testicular function is to be maintained. This is probably why the intertubular spaces of the testes of most species contain abundant *interstitial fluid* (IF) (1), as it is this fluid that must transport factors from the bloodstream to the seminiferous tubules, Leydig cells, etc. However, IF cannot deliver nutrients and other factors directly to most of the developing germ cells because these are sequestered behind the "closed doors" of the inter-Sertoli cell tight junctions. Therefore, another delivery system, *seminiferous tubule fluid* (STF), is brought into play and is responsible for the transport of most factors from the Sertoli cells to the germ cells as well as the transport of spermatozoa out of the testis. There is also a fourth transport highway, testicular lymph, although its precise functions in the testis are not very clear (2).

For certain molecules, specific transporter systems exist. For example, iron is bound to transferrin for its transport via the bloodstream. Within the testis, this complex passes into IF and is then taken up by Sertoli cells, which then reexport transferrin-bound iron to the adluminal germ cells (3). However, even though molecules such as iron may have specific carrier molecules, their transport and delivery to sites of action or requirement in the testis are completely dependent upon the main transport highways of the testis. Therefore, this short overview focuses on the regulation of the latter transport systems, as the intercellular movement of all molecules within the testis is absolutely dependent on one or more of these, irrespective of the origin and destination of the molecule in question.

Interdependence of the Transport Highways of the Testis

Transport means movement, and the extracellular fluids of the testis are in constant motion, a fact that tends to be forgotten when viewing a section of testis. Blood enters and leaves the testis via the vasculature, but within the testis IF is constantly being formed as an exudate of blood plasma from the capillaries (Fig. 16.1), and both have a very similar composition (2). Formation of IF has to be balanced by removal or return of this fluid to the bloodstream, and this occurs either via resorption into venules within the testis or return via the lymphatic drainage (Fig. 16.1). In turn, fluid is taken up from IF by Sertoli cells and is then resecreted adluminally as STF (Fig. 16.1), which has a markedly different composition from that of IF and blood plasma (2). STF is transported via peristaltic-like contractions of the seminiferous tubules to the rete testis and from there to the head of the epididymis via the efferent ducts. Much of the STF is reabsorbed in the latter two sites (2), and recent evidence also suggests that the rete testis is another important site of resorption of STF (see below). There are therefore two important points to consider. First, IF formation is dependent upon the

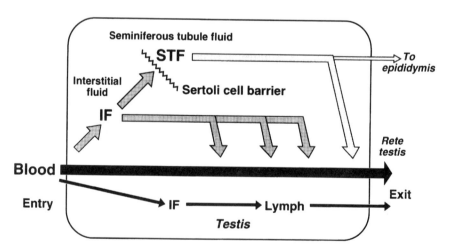

FIGURE 16.1. Diagrammatic representation of the four transport highways of the testis to illustrate their interdependence.

blood supply, and STF formation is, in turn, dependent upon IF formation and thus, indirectly, upon the blood supply. Second, the formation and resorption of IF and STF must be balanced if the testis is to function normally, and this implies close regulation of these events. As detailed below, the same factors appear to be involved in regulating all three main transport highways in the testis.

Regulation of Testicular Transport Highways by Testosterone

Blood flow to the adult testis is regulated to a considerable extent by testosterone (4), and this hormone also controls vasomotion (5). The latter describes episodic variations in high and low blood flow in capillaries (Fig. 16.2), which are generated by rhythmical contractions of precapillary arterioles (6). The latter contractions are regulated by testosterone, which acts via androgen receptors in the muscular layer of the arterioles (Fig. 16.3). The rate of formation and resorption of IF is largely dependent upon vasomotion, with IF being generated during the periods of high blood flow and then resorbed on the venous side during the intervening periods of low blood flow (Fig. 16.2).

Because testosterone regulates both blood flow and vasomotion, it also regulates IF formation (Fig. 16.4). Thus, induction of complete testosterone withdrawal in adult rats by destruction of the Leydig cells with *ethane dimethane sulfonate* (EDS) results in abolition of vasomotion (5) and a 50% decrease in testicular IF volume (7) within 6 days. In the same animals, the volume of STF declines significantly (8), demonstrating that the formation of STF is also androgen dependent (Fig. 16.4), as previous studies have indicated (e.g., 9). However, in the case of STF there is a further intriguing aspect to its regulation by testosterone, namely its apparent stage-dependent production. In the rat, seminiferous tubules at stages VII and VIII have lumina that are substantially larger than those at earlier and later stages of the spermatogenic cycle (10, 11) (Fig. 16.5). This difference disappears at 6 days after EDS-induced testosterone withdrawal, coincident with the reduction in STF volume (8). This finding, along with other evidence (reviewed in 8, 12), suggests that the androgen dependence of STF production may center on stages VII and VIII, with STF production by seminiferous tubules at other stages being largely androgen independent (8). The fact that the biological effects of testosterone on spermatogenesis (7, 13) and immunoexpression of the androgen receptor in Sertoli cell nuclei (14) also center on stages VII and VIII strongly supports this interpretation.

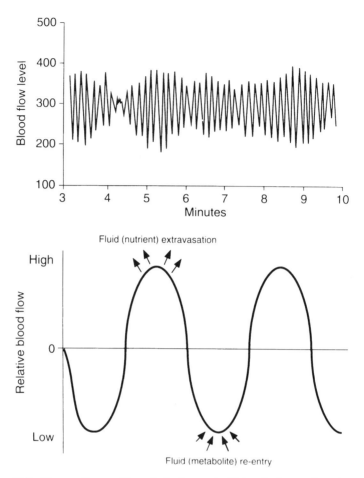

FIGURE 16.2. Vasomotion and its role in the testis. Episodic fluctuations in capillary blood flow in the adult rat testis, as recorded using laser Doppler flowmetry (top) (courtesy of Professor Anders Bergh), and on a magnified scale (bottom). The alternating periods of high and low blood flow, characteristic of vasomotion, are important for the transport of fluid and nutrients into and from interstitial fluid.

Regulation of Testicular Transport Highways by Elongate Spermatids

One other factor has been shown to exert a modulatory effect on the major transport systems of the testis, namely *elongate spermatids* (ESs). These data derive from studies in which selective depletion of particular germ cell types has been achieved either by X-irradiation (to deplete replicating spermatogonia) or by the administration of *methoxyacetic acid* (MAA) to deplete pachytene spermatocytes. In both cases, sampling of animals at

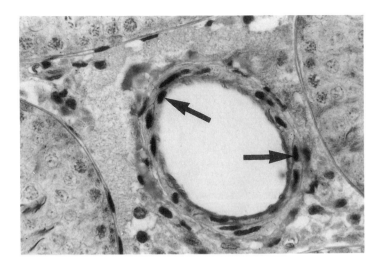

FIGURE 16.3. Immunolocalization of androgen receptors (arrows) in the nuclei of smooth muscle cells surrounding arterioles in the adult rat testis. Also evident is immunostaining of the nuclei of Leydig cells and peritubular myoid cells. Magnification ×450.

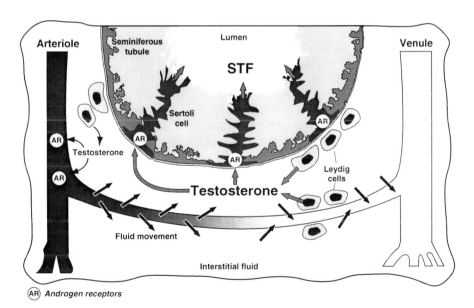

FIGURE 16.4. Diagrammatic representation of the central role of testosterone in regulating the formation of both testicular interstitial fluid, by controlling vasomotion via effects on precapillary arterioles, and seminiferous tubule fluid (STF) via effects on the Sertoli cells.

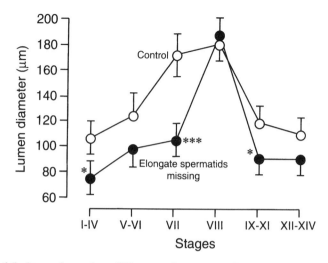

FIGURE 16.5. Stage-dependent differences in cross-sectional lumen diameter (mean ± SD) of seminiferous tubules in the adult rat testis and the modulatory effect of selectively depleting the most mature spermatids by pretreatment with methoxyacetic acid. In the latter study, note that the germ cell complement at stage VIII was normal and included elongate (step 19) spermatids, which is why no decrease in lumen diameter was evident at this stage. Adapted with permission from Sharpe (11). * $P < 0.05$, *** $P < 0.001$, in comparison with corresponding stage(s) in controls.

defined periods posttreatment enables the generation of testes depleted selectively of particular germ-cell types as a result of maturation depletion. Such studies have shown that depletion of ES, but not of earlier germ-cell types, results in decreased lumen size and abolition of the normal stage-dependent increase in lumen size at stage VII (Fig. 16.5) (11), and other studies have shown a parallel reduction in STF volume (12). In contrast, depletion of ES results in a significant increase in testicular IF volume (15, 16), a change that probably results from disruption of the normal pattern of vasomotion; thus, depletion of ES results in exaggeration of the periods of high testicular blood flow without compensatory changes in the alternating periods of low blood flow (5), a pattern that would be expected to increase the rate of IF formation (see Fig. 16.2).

It is not known how ESs exert their modulatory effects on the fluid dynamics of the testis, but it is clearly not by modulation of testosterone levels (see references cited above). It seems most likely that the ESs exert their effect via the Sertoli cells, either by directly altering STF formation or by altering vasomotion by the release of one or more vasoactive factors by the Sertoli cells. It is also possible, although less likely, that the ESs release vasoactive factors themselves that are subsequently resorbed from the rete testis into the bloodstream and are eventually circulated back to the testis to exert specific effects on the vasculature (see below).

Resorption of Testicular Fluids and Their Regulation

Testicular IF is returned to the bloodstream either via the lymphatic system or by resorption into venules within the testis. The latter process has not been studied in detail but is clearly a passive event that is influenced by a variety of factors such as vasomotion, oncotic pressure, etc. (17). The majority of STF is also resorbed, as can be judged by the dramatic increase in protein and sperm concentration that occurs during the passage of this fluid from the rete testis to the head of the epididymis (Fig. 16.6). Traditionally, it has been considered that this resorption occurs in the efferent ducts and in the head of the epididymis (2), but the epithelial cells of the rete testis exhibit classic cytological features of cells involved in both absorptive and bulk fluid endocytosis (18). Surrounding or overlying the rete testis is a major venous plexus, termed the *mediastinal venous plexus* (MVP). The close apposition of this plexus to the rete raises the possibility that fluid is absorbed from the rete into the bloodstream via the MVP. Evidence to support this possibility comes from our unpublished finding that administration of a chemical that reduces blood flow through the MVP results rapidly in distention of the rete testis and seminiferous tubules due to the

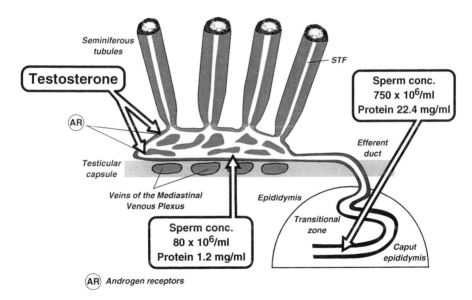

FIGURE 16.6. Diagrammatic representation of the anatomical relationship between the rete testis and the overlying mediastinal venous plexus in the adult rat testis. Resorption of fluid from the rete testis into this plexus is thought to occur, as well as from the efferent ducts and the head of the epididymis. This accounts for the indicated increase in sperm and protein concentration.

accumulation of STF. This appears to suggest that the rete is an important site of resorption of STF, although there are earlier studies that would not support this contention (19). However, if the rete is a site of fluid resorption, an important question is, What normally regulates this process? In the epididymis, testosterone has been shown to regulate fluid resorption (20), and the abundant immunoexpression of androgen receptors in the nuclei of rete epithelial cells (Fig. 16.7) is consistent with a similar role for testosterone in regulating fluid resorption from the rete testis. That spermatozoa might also influence fluid resorption in this area, analogous to the role of elongate spermatids in regulating the formation of IF and STF within the testis, is an intriguing but unexplored possibility.

Transport Role of the Mediastinal Venous Plexus

As indicated above, the MVP may play a role in resorption of fluid from the rete testis, but there is good evidence that it may also be involved in the transport of specific molecules from rete testis fluid to the bloodstream. One such molecule is α-inhibin, which is secreted by the Sertoli cells. Measurement of α-inhibin levels in venous blood collected before passage through the MVP and comparison with the levels in blood collected at the top of the spermatic cord show an increase in α-inhibin levels, due to its resorption from rete testis fluid (Fig. 16.8) (21). This increase is all the more

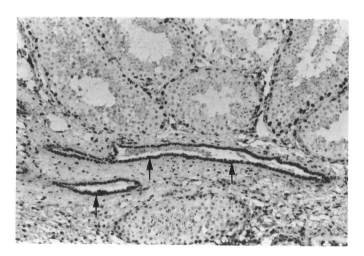

FIGURE 16.7. Immunolocalization of androgen receptors (arrows) in the nuclei of rete epithelial cells in the ram testis. Note that in this species, the rete testis lies within the body of the testis rather than just under the tunica albuginea as in the rat. Note also the pronounced immunostaining in Sertoli cell nuclei in neighboring seminiferous tubules. Magnification ×90.

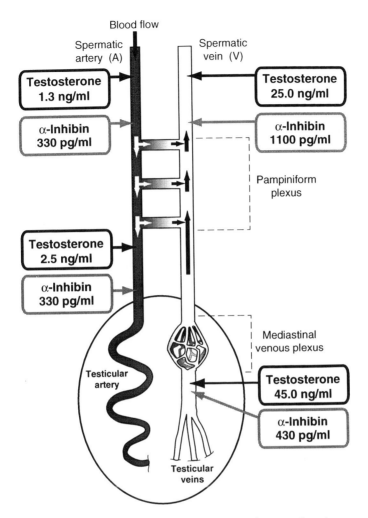

FIGURE 16.8. Diagrammatic representation of the major vascular elements of the adult rat testis. Note the differences in blood levels of testosterone and α-inhibin, according to where the blood sample is obtained (see text for explanation). Note also the anastomoses between the spermatic artery and vein within the pampiniform plexus.

remarkable when it is compared with what happens to testosterone levels, which decrease by around 40% (Fig. 16.8) (22). The latter change is due to the dilution of outgoing testicular venous blood by incoming arterial blood, which is shunted across the *arteriovenous* (A-V) anastomoses in the pampiniform plexus (Fig. 16.8). This shunting of arterial blood probably facilitates countercurrent heat exchange and may aid in reducing the pulsatility and pressure of incoming arterial blood to the testis, factors that may be important in the control of IF formation and resorption in the testis (2, 17). It is presumed that molecules other than α-inhibin, originating from either the Sertoli or germ cells, may also be resorbed selectively from the rete testis into blood (18) and may have effects on the vasculature of the testis or spermatic cord or perhaps at other sites in the body.

Conclusion

This brief overview has outlined what is known about the regulation of the major transport systems of the testis. All molecules that enter or leave the testis or move between cells within the testis must utilize one or more of these transport systems. In view of the critical dependence of normal testicular function on the successful working of these transport highways, it is essential that they are closely regulated and balanced. It is therefore not surprising that testosterone and elongate spermatids, the two principal products of the testis, are the key factors involved in this regulation. However, perhaps the most remarkable thing about these transport systems is how little they have been studied. In an age when in vitro studies predominate, it is worth remembering that these transport systems can only be studied in vivo. Moreover, nearly all in vitro experiments are static and thus do not model the in vivo situation, where all extracellular fluids are in constant movement. Disorder of any aspect of the transport highways, whether vasomotion, IF formation, or STF production and resorption, will have major adverse consequences, and it may well prove that many cases of male subfertility have their origins in such disorders. They therefore merit considerably more research interest than is the case currently.

References

1. Fawcett DW, Neaves WB, Flores MM. Comparative observations on the intertubular lymphatics and the organization of the interstitial tissue of the mammalian testis. Biol Reprod 1973;9:500–32.
2. Setchell BP, Maddocks S, Brooks DE. Anatomy, vasculature, innervation and fluids of the male reproductive tract. In: Knobil E, Neill JD, eds. The physiology of reproduction, 2nd ed. New York: Raven Press, 1994:1063–175.
3. Sylvester SR, Griswold MD. Molecular biology of iron transport in the testis. In: de Kretser DM, ed. Molecular biology of the male reproductive system. New York: Academic Press, 1993:311–26.
4. Damber J-E, Maddocks S, Widmark A, Bergh A. Testicular blood flow and vasomotion can be maintained by testosterone in Leydig cell-depleted rats. Int J Androl 1992;15:385–93.
5. Collin O, Bergh A, Damber J-E, Widmark A. Control of testicular vasomotion by testosterone and tubular factors in rats. J Reprod Fertil 1993;97:115–21.
6. Bergh A, Damber J-E. Vascular controls in testicular physiology. In: de Kretser

DM, ed. Molecular biology of the male reproductive system. New York: Academic Press, 1993:439–68.

7. Sharpe RM, Maddocks S, Millar MR, Saunders PTK, Kerr JB, McKinnell C. Testosterone and spermatogenesis: identification of stage-dependent, androgen-regulated proteins secreted by adult rat seminiferous tubules. J Androl 1992;13:172–84.

8. Sharpe RM, Kerr JB, McKinnell C, Millar MR. Temporal relationship between androgen-dependent changes in the volume of seminiferous tubule fluid, lumen size and seminiferous tubule protein secretion in rats. J Reprod Fertil 1994;101:193–8.

9. Jégou B, Le Gac F, Irby DC, de Kretser DM. Studies on seminiferous tubule fluid production in the adult rat: effect of hypophysectomy and treatment with FSH, LH and testosterone. Int J Androl 1983;6:249–60.

10. Wing T-Y, Christensen AK. Morphometric studies on rat seminiferous tubules. Am J Anat 1982;165:13–25.

11. Sharpe RM. Possible role of elongated spermatids in control of stage-dependent changes in the diameter of the lumen of the rat seminiferous tubule. J Androl 1989;10:304–10.

12. Sharpe RM. Regulation of spermatogenesis. In: Knobil E, Neill JD, eds. The physiology of reproduction, 2nd ed. New York: Raven Press, 1994:1363–434.

13. Sharpe RM, McKinnell C, McLaren TT, Millar MR, West AP, Maguire S, et al. Interactions between androgens, Sertoli cells and germ cells in the control of spermatogenesis. In: Verhoeven G, Habenicht U-F, eds. Molecular and cellular endocrinology of the testis: Ernst Schering Research Foundation Workshop, Supplement 1. Berlin: Springer-Verlag, 1994:115–42.

14. Bremner WJ, Millar MR, Sharpe RM, Saunders PTK. Immunohistochemical localization of androgen receptors in the rat testis: evidence for stage-dependent expression and regulation by androgens. Endocrinology 1994;135:1227–34.

15. Jégou B, Laws AO, de Kretser DM. Changes in testicular function induced by short-term exposure of the rat testis to heat: further evidence of interaction of germ cells, Sertoli cells and Leydig cells. Int J Androl 1984;7:244–57.

16. Sharpe RM, Bartlett JMS, Allenby G. Evidence for the control of testicular interstitial fluid volume in the rat by specific germ cell types. J Endocrinol 1991;128:359–67.

17. Sweeney T, Rozum JS, Desjardins C, Gore RW. Microvascular pressure distribution in the hamster testis. Am J Physiol 1991;260:H1581–9.

18. Morales C, Hermo L, Clermont Y. Endocytosis in epithelial cells lining the rete testis of the rat. Anat Rec 1984;209:185–95.

19. Dym M. The mammalian rete testis—a morphological examination. Anat Rec 1976;186:493–524.

20. Wong PYD, Yeung CH. Hormonal regulation of fluid reabsorption in isolated rat cauda epididymidis. Endocrinology 1977;101:1391–7.

21. Maddocks S, Sharpe RM. The route of secretion of inhibin from the rat testis. J Endocrinol 1989;120:R5–R8.

22. Maddocks S, Hargreave TB, Reddie K, Fraser HM, Kerr JB, Sharpe RM. Intratesticular hormone levels and the route of secretion of hormones from the testis of the rat, guinea pig, monkey and human. Int J Androl 1993;16:272–8.

Part V

Cell and Molecular Biology
of the Leydig Cell

17

Hormonal Regulation of the Differentiation of Leydig Cells from Mesenchymal-Like Progenitors During Puberty

Li-Xin Shan, Hui-Bao Gao, and Matthew P. Hardy

Adult Leydig cells originate within the testis postnatally. They form through a continuum of intermediate stages in which precursor cells gradually transform into more mature cells during puberty. Development of adult Leydig cells is achieved by proliferation, morphological differentiation, and acquisition of the capacity for testosterone production. Analysis of the developmental process was facilitated by the identification of three separate stages of the differentiating Leydig cell: progenitor, immature, and adult (1–3). Recognition of the distinct properties of the three stages has led to a new understanding of the hormonal control of Leydig cell differentiation. It is now clear that differentiation results from the interplay of hormonal factors, their concentrations, and the nature of the responses in each targeted Leydig cell stage. This chapter focuses on these issues, emphasizing studies of pubertal differentiation of Leydig cells in the rat.

A Three-Stage Model of Leydig Cell Differentiation

Leydig Cell Progenitors (Days 14 to 28)

The ultimate beginning of the Leydig cell lineage is a primitive stem cell. The embryonic origin of the stem cell remains unclear, although mesonephrogenic mesenchyme (4) and neuroectoderm (5) are the most likely sources. The stem cells proliferate in the interstitium neonatally and become committed to the Leydig cell lineage by day 14 postpartum. Progenitor cells result from the commitment of the stem cells and are recognizable members of the Leydig cell lineage because they express specific markers, such as *luteinizing hormone* (LH) receptor and *3β-hydroxysteroid dehydrogenase* (3β-HSD) histochemical activity, and produce low levels of androgen. Morphologically, however, the progenitor cell retains the features of a mesenchymal-like stem cell, having a spindle shape and possessing little smooth *endoplasmic reticulum* (ER).

Immature Leydig Cells (Days 28 to 56)

Leydig cell progenitors undergo morphological differentiation during days 14–28, transforming into immature Leydig cells. In contrast to progenitors, immature Leydig cells are round, have numerous lipid droplets, and possess an abundant smooth ER that contains the steroidogenic enzymes. The levels of 3β-HSD (6–8), cholesterol-side-chain-cleavage enzyme (P-450scc) (9), and 17α-hydroxylase (9) increase in tandem with the expansion of the smooth ER. Increased testosterone production, however, depends not only on higher levels of androgen biosynthetic enzyme activity, but also on a decline in testosterone metabolizing enzymes (10, 11). Metabolism predominates during the immature stage and androstane-3α,17β-diol, rather than testosterone, is the predominant androgen produced because of high activity levels of 3α-hydroxysteroid dehydrogenase (3α-HSD) (9) and 5α-reductase (8). The developmental trends of these enzymes are reflected by their steady-state *messenger RNA* (mRNA) levels in whole testis. Examples of these trends are seen in Figure 17.1: P-450scc mRNA rises dramatically with sexual maturity (on day 90), while 3α-HSD peaks during puberty and is lower in the adult.

Adult Leydig Cells (Day 56 Onward)

Adult Leydig cells arise from the immature stage by day 56 postpartum. As a consequence of higher androgen biosynthetic enzyme activities and declines in 3α-HSD and 5α-reductase, the capacity for testosterone production by adult Leydig cells is 5 times higher than that of immature cells (9). Adult Leydig cells also possess few lipid droplets and rarely divide, but they can be regenerated if destroyed. A single injection of 75 mg/kg of *ethane dimethane sulfonate* (EDS) kills all adult Leydig cells, which are completely regenerated within 7 weeks. The regeneration is dependent on the continued existence of Leydig stem cells in the interstitium (12–15).

Hormonal Regulation of Leydig Cell Differentiation

The biosynthetic pathways leading to the synthesis and metabolism of testosterone in adult Leydig cells have been delineated (16), but how these pathways are established in Leydig cells during differentiation remains unclear. The genes for the steroid biosynthesis (17, 18) and metabolism (19,

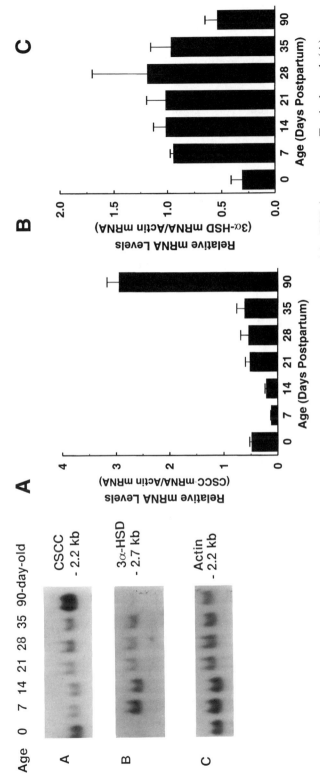

FIGURE 17.1. Age-dependent developmental changes in the levels of mRNAs for P-450scc and 3α-HSD in rat testes. Testicular poly(A) RNA samples (12 μg/lane) were isolated from rats on days 0, 7, 14, 21, 28, 35, and 90, fractionated on a formaldehyde denatured agarose gel, transferred to a nitrocellulose filter and hybridized to [32P]cDNA probes for P-450scc, 3α-HSD, and actin in succession. The intensities of mRNA signals for P-450scc (A) and 3α-HSD (B) were measured and normalized to those of actin mRNA (C). The developmental changes of relative mRNA levels for P-450scc (CSCC) and 3α-HSD are plotted in A and B, respectively, which summarize results from three replicate preparations of poly(A) RNA. In A, the P-450scc mRNA level at day 90 was higher than day 0 through day 35. In B, the 3α-HSD mRNA level at day 7 through day 35 were higher than both day 0 and day 90, with significantly different at P < 0.05.

20) have been sequenced, as have the genes for LH (21) and androgen (22) receptors. It will now be possible to study the development of androgen biosynthesis with these tools. One of the more rapidly advancing topics of the last few years is paracrine and autocrine control of testicular function, and of Leydig cells in particular. This section summarizes the effects of LH, androgen, glucocorticoid, and estradiol on Leydig cell differentiation.

Luteinizing Hormone

Luteinizing hormone (LH) is indispensable for Leydig cell function because it is the principal agonist of testosterone secretion (23, 24). LH exerts a variety of effects on adult Leydig cells, such as stimulating the formation of smooth endoplasmic reticulum (25) and increasing steroidogenic enzyme activities (26, 27). However, the role of LH in pubertal differentiation of Leydig cells in the rat has been uncertain because, unlike *follicle-stimulating hormone* (FSH), serum LH levels do not rise sharply with the onset of puberty (28). LH might act by increasing the expression of its own receptor in Leydig cell development (29). Progenitor cells possess a low but significant number of LH receptors, and that number increases during the course of their differentiation into immature Leydig cells (30). Long-term deprivation of LH in adult rats causes rapid and progressive decreases in adult Leydig cell volume, but does not dramatically lower their numbers (31). This demonstrates that adult Leydig cell number is far less dependent on LH than is cell volume. When endogenous secretion of both LH and androgen is suppressed by an *LH-releasing hormone* (LHRH) antagonist (32, 33), treatment with exogenous LH restores Leydig cell structure and function. It has been shown in the immature rat that the restorative actions of LH are due in part to increased *messenger RNA* (mRNA) levels for LH and androgen receptors in Leydig cell progenitors (34). LH is probably not critical for early proliferative activity of Leydig cells, but it is required for subsequent differentiation of these cells (35, 36).

Androgen

That LH is not the only hormone to have a role in the formative stages of the Leydig cell is unremarkable. Indeed, there are four to six potential agonists of increased testosterone production by Leydig cells listed in recent reviews (37, 38). One indication that LH cannot be the only factor regulating Leydig cell differentiation was seen in rats that are transiently hypothyroid during the neonatal period. Although serum LH is permanently suppressed in these animals, causing adult Leydig cells to be hypofunctional, they are still able to differentiate (39). Androgen receptor mRNA has been shown to be present in the cytoplasm of immature Leydig cells by in situ hybridization (Fig. 17.2). The levels of androgen receptor

FIGURE 17.2. Localization of androgen receptor mRNA in Leydig cells
by in situ hybridization. A frozen
testicular section from a 35-day-old
rat was hybridized to a fluorescein-
labeled androgen receptor antisense
probe, and mRNA for androgen receptor was detected in cytoplasm of
immature Leydig cells (ILC) and Sertoli cells (SC).

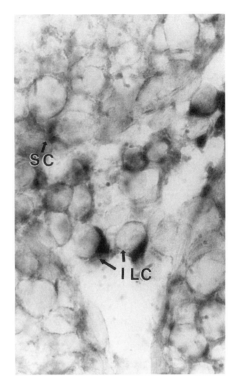

mRNA and protein are highest in immature Leydig cells and lower in adult
cells (30). The trends in the levels of androgen receptors suggest that
differentiating Leydig cells are highly sensitive to androgen and less sensitive when mature. The presence of androgen receptors in Leydig cells
indicates that androgen might act as an autocrine regulator (40–43). The
hypothesis that androgens facilitate Leydig cell differentiation in conjunction with LH is based on the fact that Leydig cell progenitors possess few
LH receptors (30) and are relatively insensitive to LH (44). Because androgen receptors outnumber LH receptors in Leydig cell progenitors, it is
possible that a requirement for androgen precedes LH-mediated events of
Leydig cell differentiation.

Several lines of evidence indicate that androgen promotes the differentiation of Leydig cells. Leydig cells of *testicular-feminized male* (Tfm) mice
and rats lack functional androgen receptors and have fewer LH receptors
than normal (45). These deficiencies in the Tfm Leydig cell probably result
from lack of androgen stimulation of progenitor cells because androgen is
necessary for the normal induction of LH receptors in Leydig cells (34, 46,
47). The Tfm mouse Leydig cell has a severely reduced capacity for testosterone production because its 17α-hydroxylase and 17-ketosteroid reductase activities are markedly lower than those of Leydig cells possessing

functional androgen receptors. This suggests that these enzymes may require androgen-receptor–mediated stimulation during development to be expressed at normal levels (48, 49).

In vivo studies of LHRH antagonists also indicate that androgen regulates Leydig cell differentiation. Testosterone replacement in LHRH antagonist-treated immature rats restored serum testosterone to normal levels and caused Leydig cell nuclei to become round, mimicking the pubertal change of Leydig cell nuclear shape in untreated animals during the transition from progenitor to immature cells (49). As with the Tfm mouse (45), testosterone replacement in the LHRH antagonist-treated animal increases the steady-state mRNA levels for LH receptors (34).

In an in vitro study, Leydig cell progenitors, when cultured for 3 days in the presence of LH plus *dihydrotestosterone* (DHT), increased their capacity for testosterone production more than 10-fold (40). Testosterone and DHT are both effective agonists of androgen-receptor–mediated action (50). This explains why suppression of 5α-reductase, which prevents the conversion of testosterone to DHT, did not affect testosterone production by Leydig cell progenitors in vitro (51). These findings are consistent with the hypothesis that action of androgen is required for differentiation of Leydig cell progenitors into immature Leydig cells.

Glucocorticoid

In all known animal species, prolonged increases in glucocorticoid secretion caused by stress and disease are accompanied by decreased testosterone production and subsequent inhibition of spermatogenesis. Glucocorticoids are known to be potent inhibitors of testosterone production, decreasing the constitutive and *adenasine 3':5'-cyclic monophosphate* (cAMP)-induced synthesis of P-450scc (52) and, 17α-hydroxylase (53). A direct action of glucocorticoid on testosterone production, independent of the hypothalamic-pituitary axis, is supported by the fact that Leydig cells possess a significant number of glucocorticoid receptors (54). The Leydig cell is not simply a target for glucocorticoids, but can oppose their action through oxidative inactivation to forms that are incapable of binding to the glucocorticoid receptor. The reaction is catalyzed by 11β-hydroxysteroid dehydrogenase (11β-HSD), which is absent from differentiating Leydig cells prior to day 25 postpartum and is most abundant in the adult Leydig cell (55). This observation indicates that the pubertal rise in testosterone production may be governed in part by a progressive decline in glucocorticoid-mediated inhibition. Consistent with this hypothesis, Leydig cells from adult adrenalectomized rats possessed an increased capacity for testosterone production (Gao et al., unpublished data). Whether levels of 11β-HSD in the Leydig cell are regulated by LH and/or androgen remains to be studied. Glucocorticoid action is probably required to maintain 11β-HSD

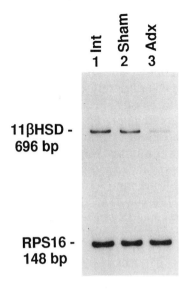

FIGURE 17.3. Detection of 11β-HSD mRNA in adult Leydig cells. Total RNA (2.5 μg) was used as a template for reverse transcription. Specific mRNAs were detected with their corresponding oligonucleotide primers after amplification by polymerase chain reaction. 11β-HSD (lane 3) in Leydig cells 7 days after adrenalectomy was lower compared to intact (lane 1) and sham-adrenalectomy (lane 2). Ribosomal protein S16 (RPS16), the internal control, was unchanged.

because an analysis of 11β-HSD mRNA (Fig. 17.3) showed that 11β-HSD mRNA levels were lower in Leydig cells after adrenalectomy compared with either intact or sham-adrenalectomy.

Estradiol

Sertoli cells are the main site of FSH binding in the testis (56), and an effect of FSH on Leydig cell differentiation is therefore mediated indirectly by Sertoli cell paracrine factors. There are certain to be paracrine signals that negatively regulate the proliferation of Leydig cells, delaying their increase in number until it is developmentally appropriate. In the immature rat, FSH stimulates the Sertoli cell to produce a protein that increases aromatase activity in Leydig cells, thereby raising the local concentration of estradiol (57, 58). Estradiol may be one of the negative regulators of Leydig cell development (59, 60). This hypothesis is dramatically supported by the observation that adult Leydig cells do not develop in rats that receive a single injection of estradiol on day 5 postpartum (61). Regeneration of adult Leydig cells following treatment with EDS is also prevented by estradiol (62). Autoradiographic studies of ³H-thymidine incorporation (63, 64) showed that estradiol inhibits Leydig cell proliferation. Unlike LH and androgen, estradiol reduces the number of LH receptors in Leydig cells (64, 65).

Suppression of endogenous levels of FSH in immature rats may facilitate the differentiation of Leydig cells by lowering estradiol. In agreement with this hypothesis, we found that anti-FSH caused a decline in testis weight but increased testosterone production by purified Leydig cell progenitors (Hardy et al., unpublished data). Estradiol production by progenitor cells was also significantly lower after anti-FSH treatment. These data are consistent with an estrogen-mediated inhibition of Leydig cell steroidogenic function (62, 66). Sertoli cells, therefore, may delay the acquisition of steroidogenic function in differentiating Leydig cells during puberty by producing a factor that increases Leydig cell aromatase activity, raising the local concentration of estradiol.

Summary

Approximately 25 million Leydig cells per testis produce the testosterone required for reproductive function in the adult male rat. Leydig cells are formed through a process of differentiation that involves three identifiable stages. The morphological and biochemical properties of the intermediate stages have been defined, providing a new understanding of the hormonal control of Leydig cell development. The first intermediate (stage 1) is a spindle-shaped Leydig cell progenitor. Leydig cell progenitor cells first differentiate from primitive stem cells in the interstitium by day 14 postpartum, and are numerous by day 21. Their differentiation is made evident by expression of low levels of Leydig cell specific proteins, such as LH receptor and 3β-HSD. The progenitor cells undergo morphological differentiation during days 14–28, transforming into immature Leydig cells (stage 2). Unlike progenitor cells, immature Leydig cells possess an abundant smooth ER providing a substratum for the steroidogenic enzymes. Although capable of steroidogenesis, immature Leydig cells produce low levels of testosterone and high levels of the 5α-reduced androgen, androstane-3α,17β-diol (from days 28 to 56). The maturation of immature Leydig cells into adult Leydig cells (stage 3) by day 56 is accompanied by increased expression of testosterone biosynthetic enzymes and decreased metabolism of testosterone by 5α-reductase and 3α-HSD. The three stages of the Leydig cell are regulated distinctly. Luteinizing hormone is required throughout differentiation, but is not the only stimulus required to induce the conversion of the Leydig cell progenitor into an immature Leydig cell. Recent studies indicate that androgen and estradiol are also involved in pubertal differentiation of the Leydig cell. We have found that progenitor cells possess high concentrations of androgen receptor and respond to androgen in vivo by increasing their steady-state levels of LH receptor and androgen receptor mRNAs. These results suggest that androgen facilitates the conversion of progenitor cells into immature Leydig cells. Suppression of endogenous FSH by treatment with anti-FSH antiserum during days 14–21 increased the capacity of Leydig cell progenitors to produce testosterone when isolated on day 21. The release of estradiol from progenitor cells declined following anti-FSH treatment. Therefore, estradiol, which is produced by Leydig cell progenitors under the influence of a Sertoli cell paracrine factor, may delay the acquisition of steroidogenic function by the differentiating Leydig cell.

Acknowledgments. The authors thank Dr. C. Wayne Bardin for support and intellectual encouragement during the course of these studies. We also thank Ms. Chantal Manon Sottas for skilled technical assistance. This work was supported in part by The Population Council and NIH Grant #1R29HD-32588.

References

1. Chemes HE, Rivarola MA, Bergada C. Effect of hCG on the interstitial cells and androgen production in the immature rat testis. J Reprod Fertil 1976;46:279–82.
2. Hardy MP, Nonneman D, Ganjam VK, Zirkin BR. Hormonal control of Leydig cell differentiation and mature function. In: Whitcomb RW, Zirkin BR, eds. Understanding male infertility: basic and clinical approaches. New York: Serono Symposia Publications from Raven Press 1993;98:125–42.
3. Teerds KJ, Veldhuizen-Tsoerkan MB, Rommerts FFG, de Rooij DG, Dorrington JH. Proliferation and differentiation of testicular interstitial cells: aspects of Leydig cell development in the (pre) pubertal and adult testis. In: Verhoeven G, Habenicht UF, eds. Molecular and cellular endocrinology of the testis. New York: Springer-Verlag, 1994:37–65.
4. Rodemer-Lenz E. On cell contribution to gonadal soma formation in quail-chick chimeras during the indifferent stage of gonadal development. Anat Embryol 1989;179:237–42.
5. Mayerhofer A, Seidl K, Lahr D, Bitter-Suermann D, Christoph A, Barthels D, Wille W, Gratz M. Leydig cells express neural cell adhesion molecules in vivo and in vitro. Biol Reprod 1992;47:656–64.
6. Haider SG, Passia D, Overmeyer G. Studies on the fetal and postnatal development of rat Leydig cells employing 3β-hydroxysteroid dehydrogenase activity. Acta Histochem 1986;32:197–202.
7. Dupont E, Luu-The V, Pelletieri G. Ontogeny of 3β-hydroxysteroid dehydrogenase $\Delta^{5,4}$ isomerase in rat testis as studied by immunocytochemistry. Anat Embryol 1993;187:583–9.
8. Murono EP. Maturational changes in steroidogenic enzyme activities metabolizing testosterone and dihydrotestosterone in two populations of testicular interstitial cells. Acta Endocrinol 1989;121:477–83.

9. Shan LX, Phillips DM, Bardin CW, Hardy MP. Differential regulation of steroidogenic enzymes during differentiation optimizes testosterone production by adult rat Leydig cells. Endocrinology 1993;133:2277–83.

10. Inano H, Hori Y, Tamaoki B. Effect of age on testicular enzymes related to steroid bioconversion. In: Wolstenholme GEW, O'Connor M, eds. Endocrinology of the testis. Boston: Little, Brown, 1967:105–19.

11. Steinberger E, Ficher M. Differentiation of steroid biosynthetic pathways in developing testes. Biol Reprod 1969;1:119–33.

12. Jackson AE, O'Leary PC, Ayers MM, de Kretser DM. The effects of ethylene dimethane sulphonate (EDS) on rat Leydig cells: evidence to support a connective tissue origin of Leydig cells. Biol Reprod 1986;35:425–37.

13. Morris ID, Phillips DM, Bardin CW. Ethylenedimethane sulfonate destroys Leydig cells in the rat testis. Endocrinology 1986;118:709–19.

14. Molenaar R, de Rooij DG, Rommerts FF, Reuvers PJ, van der Molen HJ. Specific destruction of Leydig cells in mature rats after in vivo administration of ethane dimethyl sulfonate. Biol Reprod 1985;33:1213–22.

15. Kerr JB, Donachie K, Rommerts FF. Selective destruction and regeneration of rat Leydig cells in vivo. A new method for the study of seminiferous tubular-interstitial tissue interaction. Cell Tissue Res 1985;242:145–56.

16. Hall PF. Testicular steroid synthesis: organization and regulation. In: Knobil E, Neill J, Greenwald GS, Markert CL, eds. The physiology of reproduction, vol. 1. New York: Raven Press, 1994:1335–62.

17. Rice DA, Kirkman MS, Aitken LD, Mouw AR, Schimmer BP, Parker KL. Analysis of the promoter region of the gene encoding mouse cholesterol side-chain cleavage enzyme. J Biol Chem 1990;265:11713–20.

18. Fevold HR, Lorence MC, McCarthy JL, Trant JM, Kagimoto M, Waterman MR, Mason JI. Rat P450-17α from testis: characterization of a full-length cDNA encoding a unique steroid hydroxylase capable of catalyzing both the Δ^4- and Δ^5-steroid-17,20-lyase reactions. Mol Endocrinol 1989;3:968–75.

19. Agarwal AK, Monder C, Eckstein B, White PC. Cloning and expression of rat cDNA encoding corticosteroid 11β-dehydrogenase. J Biol Chem 1989; 264:18939–43.

20. Pawlowski JE, Huizinga M, Penning TM. Cloning and sequencing of the cDNA for rat liver 3α-hydroxysteroid/dihydrodiol dehydrogenase. J Biol Chem 1991;266:8820–5.

21. McFarland KC, Sprengel R, Phillips HS, Köhler M, Rosemblit N, Nikolics K, Segaloff DL, Seeburg PH. Lutropin-choriogonadotropin receptor: an unusual member of the G protein-coupled receptor family. Science 1989;245:494–9.

22. Chang C, Kokontis J, Liao S. Structural analysis of complementary DNA and amino acid sequences of human and rat androgen receptors. Proc Natl Acad Sci USA 1988;85:7211–5.

23. Purvis K, Hansson V. Hormonal regulation of Leydig cell function. Mol Cell Endocrinol 1978;12:123–38.

24. Pakarinen P, Vihko KK, Voutilainen R, Huhtaniemi IT. Differential response of luteinizing hormone receptor and steroidogenic enzyme gene expression to human chorionic gonadotropin stimulation in the neonatal and adult rat testis. Endocrinology 1990;127:2469–74.

25. Ewing LL, Zirkin BR. Leydig cell structure and steroidogenic function. Recent Prog Horm Res 1983;39:599–632.

26. Keeney DS, Mason JI. Expression of testicular 3β-hydroxysteroid dehydrogenase/Δ^{5,4}-isomerase: regulation by luteinizing hormone and forskolin in Leydig cells of adult rats. Endocrinology 1992;130:2007–15.
27. Payne AH. Hormonal regulation of cytochrome P450 enzymes, cholesterol side-chain cleavage and 17α-hydroxylase/C17-20 lyase in Leydig cells. Biol Reprod 1990;42:399–404.
28. Dohler KD, Wuttke W. Changes with age in levels of serum gonadotropins, prolactin and gonadal steroids in prepubertal male and female rats. Endocrinology 1975;97:898–907.
29. Huhtaniemi IT, Warren DW, Catt KJ. Functional maturation of rat testis Leydig cells. Ann NY Acad Sci 1984;438:283–303.
30. Shan LX, Hardy MP. Developmental changes in levels of luteinizing hormone receptor and androgen receptor in rat Leydig cells. Endocrinology 1992; 131:1107–14.
31. Keeney DS, Mendis-Handagama SM, Zirkin BR, Ewing LL. Effect of long term deprivation of luteinizing hormone on Leydig cell volume, Leydig cell number, and steroidogenic capacity of the rat testis. Endocrinology 1988;123: 2906–15.
32. Misro MM, Ganguly A, Das RP. GnRH antagonist treatment affects nuclear size and membrane associated indentations in rat Leydig cells. Arch Androl 1991;27:25–33.
33. Huhtaniemi IT, Nikula H, Detta A, Stewart JM, Clayton RN. Blockade of rat testicular gonadotropin releasing hormone (GnRH) receptors by infusion of a GnRH antagonist has no major effects on Leydig cell function in vivo. Mol Cell Endocrinol 1987;49:89–97.
34. Shan LX, Hardy DO, Catterall JF, Hardy MP. Effects of luteinizing hormone (LH) and androgen on steady state levels of messenger ribonucleic acid for LH receptors, androgen receptors, and steroidogenic enzymes in rat Leydig cell progenitors in vivo. Endocrinology 1995;136:1686–93.
35. Teerds KJ, Rooij DG, Rommerts FFG, Hurk RVD, Wensing CJG. Proliferation and differentiation of possible Leydig cell precursors after destruction of the existing Leydig cells with ethane dimethyl sulphonate: the role of LH/hCG. J Endocrinol 1989;122:689–96.
36. Savage GN, Kerr JB. Effect of seminiferous tubule size on hCG-induced regeneration of peritubular Leydig cells in hypophysectomized, EDS-treated rats. Int J Androl 1995;18:35–44.
37. Saez JM. Leydig cells: endocrine, paracrine, and autocrine regulation. Endocr Rev 1994;15:574–626.
38. Skinner MK. Cell-cell interactions in the testis. Endocr Rev 1991;12:45–77.
39. Hardy MP, Kirby JD, Hess RA, Cooke PS. Leydig cell increase their numbers but decline in steroidogenic function in the adult rat after neonatal hypothyroidism. Endocrinology 1993;132:2417–20.
40. Hardy MP, Kelce WR, Klinefelter GR, Ewing LL. Differentiation of Leydig cell precursors in vitro: a role for androgen. Endocrinology 1990;127:488–90.
41. Sar M, Lubahn DB, French FS, Wilson EM. Immunohistochemical localization of the androgen receptor in rat and human tissues. Endocrinology 1990; 127:3180–6.
42. Bremner WJ, Millar MR, Sharpe RM, Saunders PTK. Immunohistochemical localization of androgen receptors in the rat testis: evidence for stage-

dependent expression and regulation by androgens. Endocrinology 1994; 135:1227–34.

43. Vornberger W, Prins G, Musto NA, Suarez-Quian CA. Androgen receptor distribution in rat testis: new implications for androgen regulation of spermatogenesis. Endocrinology 1994;134:2307–16.

44. Odell WD, Swerdloff RS, Bain J, Wollesen F, Grover PK. The effect of sexual maturation on testicular response to LH stimulation of testosterone secretion in the intact rat. Endocrinology 1974;95:1380–4.

45. Purvis K, Calandra R, Naess O, Attramadal A, Torjesen PA, Hansson V. Do androgens increase Leydig cell sensitivity to luteinising hormone? Nature 1977;265:169–70.

46. Bardin CW, Bullock LP, Sherins RJ, Mowszowicz I, Blackburn WR. Part II. Androgen metabolism and mechanism of action in male pseudohermaphroditism: a study of testicular feminization. Recent Prog Horm Res 1973;29:65–110.

47. Murphy L, O'Shaughnessy PJ. Testicular steroidogenesis in the testicular feminized (Tfm) mouse: loss of 17α-hydroxylase activity. J Endocrinol 1991; 131:443–9.

48. Murphy L, Jeffcoate IA, O'Shaughnessy PJ. Abnormal Leydig cell development at puberty in the androgen-resistant Tfm mouse. Endocrinology 1994;135:1372–7.

49. Misro MM, Ganguly A, Das RP. Is testosterone essential for maintenance of normal morphology in immature rat Leydig cells. Int J Androl 1993;16:221–6.

50. Deslypere JP, Young M, Wilson JD, McPhaul MJ. Testosterone and 5α-dihydrotestosterone interact differently with the androgen receptor to enhance transcription of the MMTV-CAT reporter gene. Mol Cell Endocrinol 1992;88:15–22.

51. Murono EP, Washburn AL, Goforth DP. Enhanced stimulation of 5α-reductase activity in cultured Leydig cell precursors by human chorionic gonadotropin. J Steroid Biochem 1994;48:377–84.

52. Hales DB, Payne AH. Glucocorticoid mediated repression of P450scc mRNA and de novo synthesis in cultured Leydig cells. Endocrinology 1984;124:2089–104.

53. Bambino TH, Hsueh AJW. Direct inhibitory effect of glucocorticoids upon testicular luteinizing hormone receptor and steroidogenesis in vivo and in vitro. Endocrinology 1981;108:2142–8.

54. Welsh TH, Bambino TH, Hsuch AJW. Mechanism of glucocorticoid-induced suppression of testicular androgen biosynthesis in vitro. Biol Reprod 1982;27:1138–46.

55. Phillips DM, Lakshami V, Monder C. Corticosteroid 11β-dehydrogenase in rat testis. Endocrinology 1989;125:209–16.

56. Bardin CW, Cheng CY, Musto NA, Gunsalus GL. The Sertoli cell. In: Knobil E, Neill JD, Greenwald GS, Markert CL, eds. The physiology of reproduction, vol. 1. New York: Raven Press, 1994:1291–333.

57. Canick JA, Makris A, Gunsalus GL, Ryan KJ. Testicular aromatization in immature rats: localization and stimulation after gonadotropin administration in vivo. Endocrinology 1979;104:285–8.

58. Valladares LE, Payne AH. Effects of hCG and cyclic AMP on aromatization in purified Leydig cells of immature and mature rats. Biol Reprod 1981;25:752–8.

59. Jégou B, Sharpe RM. Paracrine mechanisms in testicular control. In: de Kretser D, ed. Molecular biology of the male reproductive system. New York: Academic Press, 1993:271–310.
60. Sharpe RM. Experimental evidence for Sertoli-germ cell and Sertoli-Leydig cell interactions. In: Russell LD, Griswold MD, eds. The Sertoli cell. Clearwater, FL: Cache River Press, 1993:392–418.
61. Dhar JD, Setty BS. Epididymal response to exogenous testosterone in rats sterilized neonatally by estrogen. Endokrinologie 1976;68:14–21.
62. Abney TO, Myers RB. 17β-estradiol inhibition of Leydig cell regeneration in the ethane dimethylsulfate-treated mature rat. J Androl 1991;12:295–304.
63. Abney TO, Carswell LS. Gonadotropin regulation of Leydig cell DNA synthesis. Mol Cell Endocrinol 1986;45:157–65.
64. Saez JM, Haour F, Loras B, Sanchez P, Cathiard AM. Oestrogen induced Leydig cell refractoriness to gonadotrophin stimulation. Acta Endocrinol 1978;89:379–92.
65. Katikineni M, Davies TF, Huhtaniemi IT, Catt KJ. Luteinizing hormone-receptor interaction in the testis: progressive decrease in reversibility of the hormone-receptor complex. Endocrinology 1980;107:1980–8.
66. Papadopoulos V, Kamtchouing P, Drosdowsky MA, Carreau S. Spent media from immature seminiferous tubules and Sertoli cells inhibit adult rat Leydig cell aromatase activity. Horm Metab Res 1987;19:62–4.

18

Developmental and cAMP-Dependent Regulation of *CYP*17 Gene Expression

MICHAEL R. WATERMAN AND DIANE S. KEENEY

17α-Hydroxylase/17,20 lyase cytochrome P-450 (P-450c17), product of the *CYP*17 gene (1), serves as the key crossroad enzyme in steroidogenic pathways. It is a crossroad enzyme because of its ability to catalyze two separate reactions. In the glucocorticoid biosynthetic pathway leading from cholesterol to cortisol, P-450c17 catalyzes the conversion of pregnenolone or progesterone to their 17α-hydroxy forms, 17α-hydroxypregnenolone and 17α-hydroxyprogesterone. In the sex hormone biosynthetic pathways leading from cholesterol to testosterone and estrogen, P-450c17 also catalyzes the 17,20-lyase reaction, converting these 17α-hydroxylated C21 steroids to their respective C19 androgens, dehydroepiandrosterone and androstenedione. Thus, in the adrenal cortex, where cortisol is produced, the 17α-hydroxylase activity associated with P-450c17 is most important, while in the gonads, where sex hormones are produced, both activities are important (Fig. 18.1).

P-450c17 is a typical microsomal form of cytochrome P-450 (2). The human enzyme contains 508 amino acids (3) and a single heme group, and requires the ubiquitous microsomal flavoprotein *reduced nicotinamide adenine dinucleotide phosphate* (NADPH)-cytochrome P-450 reductase to transfer electrons from NADPH to the P-450c17 heme. The enzyme is anchored in the endoplasmic reticulum by a hydrophobic amino terminal sequence (4) and is synthesized through the signal recognition particle pathway. In the adrenal cortex, both C21 17α-hydroxysteroids that serve as intermediates in cortisol biosynthesis and C19 androgens (dehydroepiandrosterone and androstenedione) are produced. This suggests that the products of the P-450c17 17α-hydroxylase activity leave the active site and that some fraction of these 17α-hydroxy steroids rebind in a new configuration in the same active site for the 17,20-lyase activity to occur (5). Since P-450c17 expressed in testis and ovary is identical to that in the

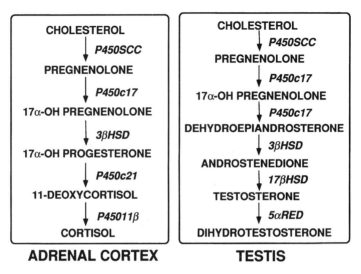

FIGURE 18.1. Steroidogenic pathways for biosynthesis of cortisol in the adrenal cortex and testosterone in the testis.

adrenal cortex, it is presumed that the same catalytic mechanism is followed, even though no cortisol is produced in the gonads. Thus, 17α-hydroxylase is the primary P-450c17 activity associated with steroidogenesis in the adrenal cortex because the majority of the products of this reaction are swept into the cortisol biosynthetic pathway. 17,20-Lyase is the primary P-450c17 activity associated with steroidogenesis in the testis and ovary because there is no other pathway to utilize 17α-hydroxysteroids.

While the emphasis in this chapter is on P-450c17 in the testis and its role in testosterone production, the major body of work on *CYP*17 and P-450c17 has been carried out in adrenal cells. Out of necessity, then, this chapter describes results obtained with both steroidogenic systems in order to provide a detailed view of regulation of *CYP*17 expression and P-450c17 activity.

Developmental Expression of *CYP*17

The essential role of *CYP*17 expression during fetal development is graphically evident from studies of the rare form of congenital adrenal hyperplasia in humans, 17α-hydroxylase/17,20-lyase deficiency. This defect has been found to be a result of genetic mutations in the coding region of the *CYP*17 gene leading to faulty forms of P-450c17 having little or no activity (6). In the case of the male genotype (46XY), development of male secondary sex characteristics, which identify the male phenotype, is either blocked or altered. In the case of a complete block, the external genitalia are female, while in the case of reduced activity the external genitalia are sometimes ambiguous. Thus, the ability of the fetal testis to produce testosterone early in fetal life is crucial in maintaining the reproductive capacity of all mammalian species. The developmental profile of expression of *CYP*17 has been examined in a few species, including human, cow, sheep, and rodents. In the human, *CYP*17 expression occurs relatively early in gestation and continues throughout fetal life in both the adrenal and testis (7). The physiological requirement for this expression is largely the demand for development of the male genital tract, without which reproduction cannot normally ensue.

Fetal steroidogenesis seems also to be important in other developmental paradigms. For example, adrenal glucocorticoids play a role in the functional differentiation of the adrenal medulla (8). However, it is not certain that P-450c17 is essential since one glucocorticoid, corticosterone, can be produced in its absence and might meet requirements for maturation events. In cows and sheep, *CYP*17 expression in the testis occurs early and persists throughout gestation. In the adrenal, however, *CYP*17 expression is on early in gestation, absent in the middle third of gestation, and back on during the latter third of gestation (9, 10). As will be described later, *CYP*17 expression during adult life relies heavily on the action of peptide hormones from the anterior pituitary that enhance intracellular levels of *adenosine 3':5'-cyclic monophosphate* (cAMP). During the period of absence of adrenal *CYP*17 expression in the bovine embryo, fetal production of *adrenocorticotropic hormone* (ACTH) is also absent, although it is observed both early and late in gestation (9). Probably the absence of adrenal *CYP*17 expression in the mid-trimester is due to the absence of ACTH in the fetal circulation. Thus, in the fetal cow and sheep, the absence of ACTH secretion, adrenal *CYP*17 expression, and cortisol production during a specific period in development must be important. On the other hand, *CYP*17 expression in the testis is important throughout gestation in these same species.

While *CYP*17 is expressed in the gonads for sex hormone biosynthesis, it is not expressed in the adrenal of adult rodents. Hence, in rodents corticosterone is the major glucocorticoid throughout life. However, during fetal life in the mouse, *Cyp*17 is expressed in the adrenal cortex, leading to an active enzyme and potential for cortisol biosynthesis (11). Expression seems limited to specific groups of cells in the adrenal cortex and disappears shortly after birth. Whether limited cortisol production is required in rodents during fetal life is not clear, but if so, this requirement is only transient.

Thus, the pattern of expression of *CYP*17 in the testis is consistent among species and begins quite early in gestation, at the time when the fetal testis is first discernible (12). In the adrenal cortex, however, considerable species variation in *CYP*17 expression is observed. It seems then that the physiological requirement for testosterone production in fetal life is important and invariant among species, whereas that for cortisol is species specific and far less profound than that for testosterone.

The developmental and tissue-specific regulation of *CYP*17 gene expression represents a very interesting problem. P-450c17 activity as noted above is necessary early in development, and therefore a regulatory system must exist for the timely onset of expression of this gene. However, *CYP*17 expression is limited to a few steroidogenic sites: adrenal cortex, testis, ovary, and placenta (in some species). Therefore, the developmental regulatory system should include a tissue-specific component. *CYP*17 expression is probably not limited to traditional steroidogenic cells, since it has recently been observed in rat stomach (13) and rat and mouse brain (14). Overall, however, expression in nonsteroidogenic tissues can be expected to be limited. It has recently been found that all steroid hydroxylase genes contain one or more copies of a DNA sequence near their promoters that binds to an orphan nuclear receptor (zinc-finger DNA-binding motif) called *steroidogenic factor-1* (SF-1) (15) or *Ad4-binding protein* (AD4BP) (16). As will be described elsewhere in this volume, SF-1 binds to a consensus DNA sequence (AGGTCA) and is expressed in mouse fetal adrenals and gonads prior to steroid hydroxylase *messenger RNA* (mRNA) (12). Further, SF-1 expression is limited to a relatively small number of cells in mice, including steroidogenic cells in adrenal, testis, and ovary. These observations have led to the hypothesis that SF-1 is important in both the developmental and tissue-specific regulation of *CYP*17 expression as well as that of the other steroid hydroxylase genes. The recent disruption of SF-1 gene expression (17) indicates a more profound role for this transcription factor, since the homozygous knockout mice have no adrenals or gonads. Nevertheless, it is reasonable to believe that in addition to its role in development of steroidogenic organs, SF-1 participates in signaling *CYP*17 expression.

The coupling of SF-1 and steroid hydroxylase expression is likely cause and effect. Nevertheless, SF-1 alone is not sufficient to regulate *CYP*17 gene expression. In the fetal mouse adrenal, P-450c17 mRNA is present in a limited set of cells and then disappears even though SF-1 is present. In the fetal bovine adrenal, where SF-1 has not yet been measured, *CYP*17 expression and fetal ACTH secretion are transiently turned off in mid-trimester at a time when SF-1 would be predicted to be present. Thus, while SF-1 may turn on the switch, other regulatory factors seem to be essential for continued expression during fetal and adult life. In the testis such factors must be present continuously from the first morphological appearance of the organ and throughout adult life.

cAMP-Dependent Regulation of *CYP*17 Expression

Peptide hormones from the anterior pituitary regulate both gene transcription and enzymatic activities of steroid hydroxylases. For example, ACTH in the adrenal cortex and *luteinizing hormone* (LH) in the testis bind to specific cell-surface receptors, activating adenylate cyclase and leading to elevated levels of intracellular cAMP. cAMP has two actions on steroidogenic cells that can be separated temporally (18). Acutely, cAMP activates the movement of cholesterol from lipid stores to the inner mitochondrial membrane in the vicinity of cholesterol *side-chain cleavage cytochrome P-450* (P-450scc) (19). This rapidly activates steroid hormone biosynthesis. Chronically, cAMP activates transcription of genes encoding steroid hydroxylases and related enzymes (20). This assures optimal steroidogenic capacity within steroidogenic organs so that steroid hormones can be produced on demand.

It has been known for more than 20 years that upon hypophysectomy, levels of steroid hydroxylases decline in testis and adrenal and can be restored by treatment of hypophysectomized animals with pharmacological doses of *human chorionic gonadotropin* (hCG) and ACTH, respectively (21, 22). Subsequently it has been shown that, in primary cultures of bovine adrenocortical cells, the chronic action of cAMP is at the transcriptional level (20). Promoter-bashing analysis of the 5′-flanking region of steroid hydroxylase genes including *CYP*17 has shown that different genes contain different *cAMP-response sequences* (CRSs) (23). The bovine *CYP*17 gene contains two CRS elements (24) shown in Table 18.1. Like other CRS elements in other steroid hydroxylase genes, these are distinct from the consensus cAMP response element CRE, which binds the transcription factor CREB and regulates cAMP-dependent transcription in a number of different genes (25). Experiments are now under way to purify the nuclear proteins (putative transcription factors) that bind to these CRS elements.

CRS2 in bovine *CYP*17 binds as many as three nuclear proteins (26). Included within this region are overlapping binding sites for SF-1 and the transcription factor COUP-TF1. Apparently these two proteins bind CRS-2 in a mutually exclusive manner. In vitro studies using cotransfection of an SF-1 expression plasmid and a CRS-2 reporter construct into nonsteroidogenic cells indicate that cAMP-dependent protein kinase stimulates SF-1–dependent transcription. Coexpression of COUP-TF1 partially blocks transcription in this system. Thus, the function of CRS-2 in cAMP-dependent *CYP*17 transcription is positively activated by SF-1 and negatively regulated by COUP-TF1.

TABLE 18.1. cAMP-responsive sequences in bovine *CYP*17.

	−243	−225
CRS-1	TTGATGGACAGTGAGCAAG	
	−76	−40
CRS-2	TGAGCATTAACATAAAGTCAAGGAGAAGGTCAGGGG	
CONSENSUS CRE	TGACGTCA	

The CRS-1 of bovine *CYP*17 also participates in the activation of cAMP-dependent transcription in steroidogenic cells, including mouse adrenal Y1 tumor cells, but does not mediate such transcription in nonsteroidogenic cells (27). Using an in vitro transcription assay, it has been found that addition of partially purified CRS-1–binding proteins from Y1 adrenal tumor cell nuclear extracts to an in vitro transcription system from nonsteroidogenic cells enhances transcription in this system previously inert to CRS-1–mediated expression (28). Purification of the CRS-1–binding proteins to homogeneity has revealed a complex of four proteins: a 60-kd protein, two 53-kd proteins, and a 43-kd protein (29). The 43-kd protein and one of the 53-kd proteins are members of the *PBX* gene family. These DNA-binding proteins contain a homeodomain (helix-turn-helix) DNA-binding motif and are present in most tissues, including steroidogenic cells. The other 53-kd protein and the 60-kd protein remain unknown. Cotransfection of an expression plasmid encoding *PBX* and a CRS-1–reporter gene construct shows enhanced cAMP-dependent transcription beyond that observed with endogenous *PBX* (29). Also, in a cell line such as HepG2 which does not express this *PBX*, a cotransfection experiment leads to a more profound increase in cAMP-dependent CRS-1–mediated transcription (30). These results indicate that *PBX* plays an important role in CRS-1–dependent *CYP*17 transcription. It is not yet clear, however, whether *PBX* is sufficient for this function. It is certainly possible that the unknown 60-kd protein is an obligatory partner for *PBX*-enhanced transcription.

Based on the concomitant loss of P-450c17 in bovine fetal adrenal and fetal ACTH secretion during the middle trimester (9) and the disappearance of P-450c17 mRNA from cultured bovine adrenocortical cells maintained in the absence of ACTH (2, 31), it is concluded that bovine adrenal *CYP*17 transcription is solely dependent on cAMP. This is not true for other bovine steroid hydroxylases whose transcription has a cAMP-independent regulatory component as well (31). cAMP-independent regulation could include the action of growth factors and cytokines. While it has not yet been studied in testis, it is reasonable to conclude that *CYP*17 expression in bovine testis, as in the bovine adrenal cortex, is solely dependent on cAMP. In testis, LH regulates cAMP levels.

There is considerable species variation associated with cAMP-dependent regulation of *CYP*17 (23). Deletion analysis of the human *CYP*17 promoter region indicates that the functional CRS in this gene has no sequence homology to bovine CRS-1 or CRS-2 (32). The CRS in the mouse *Cyp*17 gene is unrelated either to that in human *CYP*17 or to CRS-1 and CRS-2 of bovine *CYP*17 (33). Despite these species variations in *CYP*17 gene regulation, it is reasonable to believe that within a species the same biochemical systems function in both adrenal and testis, mediated by ACTH and LH, respectively.

Regulation of P-450c17 Enzymatic Activities by Cytochrome b$_5$

In addition to species variation in the regulation of gene expression of steroidogenic enzymes, species variation in enzymatic activities themselves is also well known. For example, human and bovine P-450c17 function poorly at converting 17α-hydroxyprogesterone to androstenedione (34), while the rat, chicken, and trout enzymes readily catalyze this conversion (35). This observation raised an important question regarding testosterone biosynthesis in the human testis. Testis 3β-hydroxysteroid dehydrogenase can convert pregnenolone and 17α-hydroxypregnenolone to their Δ4 derivatives. However, the purified human P-450c17 can convert progesterone only to 17α-hydroxyprogesterone and not on to androstenedione. Thus, it seemed that 17α-hydroxyprogesterone would be a dead-end product in the human testis because of the inability of P-450c17 to catalyze the Δ4 17,20-lyase reaction. That is to say, since purified human P-450c17 does not catalyze the conversion of 17α-hydroxyprogesterone to androstenedione, production of Δ4 steroids by 3β-hydroxy steroid dehydrogenase in human testis would lead nowhere. It has been reported that both the Δ4-hydroxylase and Δ4-lyase activities of pig P-450c17 are enhanced by cytochrome b$_5$ (36). Furthermore, human testis microsomes contain high levels of cytochrome b$_5$ relative to P-450 compared with other species (37). Using purified, bacterially expressed human P-450c17 and purified cytochrome b$_5$ from either human or rat, it has recently been found that, in in vitro enzymatic assays, cytochrome b$_5$ enhances >10-fold both the Δ4 and Δ5 17,20-lyase activities (38). 17α-hydroxylase activities were much less affected by cytochrome b$_5$. It is suggested from these observations that cytochrome b$_5$ has a profound effect to optimize sex hormone production in human testis. Importantly, 17α-hydroxyprogesterone is not a dead-end product in testosterone production, because a relatively high concentration of cytochrome b$_5$ in human testis assures that both the Δ4 and Δ5 steroidogenic pathways lead to testosterone production.

Summary

The pathways for testosterone biosynthesis in the Leydig cell involve different steroid hydroxylases and dehydrogenases (Fig. 18.2). P-450c17 plays an important role in these pathways by producing the androgens essential for sex hormone production. While regulation of expression of the genes involved in these pathways is generally poorly understood, some detail of the biochemical mechanisms involved in both developmental regulation and continued maintenance of *CYP*17 transcription is emerging. The zinc-finger orphan receptor SF-1, which is required for testis organogenesis, also plays

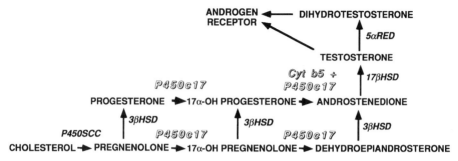

FIGURE 18.2. Roles of P-450c17 in testosterone biosynthesis.

a key role in Leydig cells in initiating transcription of *CYP*17 and *CYP*11A and the other steroid hydroxylase genes active in these cells. It will be interesting to determine which genes encoding other enzymes in the pathways in Figures 18.1 and 18.2 also are developmentally activated by SF-1. Once *CYP*17 transcription is turned on by the action of SF-1, other regulatory mechanisms are obviously important in maintenance of its transcription throughout fetal and adult life. Based on studies in a limited number of species, it can be predicted that in all mammalian Leydig cells, *CYP*17 expression is initiated early in fetal life and remains on throughout fetal and adult life. cAMP plays a key role in this process, and in some species such as cows and sheep cAMP may be the only regulator. The levels of cAMP in Leydig cells are controlled by luteinizing hormone from the anterior pituitary. In maintaining transcription of *CYP*17, cAMP functions through protein kinase A to activate specific transcription factors that bind to specific DNA sequences in the 5'-flanking region of *CYP*17. Based on a relatively limited number of studies in the adrenal, it appears that different species utilize different transcription systems. The reason for such variation is not yet known but might be related to variation in physiological requirements for adrenal steroid hormones.

In Leydig cells, there is no clear evidence yet as to what cAMP-dependent transcription systems function in *CYP*17 expression. Based on studies with hypophysectomized animals it is clear, however, that reduction in cAMP levels, which results from absence of peptide hormones, leads to reduction in levels of steroidogenic enzyme activities. Accordingly, it is not unreasonable to predict that the same biochemical systems will function to regulate *CYP*17 expression in adrenal and testis. If this presumption is correct, then species variation will also be found in cAMP-dependent regulation of *CYP*17 expression in the testis. What could be the physiological basis of such variation in this organ? Is the demand for testosterone quite different among species? Or is it simply a matter of convenience that the same system functions to regulate *CYP*17 expression in all steroidogenic organs within a species, and variation between species is guided by physiological requirements for adrenal steroids? To begin to answer these questions it will be necessary to study in detail the biochemical requirements for *CYP*17 transcription in Leydig cells.

Acknowledgment. Investigation of *CYP*17 regulation in this laboratory is supported by USPHS grant DK28350.

References

1. Nelson DR, Kamataki T, Waxman DJ, Guengerich FP, Estabrook RW, Feyereisen R, et al. The P450 superfamily: update on new sequences, gene mapping, accession numbers, early trivial names of enzymes and nomenclature. DNA Cell Biol 1993;12:1–51.
2. Zuber MX, John ME, Okamura T, Simpson ER, Waterman MR. Bovine adrenocortical cytochrome P45017α: regulation of gene expression by ACTH and elucidation of primary sequence. J Biol Chem 1986;261:2475–82.
3. Picado-Leonard J, Miller WL. Cloning and sequence of the human gene for P450c17 (steroid 17α-hydroxylase/17,20 lyase): similarity with the gene for P450c21. DNA 1987;6:439–48.
4. Clark BJ, Waterman MR. Functional expression of bovine 17α-hydroxylase in COS 1 cells is dependent upon the presence of an amino-terminal signal anchor sequence. J Biol Chem 1992;267:24568–74.
5. Kühn-Velten WN, Bunse T, Förster EC. Enzyme kinetic and inhibition analyses of cytochrome P450XVII, a protein with a bifunctional catalytic site. J Biol Chem 1991;266:6291–301.
6. Yanase T, Simpson ER, Waterman MR. 17α-hydroxylase/17,20-lyase deficiency: from clinical investigation to molecular definition. Endocr Rev 1991; 12:91–108.
7. Voutilainen R, Miller WL. Developmental expression of genes for the steroidogenic enzymes P450scc (20,22-desmolase), P-450c17 (17α-hydroxylase/ 17,20-lyase), and P450c21 (21-hydroxylase) in the human fetus. J Clin Endocrinol Metab 1986;63:1145–50.
8. Margolis FL, Rofet J, Jost A. Norepinephrine methylation in fetal rat adrenals. Science 1966;154:275–6.
9. Lund J, Faucher DJ, Ford SP, Porter JC, Waterman MR, Mason JI. Developmental expression of bovine adrenocortical steroid hydroxylases: regulation of P45017α expression leads to episodic fetal cortisol production. J Biol Chem 1988;263:16195–201.
10. Tangalakis K, Coghlan JR, Connell J, Crawford R, Darling P, Hammond VE, et al. Tissue distribution and levels of gene expression of three steroid hydroxylases in ovine fetal adrenal glands. Acta Endocrinol 1989;120:225–32.
11. Keeney DS, Jenkins CM, Waterman MR. Differential patterns of expression of corticosteroid and mineralocorticoid biosynthetic enzymes in the murine fetal adrenal gland. Endocrinology 1995;136:4872.9.
12. Ikeda Y, Shen W-H, Ingraham HA, Parker KL. Developmental expression of mouse steroidogenic factor-1, an essential regulator of steroid hydroxylases. Mol Endocrinol 1994;8:654–62.

13. Vianello S, Valle LD, Ramina A, Malocco C, Belvedere P, Colombo L. Expression of steroid biosynthetic enzymes in rat liver and digestive tract. Program of the IX International Congress on Hormonal Steroids, Dallas, TX, 1994:95 (abstract).

14. Strömstedt M, Waterman MR. Messenger RNAs encoding steroidogenic enzymes are expressed in rodent brain. Mol Brain Res 1995;34:75–88.

15. Lala DS, Rice DA, Parker KL. Steroidogenic factor 1, a key regulator of steroidogenic enzyme expression, is the mouse homolog of *fushi tarazu*-factor 1. Mol Endocrinol 1992;6:1249–58.

16. Morohashi K, Honda S, Inomata Y, Handa H, Omura T. A common transacting factor, Ad4-binding protein, to the promoters of steroidogenic P450s. J Biol Chem 1992;267:17913–9.

17. Luo X, Ikeda Y, Parker KL. A cell-specific nuclear receptor is essential for adrenal and gonadal development and sexual differentiation. Cell 1994;77:481–90.

18. Simpson ER, Waterman MR. Action of ACTH to regulate the synthesis of steroidogenic enzymes in adrenal cortical cells. Annu Rev Physiol 1988;50:427–40.

19. Jefcoate CR, McNamara BC, Artemenko I, Yamazaki T. Regulation of cholesterol movement to mitochondrial cytochrome P450scc in steroid hormone synthesis. J Steroid Biochem Mol Biol 1992;43:751–67.

20. John ME, John MC, Boggaram V, Simpson ER, Waterman MR. Transcriptional regulation of steroid hydroxylase genes by ACTH. Proc Natl Acad Sci USA 1986;83:4715–9.

21. Purvis JL, Canick JA, Latif SA, Rosenbaum JH, Hologgitas J, Menard RH. Lifetime of microsomal cytochrome P450 and steroidogenic enzymes in rat testis as influenced by human chorionic gonadotropin. Arch Biochem Biophys 1973;159:39–49.

22. Purvis JL, Canick JA, Mason JI, Estabrook RW, McCarthy JL. Lifetime of adrenal cytochrome P450 as influenced by ACTH. Ann NY Acad Sci 1973;212:319–42.

23. Waterman MR. Biochemical diversity of cAMP-dependent transcription of steroid hydroxylase genes in the adrenal cortex. J Biol Chem 1994;269:27783–6.

24. Lund J, Ahlgren R, Wu D, Kagimoto M, Simpson ER, Waterman MR. Transcriptional regulation of the bovine *CYP17* (P45017α) gene. Identification of two cAMP regulatory regions lacking the consensus CRE. J Biol Chem 1990;265:3304–12.

25. Roesler WJ, Vandenbar GR, Hanson RW. Cyclic AMP and the induction of eucaryotic gene transcription. J Biol Chem 1988;263:9063–6.

26. Lund J, Bakke M. Transcriptional regulation of the bovine *CYP17* gene in adrenocortical cells. Program of the IX International Congress on Hormonal Steroids, Dallas, TX, 1994:67 (abstract).

27. Zanger UM, Kagawa N, Lund J, Waterman MR. cAMP-dependent transcription of *CYP17* and *CYP21* involves distinct biochemical mechanisms. FASEB J 1992;6:719–23.

28. Zanger UM, Lund J, Simpson ER, Waterman MR. Activation of transcription in cell-free extracts by a novel cAMP responsive sequence from the bovine *CYP17* gene. J Biol Chem 1991;266:11417–20.

29. Kagawa N, Ogo A, Takahashi Y, Iwamatsu A, Waterman MR. A cAMP-responsive sequence (CRS-1) of *CYP*17 is a cellular target for the homeo-domain protein Pbx1. J Biol Chem 1994;269:18716–9.

30. Ogo A. Unpublished observation.

31. Waterman MR, Simpson ER. Regulation of steroid hydroxylase gene expression is multifactorial in nature. Recent Prog Horm Res 1989;45:533–66.

32. Brentano ST, Picado-Leonard J, Mellon SH, Moore CCD, Miller WL. Tissue-specific, cyclic adenosine 3′,-5′-monophosphate-induced, and phorbol ester-repressed transcription from the human P450c17 promoter in mouse cells. Mol Endocrinol 1990;4:1972–9.

33. Youngblook GL, Payne AH. Isolation and characterization of the mouse P450 17α-hydroxylase/C17-20-lyase gene (*CYP*17): transcriptional regulation of the gene by cyclic adenosine 3′,5′-monophosphate in MA-10 Leydig cells. Mol Endocrinol 1992;6:927–34.

34. Imai T, Globerman H, Gertner J, Kagawa N, Waterman MR. Expression and purification of functional human 17α-hydroxylase/17,20-lyase (P45017α) in *Escherichia* coli: use of this system for study of a novel form of combined 17α-hydroxylase/17,20-lyase deficiency. J Biol Chem 1993;268:19681–9.

35. Fevold HR, Lorence MC, McCarthy JL, Trant JM, Kagimoto M, Waterman MR, et al. Rat testis P45017α: characterization of a full-length cDNA encoding a unique steroid hydroxylase capable of catalyzing both Δ4 and Δ5-17,20-lyase reactions. Mol Endocrinol 1989;3:968–76.

36. Onoda M, Hall PF. Cytochrome b_5 stimulates purified testicular microsomal cytochrome P450 (C-21 side-chain cleavage). Biochem Biophys Res Commun 1982;108:454–60.

37. Mason JI, Estabrook RW. Testicular cytochrome P-450 and iron-sulfur protein as related to steroid metabolism. Ann N Y Acad Sci 1973;212:406–19.

38. Katagiri M, Kagawa N, Waterman MR. The role of cytochrome b_5 in the biosynthesis of androgens by human P450c17. Arch Biochem Biophys 1995;317:343–7.

19

A Cell-Specific Nuclear Receptor Plays Essential Roles in Reproductive Function

XUNRONG LUO, YAYOI IKEDA, AND KEITH L. PARKER

Steroid hormone biosynthesis requires the cytochrome P-450 steroid hydroxylases, which act sequentially to convert cholesterol to physiologically active steroid hormones (reviewed in 1). Expression of these enzymes is generally limited to steroidogenic cells and, within these cells, is coordinately induced by trophic hormones, raising the possibility that their expression is controlled by a shared transcriptional regulator. Studies analyzing promoter activity of the 5'-flanking regions of these genes in cell lines derived from steroidogenic cells showed that multiple promoter elements were needed for full levels of expression. Notably, each gene was regulated by elements that matched the AGGTCA "half-site" motif for nuclear receptor family members (2, 3). Recent studies described here indicate that these elements interact with a cell-selective nuclear receptor, *steroidogenic factor-1* (SF-1), that is essential for adrenal and gonadal development and that also plays key roles at the hypothalamic and pituitary levels of the reproductive axis.

Results

Isolation and Characterization of SF-1

The similar sequences of the steroidogenic regulatory elements suggested that the same regulatory protein interacted with these sequences to coordinate the expression of the steroid hydroxylases (2, 3). Because the protein that formed this complex was restricted to steroidogenic cell lines, we designated it steroidogenic factor-1 (SF-1). When a *complementary DNA* (cDNA) encoding SF-1 was isolated (4), several important features became apparent. First, SF-1 was clearly a member of the nuclear hormone receptor family, a diverse group of structurally related proteins that mediate transcriptional activation by various steroid hormones, vitamin D, thyroid hormone, and retinoids (reviewed in 5). The most striking match was to a cDNA isolated from embryonal carcinoma cells and designated *embryonal long terminal repeat–binding protein* (ELP) due to its ability to inhibit transcription of retroviral *long terminal repeats* (LTRs) (6). Isolation and characterization of genomic sequences encoding SF-1 ultimately showed that both SF-1 and ELP arise from the same structural gene by alternative promoter usage and 3′ splicing (7). This gene was designated *Ftz-F1* because it also resembles a *Drosophila* nuclear receptor that encodes two developmentally regulated nuclear receptors, one of which regulates the *fushi tarazu* (*ftz*) homeobox gene (8, 9).

Developmental Regulation of SF-1

Based on the essential roles of steroid hormones in male sexual differentiation, we analyzed the developmental profile of SF-1 in mouse embryos by an in situ hybridization approach. As summarized in Table 19.1, these analyses of SF-1 expression provided intriguing insights into its possible role in steroidogenic organ development (10). SF-1 transcripts were present in the adrenal primordium from the inception of adrenal formation at approximately embryonic day 10.5 (E10.5). Later, as the neural crest-derived sympathoadrenal cells migrated into the adrenal gland to form the medulla, SF-1 expression was confined to the cortical region where steroidogenesis occurs. SF-1's expression at the earliest stages of adrenal differentiation suggested a key role in adrenal development. Similarly, SF-1 was expressed at very early stages of gonadogenesis, beginning at E9; this expression was seen in both male and female embryos. At this developmental stage, the gonads of males and females are indistinguishable and

TABLE 19.1. Ontogeny of SF-1 expression during mouse embryogenesis.

Adrenal gland
  Expressed from earliest stages of adrenal development (E10.5)
  Localizes to outer cortical regions as chromaffin cell precursors invade adrenal from
    neural crest (~E13)

Gonads
  Expressed from earliest stages of gonadogenesis (indifferent gonad) in both testis and
    ovary (E9)
  In testis, expression persists after sexual differentiation (E12.5) in both interstitial region
    (Leydig) and testicular cords (Sertoli)
  In ovary, expression decreases coincident with sexual differentiation (E12.5)

Other sites
  Expressed in ventral diencephalon (hypothalamic precursor)
  Expressed in anterior pituitary, later localizes to gonadotropes

are therefore termed indifferent or bipotential gonads. At E12.5, as morphologic sexual differentiation is occurring, SF-1 expression persisted in the testes but was extinguished in ovaries. Moreover, SF-1 was expressed in both compartments of the fetal testes: the interstitial region, which contains the fetal Leydig cells that produce androgens, and the testicular cords, which contain fetal Sertoli cells and primordial germ cells. The expression of SF-1 in the Sertoli cells and its sexually dimorphic pattern suggested that SF-1's role in the gonadal development extended beyond regulating the steroidogenic enzymes.

Finally, SF-1 was expressed in discrete regions of the embryonic ventral diencephalon and anterior pituitary (11). Intriguingly, the ventral diencephalon ultimately contributes to the endocrine hypothalamus, whereas the anterior pituitary includes the gonadotropes that produce the predominant regulators of gonadal steroidogenesis—the gonadotropins. These findings suggested that SF-1 also functions at additional levels of the hypothalamic-pituitary-steroidogenic tissue axis.

The Gene-Encoding SF-1 Is Essential for Adrenal and Gonadal Development

To define the role of SF-1 in vivo, we used the technique of targeted gene disruption to knock out the mouse *Ftz-F1* gene that encodes SF-1 (12). The strategy employed (Fig. 19.1) abolished both ELP and SF-1 activity. In matings of heterozygous *Ftz-F1*–disrupted mice, −/− animals were born at about the expected frequency of 25%, indicating that neither ELP nor SF-1 is required for embryonic survival. As summarized in Table 19.2, all knockout animals died shortly after birth; all had depressed corticosterone levels, consistent with a pronounced impairment of corticosteroid biosynthesis, and all had female external genitals irrespective of genetic sex, consistent with a failure to produce testicular androgens. To our considerable surprise, the *Ftz-F1*–disrupted animals also lacked adrenal glands and gonads, demonstrating the essential role of SF-1 in adrenal and gonadal development.

The *Ftz-F1* Gene Also Plays Important Roles in Pituitary Gonadotropes and the Ventromedial Hypothalamic Nucleus.

TABLE 19.2. Features of *Ftz-F1*–disrupted mice.

Make up 25% of live births, indicating that the *Ftz-F1* gene is not required for embryos to survive

Appear normal, although all animals have female external genitalia irrespective of genetic sex

Fail to gain weight despite normal suckling

Die shortly after birth unless rescued by treatment with corticosteroids

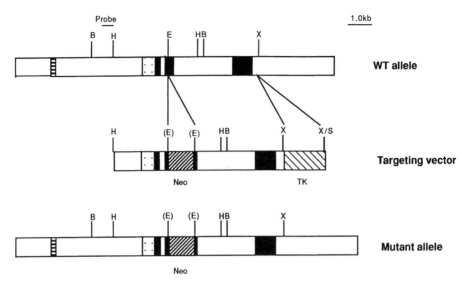

FIGURE 19.1. A schematic summary of the strategy used to disrupt the mouse *Ftz-F1* gene. Solid areas indicate shared exons, horizontally lined areas denote SF-1–specific exons, and stippled areas denote ELP-specific exons. The Neo selectable marker and thymidine kinase (TK) gene were inserted into a plasmid containing the indicated *Ftz-F1* genomic sequences. The Neo gene disrupts the second zinc finger region required for DNA binding. Restriction endonuclease sites include B, BglII; X, XhoI; H, HindIII; E, Eco47 III. The position of the probe used for Southern blotting analyses is indicated.

As noted above, SF-1 was also expressed in the ventral diencephalon and the anterior pituitary, suggesting that it might act at additional levels of the hypothalamic-pituitary-steroidogenic organ axis. Consistent with this model, the *Ftz-F1*–disrupted mice were selectively deficient in their pituitary expression of multiple markers of gonadotropes, including the α-subunit of glycoprotein hormones, luteinizing hormone, follicle-stimulating hormone, and the gonadotropin-releasing hormone receptor (11). They also lacked the ventromedial hypothalamic nucleus (13), a region of the hypothalamus containing high concentrations of estrogen, progesterone, and androgen receptors that has been implicated in reproductive behavior (14).

Discussion

The central focus of our laboratory has been to define the mechanisms that regulate gene expression of the steroid hydroxylases, initially in the adrenal cortex and more recently in gonads. These studies implicated SF-1 as an essential regulator of steroid hydroxylase gene expression; more important, the role of SF-1 has recently been extended considerably with the demonstration that the *Ftz-F1* gene is essential for adrenal and gonadal development and also plays key roles in the pituitary and hypothalamus. These *Ftz-F1*-disrupted animals provide an excellent model system in which to ascertain the target genes through which SF-1 exerts its actions in steroid organ development. For example, gonadal agenesis also accompanies disruption of the Wilms' tumor–related gene WT-1 (15). Preliminary analyses in E11 *Ftz-F1*-disrupted embryos indicate that WT-1 expression is maintained in the absence of SF-1; similarly, SF-1 expression is maintained in the WT-1 null mice (Y. Ikeda, unpublished observation). These results suggest that, although they are both essential for gonadal development, WT-1 and SF-1 act independently in parallel pathways in gonadal development.

Similarly, analyses of the 5′-flanking region of the gene encoding *Müllerian inhibiting substance* (MIS) have identified a potential SF-1-responsive element and have shown a temporal correlation between SF-1 and MIS gene expression (16). If functional studies can support a role for this element in MIS gene expression, it will directly implicate SF-1 in both critical arms of male sexual development: androgen production by fetal Leydig cells and MIS production in fetal Sertoli cells.

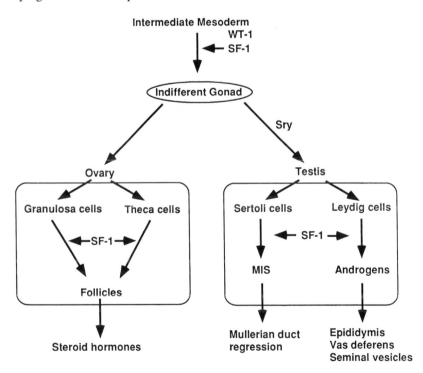

FIGURE 19.2. The roles of SF-1 in gonadal development and function. A model of gonadal development is shown, including sites at which SF-1 is believed to play important roles.

Based on these studies, SF-1 apparently acts at several positions within the hierarchy of gonadal development (Fig. 19.2). Based on its early expression in both male and females at the bipotential gonad stage, and the absence of gonads in both sexes, it seems probable that SF-1 participates in critical early developmental events in the bipotential gonad. As SF-1 is expressed in both males and females with a time course that precedes the onset of Sry expression, it seems highly unlikely that Sry directly regulates SF-1 expression. It nonetheless remains possible that Sry indirectly regulates SF-1, perhaps by inhibiting a negative regulator that silences SF-1 expression in the ovary. As male sexual determination and differentiation take place, SF-1 is expressed in both the interstitial region and the testicular cords, where it is postulated to regulate androgen production and MIS biosynthesis, respectively. In the ovary, SF-1 expression decreases at critical periods of sex differentiation, and high levels are not seen until after birth. In the adult ovary, SF-1 is expressed in both theca and granulosa cells and is again proposed to be a key regulator of steroid hydroxylase gene expression.

Acknowledgments. This work was supported by the Howard Hughes Medical Institute and the National Institutes of Health. We thank Drs. Douglas Rice, Andrea Mouw, and Deepak Lala for their key contributions to early studies of SF-1, and Dr. Beverly Koller for invaluable assistance in preparing the *Ftz-F1*–disrupted mice.

References

1. Miller WL. Molecular biology of steroid hormone biosynthesis. Endocr Rev 1988;9:295–318.
2. Rice DA, Mouw AR, Bogerd A, Parker KL. A shared promoter element regulates the expression of three steroidogenic enzymes. Mol Endocrinol 1991;5:1552–61.
3. Morohashi K, Honda S, Inomata Y, Handa H, Omura T. A common trans-acting factor, Ad4BP, to the promoters of steroidogenic P450s. J Biol Chem 1992;267:17913–19.
4. Lala DS, Rice DA, Parker KL. Steroidogenic factor I, a key regulator of steroidogenic enzyme expression, is the mouse homolog of fushi tarazu-factor I. Mol Endocrinol 1992;6:1249–58.
5. Evans RM. The steroid and thyroid hormone receptor superfamily. Science 1988;240:889–95.
6. Tsukiyama T, Ueda H, Hirose S, Niwa O. Embryonal long terminal repeat-binding protein is a murine homolog of FTZ-F1, a member of the steroid receptor superfamily. Mol Cell Biol 1992;12:1286–91.
7. Ikeda Y, Lala DS, Luo X, Kim E, Moisan M-P, Parker KL. Characterization of the mouse FTZ-F1 gene, which encodes an essential regulator of steroid hydroxylase gene expression. Mol Endocrinol 1993;7:852–60.

8. Lavorgna G, Ueda H, Clos J, Wu C. FTZ-F1, a steroid hormone receptor-like protein implicated in the activation of *fushi tarazu*. Science 1991;252:848–51.
9. Lavorgna G, Karim FD, Thummel CS, Wu C. Potential role for a FTZ-F1 steroid receptor superfamily member in the control of *Drosophila* metamorphosis. Proc Natl Acad Sci USA 1993;90:3004–8.
10. Ikeda Y, Shen W-H, Ingraham HA, Parker KL. Developmental expression of mouse steroidogenic factor 1, an essential regulator of the steroid hydroxylases. Mol Endocrinol 1994;8:654–62.
11. Ingraham HA, Lala DS, Ikeda Y, Luo X, Shen W-H, Nachtigal MW, et al. The nuclear receptor SF-1 acts at multiple levels of the reproductive axis. Genes Dev 1994;8:2302–12.
12. Luo X, Ikeda Y, Parker KL. A cell specific nuclear receptor is required for adrenal and gonadal development and for male sexual differentiation. Cell 1994;77:481–90.
13. Ikeda Y, Luo X, Abbud R, Nilson JH, Parker KL. The nuclear receptor steroidogenic factor 1 is essential for the formation of the ventromedial hypothalamic nucleus. Mol Endocrinol 1995;9:478–86.
14. Pfaff DW, Schwartz-Giblin S, McCarthy MM, Kow L-M. Cellular and molecular mechanisms of female reproductive behaviors. In: Knobil E, Neill JD, eds. The physiology of reproduction, 2nd ed. New York: Raven Press, 1994:107–220.
15. Kreidberg JA, Sariola H, Loring JM, Maeda M, Pelletier J, Housman D, Jaenisch R. WT-1 is required for early kidney development. Cell 1993;74:679–91.
16. Shen W-H, Moore CCD, Ikeda Y, Parker KL, Ingraham HA. Nuclear receptor steroidogenic factor 1 regulates MIS gene expression: a link to the sex determination cascade. Cell 1994;77:651–61.

20

Activating Mutations of the Luteinizing Hormone Receptor Gene in Familial Testotoxicosis

ANDREW SHENKER AND SHINJI KOSUGI

Heptahelical, membrane-spanning cell-surface receptors utilize heterotrimeric guanine nucleotide binding proteins (G proteins) to transmit extracellular signals to cellular effectors (1–4). Diverse stimuli, including photons, hormones, neurotransmitters, odorants, proteases, and ions, trigger conformational changes in the receptor transmembrane helices that are relayed to the cytoplasmic surface, leading to G protein activation (Fig. 20.1A).

Different *G protein–coupled receptors* (GPCRs) share significant structural homology, consisting of seven hydrophobic regions (TM 1–TM 7) that are predicted to form a compact bundle of α-helices, connected by alternating extracellular (E1-E3) and intracellular (I1-I3) loops. A conserved Cys residue in the C-terminal tail of many GPCRs serves as a potential site for palmitoylation, and this modification may serve to anchor the tail to the plasma membrane and form a fourth intracellular loop. Certain highly conserved amino acids within the transmembrane domain have been shown to play key roles in receptor expression, structure, or function (1, 5). Rhodopsin, the rod cell photoreceptor, contains a covalently bound molecule of retinal within the hydrophilic pocket formed by its membrane-spanning helices. The ligand-binding pocket of receptors for biogenic amines is similarly located in the transmembrane core, but in the case of some peptide hormone receptors residues in the N-terminal and extracellular loop domains have also been implicated in agonist binding.

Receptors for glycoprotein hormones [*luteinizing hormone* (LH)/*human chorionic gonadotropin* (hCG), *thyroid-stimulating hormone* (TSH), *follicle-stimulating hormone* (FSH)] have extended N-terminal extracellular domains (>300 amino acids) that can independently determine agonist binding affinity and specificity (6–8). It has been suggested that the glycoprotein hormone receptors and other GPCR subfamilies with unique

A. Normal

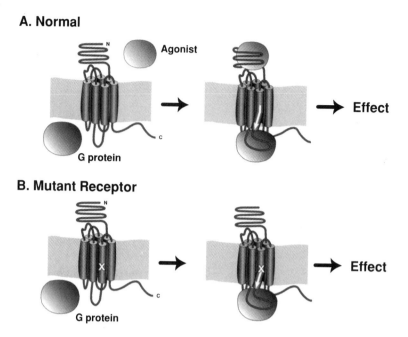

B. Mutant Receptor

FIGURE 20.1. (*A*) Normal agonist-mediated activation of a G protein–coupled signaling pathway. Binding of agonist triggers a conformational change in the receptor transmembrane bundle that is relayed to the cytoplasmic domain, exposing sites necessary for G protein coupling. Several cytoplasmic regions, including the C-terminus of the I3 loop, are involved in G protein activation. (*B*) Certain mutations encode amino acid substitutions (X) that enable the receptor to adapt a partially activated conformation and activate G proteins in the absence of agonist.

N-terminal domains may have originated as the result of recombination between a gene encoding a simple heptahelical membrane bundle and one encoding a specialized binding protein (6, 9, 10). This evolutionary mechanism could serve to promote the creation of hybrid GPCRs with novel signaling functions.

Receptor Activation Mechanisms

In the case of rhodopsin, a change in the shape of retinal upon photoisomerization apparently imposes a strain on the binding pocket that drives structural rearrangement, disruption of a key interhelical salt bridge, lateral expansion of the receptor, and protonation of two distant residues (11, 12). Rearrangement of side chains in the transmembrane-binding pocket is also likely to be the primary event in signal transduction induced by monoamines and other small agonists (2). In contrast, activation of receptors for other types of ligands, including the large glycoprotein hormones, might be triggered wholly or partially by forces imposed on the extracellular surface of the receptor. For example, portions of the extracellular loops, including E3 (13) and a key Asp residue in E1 (14), seem necessary for signal transduction by the *thyrotropin receptor* (TSHR) and the *lutropin receptor* (LHR), respectively. Sequence comparison reveals that all glycoprotein hormone receptors lack a Pro residue found in TM 5 in most other GPCRs, but they all share a unique Pro in TM 7 (15). Because kinks caused by Pro residues have the potential to influence the pattern of interhelical packing and to participate in agonist-induced conformational transitions (16, 17), it is possible that these structural differences reflect an important difference in the mechanism by which this group of receptors undergoes agonist-induced activation.

In fact, the precise sequence of events that link agonist binding to G protein activation is not known for any GPCR. Evidence from a variety of experimental approaches indicates that the concerted action of several intracellular domains, including part of I2 and the N- and C-terminal ends of I3, are involved in determining the receptor's affinity for G proteins and for transmitting the signal produced by agonist binding. For example, small peptides based on cytoplasmic loop sequences can partially mimic the GPCR from which they were derived by binding and activating G proteins (18, 19). Detailed comparison of I3 sequences from many different GPCRs fails to reveal consensus sequences or similarities that segregate according to G protein–coupling preference, suggesting that the function of I3 depends on its three-dimensional conformation in the context of other cytoplasmic loop domains. An Asp/Glu-Arg-Tyr tripeptide motif at the junction of TM 3 and I2 is characteristic of many GPCRs, and may play a key role in the activation process (12, 20).

In the course of studying the functional anatomy of the α_{1B}-*adrenergic receptor* (AR), Lefkowitz and colleagues discovered that substitution of an Ala residue located at the junction of I3 and TM 6 with any other amino acid caused increased agonist affinity, increased sensitivity to agonist, and increased activation of G proteins in the absence of agonist (i.e., constitutive activation) (21). Furthermore, an activated mutant α_{1B}AR expressed in rodent fibroblasts was shown to be oncogenic (22). Substitution of corresponding or nearby amino acids in the β_2AR (23), the α_2AR (24), the TSHR (25), and a yeast pheromone GPCR (26) were also found to produce constitutive activation.

The discovery of GPCR mutations capable of causing agonist-independent activation led to the proposal that the function of the inactive, constrained GPCR conformation is to conceal key cytoplasmic peptide sequences and prevent them from interacting with G proteins (21, 23). This model incorporates the concept that unoccupied receptors can occasionally undergo spontaneous isomerization to the activated conformation, thereby producing some low level of "basal" activity. According to the model, agonists act to disrupt constraints and drive the receptor into an active conformation in which the newly exposed cytoplasmic residues are able to bind and activate G proteins. The activating effect of certain amino acid substitutions can be viewed as augmenting the receptor's intrinsic ability to adapt an activated conformation in the absence of agonist (Fig. 20.1B).

The discovery that artificial mutagenesis could be used to generate activated receptors raised the possibility that a naturally occurring gene mutation that led to constitutive activation of a GPCR could serve as a mechanism of human disease (21, 22). Inactivating mutations of GPCR genes were already known to cause diseases such as retinitis pigmentosa (27) and X-linked nephrogenic diabetes insipidus (28). Knowledge of the effects of activating mutations in several other classes of transmembrane receptors, including receptor tyrosine kinases (29, 30), the erythropoietin receptor (31), and bacterial chemoreceptors (32), provided additional precedent for the notion that activating gene GPCR mutations could be pathogenic in man.

Activating Mutations of the LHR in Familial Testotoxicosis

Testotoxicosis, also known as familial male precocious puberty, is a gonadotropin-independent disorder that is inherited in an autosomal-dominant, male-limited pattern (33). Testosterone secretion and Leydig cell hyperplasia occur in the context of prepubertal levels of LH, and the onset of puberty in affected boys usually occurs by age 4. It was hypothesized that testotoxicosis was due to a mutant LHR that could be activated in the presence of little or no agonist, and a heterozygous mutation that results in substitution of Asp[578] in TM 6 with Gly was indeed found in affected individuals from nine different kindreds (34, 35). The mutation created a novel recognition site for the restriction endonuclease MspI; restriction digest analysis revealed linkage of this mutation to testotoxicosis.

To assess the functional effect of the Asp[578]→Gly mutation, wild type and mutated human LHR were transiently expressed in COS-7 cells (34). In contrast to the silent wild type LHR, the mutant LHR produces a 4.5-fold increase in basal *adenosine 3′:5′-cyclic monophosphate* (cAMP) production in COS-7 cells, indicating that it is constitutively active (Fig. 20.2). Agonist-independent stimulation of cAMP production represents about 40% of the maximal stimulation produced by the agonist hCG, and is not simply due to increased receptor expression (36, 37). The mutant receptor is also capable of responding to increasing concentrations of hCG, with a *median effective concentration* (EC_{50}) and maximal hCG-stimulated cAMP production similar to that of the wild-type receptor. The mutation has no effect on

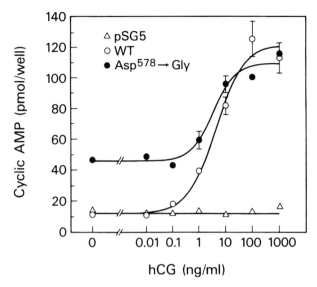

FIGURE 20.2. Asp[578]→Gly mutation of the lutropin receptor (LHR) causes constitutive activation. Basal and human chorionic gonadotropin (hCG)-stimulated cAMP accumulation in COS-7 cells transfected with pSG5 vector alone, wild type LHR DNA (WT), or Asp[578]→Gly mutant LHR DNA is shown. The mutant receptor produces a 4.5-fold increase in cAMP accumulation in the absence of agonist, but retains the ability to respond to hCG. Reprinted with permission from Shenker et al. (34) Nature 365:652–4. © 1993, Macmillan Magazines Limited.

agonist binding affinity, which is known to be determined primarily by sequences in the large N-terminal domain (36, 37). Although the wild-type LHR, like other glycoprotein hormone receptors, is characterized by the ability to couple to both the cAMP and the phosphatidylinositol hydrolysis signaling pathways, only the cAMP pathway is constitutively activated by the Asp[578]→Gly mutation (36, 37).

The Asp[578]→Gly LHR mutation is the most common cause of familial testotoxicosis, and it has also been detected in several sporadic cases of gonadotropin-independent, male precocious puberty (36, 38, 39). Different mutations of the LHR, mostly clustered in TM 6, have been found in other patients (35, 37, 39, 40). The location of activating LHR mutations is shown in Figure 20.3. Some of the newly described LHR mutations produce biochemical phenotypes similar to that of the original Asp[578]→Gly substitution, but others do not (37, 39–41). For example, an LHR mutation encoding substitution of Asp[578] with Tyr promotes much higher basal cAMP accumulation in transfected cells than that produced by the other mutations (39, 41). This mutation has been found in 2 boys with unusually early signs of puberty, suggesting that their clinical phenotypes are related to the strongly activating nature of the Asp[578]→Tyr substitution.

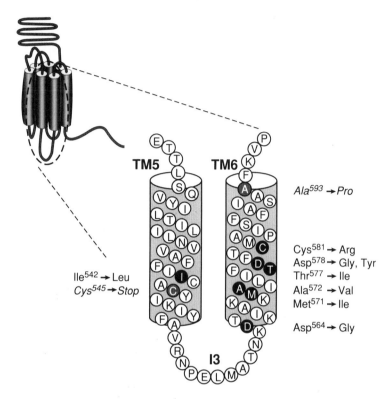

FIGURE 20.3. Naturally occurring mutations of the lutropin receptor in transmembrane helices 5 and 6. Each helix has been split and laid flat so that residues thought to face the internal receptor cavity are located along the central axis (1). Black circles denote residues that are mutated in testotoxicosis. Gray circles and italicized text denote residues that are mutated in familial Leydig cell hypoplasia.

Dominant mutations that lead to constitutive activation of the LHR-mediated cAMP signaling pathway can explain the pathophysiology of gonadotropin-independent precocious puberty in males. LHR-mediated effects, including testosterone production, are known to involve increased production of cellular cAMP (8). Intracellular cAMP accumulation triggered by unoccupied mutant receptors is apparently sufficient to cause Leydig cell hyperfunction and hyperplasia. Because LH alone is adequate to trigger steroidogenesis in Leydig cells, but both LH and FSH are required to activate ovarian steroidogenesis, inappropriate activation of LHR alone would not be expected to cause precocious puberty in females. For example, hCG-secreting germ-cell tumors cause sexual precocity in males, but not females (42). The reason why normal cellular desensitization mechanisms are apparently not adequate to compensate for the effects of constitutively activated receptors in vivo is a topic for future research.

Activating LHR mutations may help provide insight into the normal mechanism of GPCR activation. The location of most of the mutations is consistent with earlier data showing that residues at the base of TM 6 and in the adjacent C-terminal portion of I3 play a critical role in G protein coupling. When plotted on a helical net representation of the LHR (Fig. 20.3), many of the affected residues in the LHR are predicted to face inward. It is proposed that the conformation of LHR TM 6 is constrained in the inactive receptor state. When LH or hCG binds to the receptor, these constraints are broken and a conformational change ensues. Substitution of certain residues in TM 6 may cause structural changes that weaken the constraints and therefore partially mimic agonist occupancy. A model of the arrangement of the transmembrane α-helices places Asp^{578} near the middle of TM 6, oriented toward the internal cleft (1). Asp^{578} is conserved in all glycoprotein hormone receptors, and replacement of Asp with Asn in the rat LHR does not result in constitutive activation of the cAMP pathway (43). It has been suggested that the equivalent residue in the opsins and cationic neurotransmitter receptors (Phe or Tyr) undergoes a key conformational change during receptor activation (15, 17). Just as disruption of a critical interhelical electrostatic interaction appears to explain constitutive activation of certain mutant rhodopsin molecules (44–46), the activating effect of particular Asp^{578} substitutions in the LHR may be attributed to the analogous loss of a stabilizing interhelical hydrogen bond (15, 34). It is possible that the strongly activating effect of a bulky Tyr substituent at position 578, compared with that of Gly, is due to greater distortion of interhelical packing. The mechanisms by which naturally occurring substitutions at other positions in the LHR cause spontaneous activation remain to be explored. Although some GPCR substitutions appear to act by increasing the proportion of receptors in the active conformation, it is possible that other activating substitutions will be found to act primarily by increasing the affinity of the isomerized receptor for G protein, or by interfering with normal desensitization mechanisms.

Activating GPCR Mutations in Other Human Diseases

Naturally occurring missense mutations that lead to constitutive activation of other GPCRs have been described as the cause of a number of different human diseases, including severe retinitis pigmentosa (44), congenital night blindness (45, 46), autosomal dominant hypocalcemia (47), and Jansen-type metaphyseal chondrodysplasia (48). Somatic and germline mutations in the TSHR gene have been identified in sporadic hyperfunctional thyroid adenomas and autosomal dominant thyroid hyperplasia, respectively (49–52). As with the LHR mutations in testotoxicosis, many of the TSHR mutations are clustered in TM 6, but substitutions found in E1, TM 3, and TM 7 indicate that other regions of the TSHR must also participate in stabilizing the inactive receptor conformation. Most of the LHR and TSHR mutations occur at residues that are perfectly conserved in all mammalian glycoprotein hormone receptors, and some of the residues are even conserved in partially homologous invertebrate GPCRs (9, 53), suggesting that these amino acids normally serve a critical functional role.

Inactivating Mutations of the LHR in Familial Leydig Cell Hypoplasia

Male pseudohermaphroditism due to Leydig cell unresponsiveness to hCG/LH is a rare, autosomal recessive condition characterized by Leydig cell agenesis or hypoplasia in a 46,XY individual. Phenotypically, the appearance of the external genitalia may range from normal female to hypoplastic male. Because normal masculinization of the external genitalia during late fetal life depends on production of testosterone by fetal Leydig cells, it was postulated several years ago that this disorder was due to an inherited defect in the LHR, with resultant fetal testosterone deficiency (54).

A homozygous missense mutation of the LHR (Ala^{593}→Pro) was recently found in two 46,XY siblings who presented with female genitalia and primary amenorrhea, and whose parents were first cousins (55). Signaling through the mutant receptor is absent in transfected cells, at least partially because of diminished surface expression. Sisters from another family were shown to be heterozygous for an LHR gene mutation encoding a premature stop codon (Cys^{545}→Stop) (56). Whether this mutation has a dominant negative effect or whether the patients bear a different inactivating mutation on their other LHR allele remains to be defined. The location of the Ala^{593}→Pro and Cys^{545}→Stop mutations is shown in Figure 20.3. It is anticipated that other patients with Leydig cell hypoplasia and partially masculinized external genitalia will be found to have milder LHR defects that result in incomplete resistance to hCG/LH (54, 55).

Conclusion

Because data on the actual three-dimensional structure of GPCRs are limited, our present understanding of receptor structure and function has necessarily been based on a combination of biophysical measurements, molecular modeling, and pharmacological characterization of artificially mutated receptors. Even though high-resolution structural data on rhodopsin and other GPCRs will be vital, this information alone will not reveal how receptors work. Site-directed mutagenesis is time-consuming, and the number of different amino acids substituted for one suspected of being important is usually limited. Even if an investigator targets an important residue, the choice of substituents can determine what, if any, phenotype will be seen. The significance of disease-causing mutations is that they have, by definition, produced an abnormal phenotype. Thus, identification and characterization of naturally occurring receptor mutations not only has inherent value in understanding the molecular basis of disease and in highlighting the normal physiological role of different GPCR pathways, but can also accelerate progress in understanding basic receptor mechanisms. Studies of disease-causing LHR mutations should continue to provide important insights into Leydig cell development and into the structure and function of glycoprotein hormone receptors.

Acknowledgment. We are grateful to all our collaborators whose work is summarized in this chapter.

References

1. Baldwin JM. Structure and function of receptors coupled to G proteins. Curr Opin Cell Biol 1994;6:180–90.
2. Strader CD, Fong TM, Tota MR, Underwood D. Structure and function of G protein-coupled receptors. Annu Rev Biochem 1994;63:101–32.
3. Birnbaumer M. Mutations and diseases of G protein coupled receptors. J Recept Signal Transduct Res 1995;15:131–60.
4. Shenker A. G protein-coupled receptor structure and function: the impact of disease-causing mutations. Baillieres Clin Endocrinol Metab 1995;9:427–51.
5. Schwartz TW. Locating ligand-binding sites in 7TM receptors by protein engineering. Curr Opin Biotechnol 1994;5:434–44.
6. Tsai-Morris CH, Buczko E, Wang W, Dufau ML. Intronic nature of the rat luteinizing hormone receptor gene defines a soluble receptor subspecies with hormone binding activity. J Biol Chem 1990;265:19385–8.
7. Vassart G, Dumont JE. The thyrotropin receptor and the regulation of thyrocyte function and growth. Endocr Rev 1992;13:596–611.
8. Segaloff DL, Ascoli M. The lutropin/choriogonadotropin receptor . . . 4 years later. Endocr Rev 1993;14:324–47.
9. Tensen C, van Kesteren ER, Planta RJ, Cox KJA, Burke JF, van Heerikhuizen H, et al. A G protein-coupled receptor with low density lipoprotein-binding motifs suggests a role for lipoproteins in G-linked signal transduction. Proc Natl Acad Sci USA 1994;91:4816–20.
10. Conkin BR, Bourne HR. Marriage of the flytrap and the serpent. Nature 1994;367:22.
11. Nathans J. Rhodopsin: structure, function, and genetics. Biochemistry 1992;31:4923–31.
12. Arnis S, Fahmy K, Hofmann KP, Sakmar TP. A conserved carboxylic acid group mediates light-dependent proton uptake and signaling by rhodopsin. J Biol Chem 1994;269:23879–81.

13. Kosugi S, Mori T. The third exoplasmic loop of the thyrotropin receptor is partially involved in signal transduction. FEBS Lett 1994;349:89–92.
14. Ji I, Zeng H, Ji TH. Receptor activation of and signal generation by the lutropin/choriogonadotropin receptor. Cooperation of Asp[397] of the receptor and αLys[91] of the hormone. J Biol Chem 1993;268:22971–4.
15. Hoflack J, Hibert MF, Trumpp-Kallmeyer S, Bidart J-M. Three-dimensional models of gonado-thyrotropin hormone receptor transmembrane domain. Drug Des Discov 1993;10:157–71.
16. Ballesteros JA, Weinstein H. Analysis and refinement of criteria for predicting the structure and relative orientations of transmembrane helical domains. Biophys J 1992;62:107–9.
17. Trumpp-Kallmeyer S, Hoflack J, Bruinvels A, Hibert M. Modeling of G-protein-coupled receptors: application to dopamine, adrenaline, serotonin, acetylcholine, and mammalian opsin receptors. J Med Chem 1992;35:3448–62.
18. Hedin KE, Duerson K, Clapham DE. Specificity of receptor-G protein interactions: searching for the structure behind the signal. Cell Signal 1993;5:505–18.
19. Taylor JM, Neubig RR. Minireview: peptides as probes for G protein signal transduction. Cell Signal 1995;6:841–9.
20. Oliveira L, Paiva ACM, Sander C, Vriend G. A common step for signal transduction in G protein-coupled receptors. Trends Pharmacol Sci 1994;15:170–2.
21. Kjelsberg MA, Cotecchia S, Ostrowski J, Caron MG, Lefkowitz RJ. Constitutive activation of the α_{1B}-adrenergic receptor by all amino acid substitutions at a single site: evidence for a region which constrains receptor activation. J Biol Chem 1992;267:1430–3.
22. Allen LF, Lefkowitz RJ, Caron MG, Cotecchia S. G-protein-coupled receptor genes as protooncogenes: constitutively activating mutation of the α_{1B}-adrenergic receptor enhances mitogenesis and tumorigenicity. Proc Natl Acad Sci USA 1991;88:11354–8.
23. Samama P, Cotecchia S, Costa T, Lefkowitz RJ. A mutation-induced activated state of the β_2-adrenergic receptor: extending the ternary complex model. J Biol Chem 1993;268:4625–36.
24. Ren Q, Kurose H, Lefkowitz RJ, Cotecchia S. Constitutively active mutants of the α_2-adrenergic receptor. J Biol Chem 1993;268:16483–7.
25. Kosugi S, Okajima F, Ban T, Hidaka A, Shenker A, Kohn LD. Substitutions of different regions of the third cytoplasmic loop of the thyrotropin (TSH) receptor have selective effects on constitutive, TSH-, and TSH receptor autoantibody-stimulated phosphoinositide and 3′,5′-cyclic adenosine monophosphate signal generation. Mol Endocrinol 1993;7:1009–20.
26. Boone C, Davis NG, Sprague GF Jr. Mutations that alter the third cytoplasmic loop of the a-factor receptor lead to a constitutive and hypersensitive phenotype. Proc Natl Acad Sci USA 1993;90:9921–5.
27. Dryja TP, McGee TL, Hahn LB, Cowley GS, Olsson JE, Reichel E, et al. Mutations within the rhodopsin gene in patients with autosomal dominant retinitis pigmentosa. N Engl J Med 1990;323:1302–7.
28. Rosenthal W, Seibold A, Antaramian A, Lonergan M, Arthus M-F, Hendy GN, et al. Molecular identification of the gene responsible for congenital nephrogenic diabetes insipidus. Nature 1992;359:233–5.

29. Bargmann CI, Hung M-C, Weinberg RA. Multiple independent activations of the *neu* oncogene by a point mutation altering the transmembrane domain of p185. Cell 1986;45:649–57.
30. Mulligan LM, Kwok JBJ, Healey CS, Elsdon MJ, Eng C, Gardner E, et al. Germ-line mutations of the *RET* proto-oncogene in multiple endocrine neoplasia type 2A. Nature 1993;363:458–60.
31. de la Chapelle A, Träskelin A-L, Juvonen E. Truncated erythropoietin receptor causes dominantly inherited benign human erythrocytosis. Proc Natl Acad Sci USA 1993;90:4495–9.
32. Yaghmai R, Hazelbauer GL. Ligand occupancy mimicked by single residue substitutions in a receptor: transmembrane signaling induced by mutation. Proc Natl Acad Sci USA 1992;89:7890–4.
33. Holland FJ. Gonadotropin-independent precocious puberty. Endocrinol Metab Clin North Am 1991;20:191–210.
34. Shenker A, Laue L, Kosugi S, Merendino JJ Jr, Minegishi T, Cutler GB Jr. A constitutively activating mutation of the luteinizing hormone receptor in familial male precocious puberty. Nature 1993;365:652–4.
35. Kremer H, Mariman E, Otten BJ, Moll GW Jr, Stoelinga GBA, Wit JM, et al. Cosegregation of missense mutations of the luteinizing hormone receptor gene with familial male-limited precocious puberty. Hum Mol Genet 1993;2:1779–83.
36. Yano K, Hidaka A, Saji M, Polymeropoulos MH, Okuno A, Kohn LD, et al. A sporadic case of male-limited precocious puberty has the same constitutively activating point mutation in luteinizing hormone/choriogonadotropin receptor gene as familial cases. J Clin Endocrinol Metab 1994;79:1818–23.
37. Kosugi S, Van Dop C, Geffner ME, Rabl W, Carel J-C, Chaussain J-L, et al. Characterization of heterozygous mutations causing constitutive activation of the luteinizing hormone receptor in familial male precocious puberty. Hum Mol Genet 1995;4:183–8.
38. Boepple P, Crowley WF Jr, Albanese C, Jameson JL. Activating mutations of the LH receptor in sporadic male gonadotropin-independent precocious puberty [abstract]. Program and Abstracts, The Endocrine Society 76th Annual Meeting 1994;494.
39. Laue L, Chan W-Y, Hsueh AJW, Kudo M, Hsu SY, Wu S-M, et al. Genetic heterogeneity of constitutively activating mutations of the human luteinizing hormone receptor in familial male-limited precocious puberty. Proc Natl Acad Sci USA 1995;92:1906–10.
40. Yano K, Saji M, Hidaka A, Moriya N, Okuno A, Kohn LD, et al. A new constitutively activating point mutation in the luteinizing hormone/choriogonadotropin receptor gene in cases of male-limited precocious puberty. J Clin Endocrinol Metab 1995;80:1162–68.
41. Müller J, Kosugi S, Shenker A. A severe, non-familial case of testotoxicosis associated with a new mutation (Asp[578] to Tyr) of the lutropin receptor (LHR) gene [abstract]. Horm Res 1995;44(Suppl):13.
42. Sklar CA, Conte FA, Kaplan SL, Grumbach MM. Human chorionic gonadotropin-secreting pineal tumor: relation to pathogenesis and sex limitation of sexual precocity. J Clin Endocrinol Metab 1981;53:656–60.
43. Ji I, Ji TH. Asp[383] in the second transmembrane domain of the lutropin receptor is important for high affinity hormone binding and cAMP production. J Biol Chem 1991;266:14953–7.

44. Robinson PR, Cohen GB, Zhukovsky EA, Oprian DD. Constitutively active mutants of rhodopsin. Neuron 1992;9:719–25.
45. Dryja TP, Berson EL, Rao VR, Oprian DD. Heterozygous missense mutation in the rhodopsin gene as a cause of congenital stationary night blindness. Nat Genet 1993;4:280–3.
46. Rao VR, Cohen GB, Oprian DD. Rhodopsin mutation G90D and a molecular mechanism for congenital night blindness. Nature 1994;367:639–42.
47. Pollak MR, Brown EM, Estep HL, McLaine PN, Kifor O, Park J, et al. Autosomal dominant hypocalcemia caused by a Ca^{2+}-sensing receptor gene mutation. Nat Genet 1994;8:303–7.
48. Schipani E, Kruse K, Jüppner H. A constitutively active mutant PTH-PTHrP receptor in Jansen-type metaphyseal chondrodysplasia. Science 1995;268:98–100.
49. Parma J, Duprez L, Van Sande J, Cochaux P, Gervy C, Mockel J, et al. Somatic mutations in the thyrotropin receptor gene cause hyperfunctioning thyroid adenomas. Nature 1993;365:649–51.
50. Porcellini A, Ciullo I, Laviola L, Amabile G, Fenzi G, Avvedimento VE. Novel mutations of thyrotropin receptor gene in thyroid hyperfunctioning adenomas. Rapid identification by fine needle aspiration biopsy. J Clin Endocrinol Metab 1994;79:657–61.
51. Kopp P, Van Sande J, Parma J, Duprez L, Gerber H, Joss E, et al. Brief report: congenital hyperthyroidism caused by a mutation in the thyrotropin-receptor gene. N Engl J Med 1995;332:150–4.
52. Vassart G, Parma J, Van Sande J, Dumont JE. The thyrotropin receptor and the regulation of thyrocyte function and growth: update 1994. In: Braverman LE, Refetoff S, eds. Endocrine Reviews Monographs 3. Clinical and molecular aspects of diseases of the thyroid. Bethesda, MD: Endocrine Society Press, 1994:77–80.
53. Nothacker H-P, Grimmelikhuijzen CJP. Molecular cloning of a novel, putative G protein-coupled receptor from sea anemones structurally related to members of the FSH, TSH, LH/CG receptor family from mammals. Biochem Biophys Res Commun 1993;197:1062–9.
54. Grumbach MM, Conte FA. Disorders of sex differentiation. In: Wilson JD, Foster DW, eds. Williams' textbook of endocrinology. Philadelphia: WB Saunders, 1992:853–951.
55. Kremer H, Kraaij R, Toledo SPA, Post M, Fridman JB, Hayashida CY, et al. Male pseudohermaphroditism due to a homozygous missense mutation of the luteinizing hormone receptor gene. Nat Genet 1995;9:160–4.
56. Laue L, Wu SM, Kudo M, Hsueh AJW, Griffin JE, Wilson JD, et al. An inactivating mutation of the human luteinizing hormone receptor (hLHR) gene in familial Leydig cell hypoplasia [abstract]. Mol Biol Cell 1994;5:68a.

Part VI

Regulation of Steroidogenesis

21

Characterization of the Protein Responsible for the Acute Regulation of Steroidogenesis in Mouse Leydig Tumor Cells

Douglas M. Stocco, Barbara J. Clark, Dong Lin,
Teruo Sugawara, Jerome F. Strauss III,
and Walter L. Miller

This chapter discusses the cellular events that rapidly occur in response to the trophic hormone stimulation of steroidogenic tissues and result in the synthesis and secretion of arguably their most important products, the steroid hormones. These rapid or acute effects of hormone stimulation can be distinguished from the slower chronic effects in that acute effects occur within minutes, whereas chronic effects are those that require a period of many hours. Further, as pointed out earlier, the acute effects result in the synthesis and secretion of steroids only, whereas chronic effects usually involve increased gene transcription and translation of the proteins involved in the biosynthesis of these steroids in addition to steroid production. While both areas have been intensely studied, the molecular events that regulate the rapid production of hormonal steroids in steroidogenic tissues in response to trophic hormone stimulation have been the subject of intense investigation for over three decades. This chapter focuses only on those studies designed to elucidate the factors and mechanisms involved in the acute regulation of steroid production in response to hormone stimulation. Overviews of the effects of chronic stimulation on steroidogenic enzymes have appeared in several excellent review articles (1–4). While the focus of this book is on recent findings in the testis, the fact that a great deal of work on the acute regulation of steroidogenesis has been performed in other steroidogenic tissues, especially the adrenal, makes it imperative that these studies be included in this chapter.

The biosynthesis of all hormonal steroids in all steroidogenic tissues studied to date begins with the enzymatic cleavage of the side chain of the substrate cholesterol to form pregnenolone. This reaction is catalyzed by the *cholesterol side-chain cleavage* (CSCC) enzyme system, which is located on the matrix side of the inner mitochondrial membrane. Therefore, in order to initiate and sustain steroidogenesis, it is necessary to provide a constant supply of this substrate to this site of cleavage. Cholesterol transport within steroidogenic cells can be thought of as occurring in two separate processes. The first part of the process is the mobilization of cholesterol from cellular stores to the outer mitochondrial membrane, while the second part consists of the transfer of cholesterol from the outer to the inner mitochondrial membrane (5). It has also been reported that in MA-10 mouse Leydig tumor cells the immediate source of cholesterol for transfer to the inner mitochondrial membrane is the plasma membrane (6). Although the rate-limiting *enzymatic* step in steroidogenesis is the conversion of the substrate cholesterol to pregnenolone by the CSCC (7–9), the *true* rate-limiting step in this process is the delivery of the substrate to the inner mitochondrial membrane and the CSCC (10–14). Thus it is the second part of this two-part process that is considered rate limiting. The CSCC system is composed of three proteins: an iron sulfur protein, adrenodoxin; a flavoprotein, adrenodoxin reductase; and lastly, *cytochrome P-450 side-chain cleavage* (P-450scc), which cleaves cholesterol to pregnenolone (15–17). The major barrier to be overcome in the translocation of cholesterol to the P-450scc is the aqueous space between the outer and inner mitochondrial membranes through which this relatively hydrophobic compound must pass. Since the aqueous diffusion of cholesterol is extremely slow (18–20) and could not provide sufficient substrate to account for the rapid and large increase in steroid production observed in steroidogenic cells, the successful stimulation of steroidogenesis would appear to require the presence of a mechanism that rapidly transports cholesterol across this barrier. Thus, in simple terms, the regulation of steroidogenesis is controlled by a set of circumstances that facilitate the translocation of cholesterol from cellular stores across the aqueous intermembrane space of the mitochondria to the inner membrane.

Role of Translation

Early studies attempting to elucidate the mechanism responsible for the acute regulation of steroidogenesis demonstrated that steroid production in response to hormone stimulation had an absolute requirement for the synthesis of new proteins. The first of such studies demonstrated that stimulation of corticoid synthesis in adrenal glands by *adrenocorticotropic hormone* (ACTH) was sensitive to the protein synthesis inhibitor puromycin (21). Subsequent studies (22) indicated that adrenocorticoid production in response to ACTH could be totally blocked by inhibition of translation but not transcription. Later, Simpson et al. (23) determined that the cycloheximide-sensitive step in this process was located in the mitochondria, but, importantly, it was also noted that protein synthesis inhibitors had no effect on the activity of the CSCC complex itself (24). The observation that de novo protein synthesis is indispensable for the acute production of steroids in response to hormone stimulation has also been made more recently in several different steroidogenic tissues (25–29). All of these observations have been elegantly confirmed in both mouse Y-1 adrenal tumor cells and MA-10 mouse Leydig tumor cells (30). These studies demonstrated that while cholesterol could be delivered to a "presteroidogenic pool" in the presence of cycloheximide, pregnenolone production did not take place until the inhibitor was removed and the cells subsequently stimulated with hormone. As a result of these and other observations, the model arose that the acute production of steroids was dependent on a rapidly synthesized, cycloheximide-sensitive, and highly labile protein that appeared in re-sponse to trophic hormone treatment. A graphic illustration of the compo-nents of the system that depicts the problem involved in the transport of cholesterol both to the mitochondria and subsequently to the CSCC is shown in Figure 21.1.

Role of Transcription

Over the years studies have been performed in order to determine whether, in a manner similar to that observed for translation, de novo transcription was also required in the acute regulation of steroidogenesis. While one such study (31) indicated that new transcription was required for the acute production of steroids in rat testicular cells in response to hormone treat-ment, the majority of such studies indicated that acute steroidogenesis could occur independently of new RNA synthesis (32–36). It has been argued that the rapidity with which steroid synthesis begins in response to hormone stimulation would make it most difficult to account for both the transcription and translation of a new protein (37). Thus, mechanisms were proposed in which either an existing, inactive protein required for steroido-genesis was rapidly converted to an active protein by the action of trophic hormone or a new protein was rapidly synthesized using a preexisting and stable *messenger RNA* (mRNA) (37). In summary, prior to this time it has not been possible to determine unequivocally whether new transcription was required for the acute production of steroids. We will present evidence later in this chapter that is based on recent observations in our laboratory and that will serve to clarify the role of transcription in the acute production of steroids. What does appear to be clear, as described above, is that based on a large volume of data using protein synthesis inhibitors (21, 22, 37–39) a newly synthesized protein is required for cholesterol transfer. Thus, any mechanism proposed for the activation of a preexisting mRNA with trophic hormone and resulting in the synthesis of a new protein would be consistent

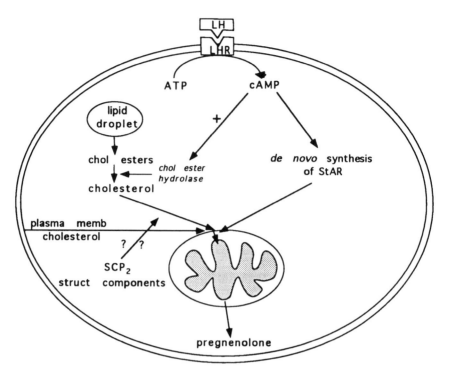

FIGURE 21.1. Effects of trophic hormone stimulation on leydig cells. This figure depicts the cellular response to tropic hormone stimulation in Leydig cells and probably in all steroidogenic cells as well. In response to tropic hormone stimulation, activation of the adenylate cyclase enzyme results in the intracellular increase in cAMP. This increase in turn results in the activation of two separate but important pathways in support of the acute production of steroids. First, activation of the cholesterol ester hydrolase by phosphorylation converts cholesterol esters to free cholesterol, which is mobilized to the outer mitochondrial membrane. Also, other mechanisms involved in the mobilization of cholesterol to the outer mitochondrial membrane may be activated by trophic hormone. These steps are necessary to assure an adequate supply of this precursor for sustained steroid biosynthesis. Second, the de novo synthesis of the 37-kd StAR precursor protein is rapidly accomplished. The synthesis and processing of the StAR precursor results in the transfer of cholesterol to the inner mitochondrial membrane, where it is cleaved to pregnenolone (and probably to progesterone by the mitochondrial 3β-hydroxystyeroid dehydrogenase). Recent results from our laboratory indicate that expression of StAR cannot result in maximal steroid production in the absence of cholesterol mobilization, but they also indicate, more importantly, that even in the presence of maximal cholesterol mobilization no steroid synthesis occurs in the absence of StAR.

with these data. In summary, it appears that while de novo protein synthesis is required for the acute regulation of steroid production in response to hormone stimulation, as we shall discuss later, de novo transcription is not.

Role of Phosphorylation

Steroidogenic cells respond to trophic hormones with the rapid production of steroids. This response is mediated through the *adenosine 3':5'-cyclic monophosphate* (cAMP) second messenger system (36, 40–43), which in turn activates cAMP-dependent protein kinase (protein kinase A). Activation of protein kinase A normally results in the phosphorylation of proteins on either threonine or serine residues (44). Thus, steroidogenesis would appear to be dependent upon the phosphorylation of a protein(s) substrate on serine or threonine residues in response to hormone stimulation. Using amino acid analogues that were incapable of being phosphorylated, it has been demonstrated that in both rat adrenal cortex cells (45) and MA-10 Leydig tumor cells (46) the phosphorylation of a protein on a threonine residue is required for steroidogenesis. The presence of newly synthesized phosphoproteins has been observed in stimulated adrenal cells (27, 47–49), in primary cultures of mouse Leydig cells (26), and in stimulated MA-10 cells (50), but a cause-and-effect relationship between the phosphorylation of these proteins and steroid production cannot be confirmed at this time. This is a most important area that requires significant attention in the immediate future.

Cellular Architecture

A number of studies have indicated that cellular architecture plays an important role in the delivery of cholesterol to the mitochondria for subsequent steroidogenesis. The transfer of cholesterol to the outer mitochondrial membrane in response to trophic hormone stimulation was found to occur in the absence of de novo protein synthesis (10, 12, 13) but was inhibited by compounds that disrupted microtubules and microfilaments (10, 38, 51–56). Thus, the cytoskeleton is believed to have an important function in steroidogenesis (53, 54, 57–59). It has also been shown that trophic hormone stimulation of human granulosa cells results in a morphological rounding of the cells, which causes a clustering of steroidogenic organelles, potentially bringing mitochondria into closer contact with pools of cholesterol (60). More recently, several studies have demonstrated the importance of the 10-nm intermediate filaments in the movement of cholesterol within Y-1 mouse adrenal tumor cells and primary cultures of bovine adrenal and rat Leydig cells (61–64). These studies demonstrated that both lipid droplets and mitochondria are co-localized on intermediate filaments and hypothesized that this co-localization was the means by which cholesterol was delivered to the mitochondria from the lipid droplet. Thus, it appears that subcellular structures such as microtubules, microfilaments, and intermediate filaments are instrumental in the delivery of cholesterol to the mitochondria. However, there is no convincing evidence that any of these structures play a role in the transfer of cholesterol from cellular stores or the outer mitochondrial membrane to the inner mitochondrial membrane where cleavage takes place.

Candidates for the Acute Regulatory Protein

Sterol Carrier Protein-2 (SCP₂)

SCP_2 is a 13-kd protein that has been found in high abundance in liver as well as in various steroidogenic tissues. Also known as nonspecific lipid transfer protein, the role of this protein in liver and adrenal cells has been reviewed by Vahouny et al. (65, 66). SCP_2 has been demonstrated to transfer cholesterol from lipid droplets to mitochondria in a 1:1 ratio (67). It has also been shown to be capable of stimulating steroid production in isolated adrenal mitochondria (67–70). Also, coexpression of SCP_2 with cholesterol side-chain cleavage enzyme and adrenodoxin in COS 7 cells resulted in a 2.5-fold increase in steroid production over that seen with expression of the steroidogenic enzyme system alone (71). Another indication of the role of SCP_2 in steroidogenesis can be found in the observation that treatment of adrenal cells with anti-SCP_2 antibody resulted in an inhibition of steroid production (72). The gene encoding SCP_2 gives rise to two transcripts: one encoding a 58-kd protein, SCPx, which has homologies to thiolases, and the other encoding a 15.3-kd protein, SCP_2, which is processed to yield a mature 13-kd polypeptide. Both SCPx and SCP_2 have carboxy terminal peroxisome targeting sequences, and SCPx/SCP_2 immunoreactivity has been localized to peroxisomes that are the sites of cholesterol synthesis (73–77). While the synthesis of SCP_2 has been shown to be under the regulation of ACTH (78), this regulation only occurred after many hours and, in fact, acute stimulation of adrenal cells with ACTH had no effect on SCP_2 levels (79). However, in rat testicular Leydig cells, acute stimulation with *luteinizing hormone* (LH) appeared to result in a redistribution of SCP_2 within the cell (80). While SCP_2 has been demonstrated to be regulated by cAMP analogues in the ovary, it is also regulated in a similar manner in a non-steroidogenic granulosa cell line, indicating that its regulation is not obligatorily coupled to steroidogenesis (81). In addition, evidence that SCP_2 is able to effectively transfer cholesterol to the inner mitochondrial membrane and the P-450scc in amounts adequate to support steroidogenesis in response to hormone stimulation is not convincing at this time. This coupled with the observation that SCP$_2$ levels do not rapidly change in response either to acute stimulation or to treatment with cycloheximide makes it unlikely that this protein has a major role in the acute regulation of steroid production; instead, it may function to maintain sterol movement within the cell in support of steroidogenesis, perhaps by affecting the utilization of peroxisome-derived cholesterol (82).

Steroidogenesis Activator Polypeptide (SAP)

Another peptide thought to play a role in the acute regulation of steroidogenesis is SAP. Originally purified as a 2.2-kd peptide from rat adrenal cells (83, 84), SAP was later determined to be a 30 amino acid (3.2-kd) peptide when it was purified from rat Leydig tumor cells (85). This peptide was found to be present only in steroidogenic cells; its levels could be acutely increased by trophic hormone stimulation, and this increase was prevented by cycloheximide (86–88). Addition of SAP to isolated mitochondria was able to increase steroid production by 4- to 5-fold in a dose-dependent manner, thus indicating that SAP may play a role in cholesterol transfer within this organelle (83, 84). SAP was found to be nearly completely identical to the carboxy terminal of a minor heat shock protein known as glucose-related protein 78 (89, 90). While a mechanism whereby SAP can transport cholesterol to the inner mitochondrial membrane has not yet been satisfactorily demonstrated, because of its reported characteristics, this small peptide must still be considered when discussing intra-mitochondrial cholesterol transport.

Peripheral Benzodiazepine Receptor (PBR); 8.2-kd Protein

A great deal of attention has been given to the possible role of the *peripheral benzodiazepine receptor* (PBR) [also called the *mitochondrial benzodiazepine receptor* (MBR)] in the acute regulation of steroidogenesis. PBRs are 18-kd proteins present in most cell types and originally found to be present in high concentrations in the outer mitochondrial membrane (91, 92). Reviews of both the characteristics of the PBRs and their potential role in steroidogenesis have recently appeared (93–96). PBRs were found to be present in especially high concentrations in the outer mitochondrial membranes of steroidogenic tissues (93, 97–99). Treatment of either MA-10 mouse Leydig tumor cells or Y-1 mouse adrenal tumor cells with PBR agonists resulted in significant increases in steroid production (96, 98–102). Stimulation of steroid production in response to PBR ligands was also observed in bovine primary adrenal cell cultures (103), human placental tissue (104), and ovarian granulosa cells (97). It was also demonstrated that the endogenous ligand for the PBR was an approximately 10-kd peptide known as the *diazepam-binding inhibitor* (DBI), also known as endozepine (105).

Subsequent studies showed that both DBI and DBI processing products were able to stimulate steroid production in rat adrenal primary cultures, Y-1 adrenal, and MA-10 Leydig cells (106–108). Furthermore, addition of the PBR ligand, endozepine, to a cholesterol side-chain cleavage reconstituted enzyme system was able to stimulate the conversion of cholesterol to pregnenolone (109). Also, a DBI antagonist was shown to inhibit the trophic hormone stimulated steroid production in both Y-1 adrenal and MA-10 Leydig cells (101). Further studies indicated that DBI and another PBR ligand, 4'-chlorodiazepam, were both able to stimulate pregnenolone production in the C6-2B glioma cell line (102, 110). An additional observation that illustrated the potential for DBI/PBR to provide cholesterol for steroidogenesis was the demonstration that removal of DBI from MA-10 Leydig cells using cholesterol-linked phosphorothioate antisense oligonucleotides to DBI resulted in a loss of trophic hormone stimulated steroid production in these cells (111).

Supporting the role of DBI/PBR in steroidogenic regulation were the studies of Yanagibashi et al. (112) in which they demonstrated that an 8.2-kd peptide purified from bovine adrenal cells was able to stimulate pregnenolone production in isolated mitochondria. The significance of this observation became apparent when the peptide was identified as des-(Gly-Ile)-endozepine (113). Thus, the 8.2-kd peptide and DBI were virtually identical. To account for the mechanism whereby the PBR/DBI system can effect the transfer of cholesterol to the inner mitochondrial membrane, recent studies have indicated that stimulation of MA-10 Leydig tumor cells with trophic hormone resulted in the induction of a higher affinity DBI binding site on the PBR, which in turn resulted in the increased transfer of cholesterol to the inner membrane (114). This group also reported that in the constitutive steroid producing cell line, the rat R2C Leydig tumor cell line, the higher affinity DBI site was continuously present and hence, a steady supply of cholesterol was available to the inner mitochondrial membrane (115). Lastly, they put forth the model that it was the association of PBR and DBI with several additional molecules in the mitochondrial membrane that formed a pore complex of approximately 140,000 MW through which cholesterol and possibly other molecules could theoretically pass to the inner mitochondrial membrane (116).

Snyder and colleagues have demonstrated that the PBR can be isolated from mitochondria as a complex of three proteins consisting of the 18-kd PBR, the 32-kd *voltage-dependent anion carrier* (VDAC), and the 30-kd *adenine nucleotide carrier* (ANC) (117). They also illustrated that ligands to the PBR were able to link this receptor to inner mitochondrial membrane ion channels at nanomolar concentrations (118). The significance of these findings is that the VDAC is associated with areas of the mitochondrial membrane known as "contact sites," where the inner and outer membranes come in close apposition to each other (119–121). The role of contact sites in the intramitochondrial transfer of cholesterol has recently been reviewed (122), and it appears that the formation of such contacts may be a necessary component for sterol transfer. Thus, PBR-ligand interactions may enhance the formation of contact sites through PBR's association with the VDAC, thus allowing cholesterol to transfer to the inner membrane.

However, several inconsistencies arise in studies dealing with the role of DBI/PBR in the acute regulation of steroidogenesis in steroidogenic cells. It was first reported (123) that the acute synthesis of des-(Gly-Ile)-DBI was rapidly increased by ACTH in adrenocortical cells and that the half-life of this protein was very short in the presence of cycloheximide, both characteristics for a potential steroidogenic regulatory protein as described by Ferguson (21), Garren et al. (22), and Stevens et al. (30). However, more recent studies have shown that DBI is not acutely regulated by trophic hormone treatment of either adrenocortical or Leydig cells and that the half-life of this protein is greater than 3 h (124). This makes it unlikely that hormonal regulation of DBI could be responsible for the acute production of steroids. In another study it was demonstrated that rat adrenal DBI and PBR levels were reduced dramatically following 9 days of hypophysectomy. ACTH administration to these hypophysectomized rats resulted in an increase in steroidogenesis that peaked within 1 h while both PBR and DBI mRNA and protein levels showed no increase for approximately 12 h, leading the authors to conclude that steroidogenesis and PBR/DBI levels were not temporally related to the acute steroidogenesis induced by ACTH and may reflect its long-term trophic action on adrenocortical cells (125). Also, it was argued that the outer mitochondrial location of the PBR provided strong evidence for its specific role in the regulation of cholesterol transfer and steroidogenesis (99). However, PBRs, while heavily concentrated on the outer mitochondrial membrane, have recently been shown to be present on the cell surface in adrenal cortex cells as well (126). Also, studies performed in one of our laboratories (J.F.S.) failed to demonstrate any stimulation of pregnenolone synthesis in COS cells cotransfected with P-450scc, adrenodoxin, and human PBR, both with and without its ligand DBI (unpublished observations). Similar cotransfections in COS cells with P-450scc, adrenodoxin, and SCP_2 resulted in a 2.5-fold increase in steroid production (71), and cotransfections with P-450scc, adrenodoxin, and the *steroidogenic acute regulatory* (StAR) protein also resulted in highly significant increases in steroid production, as will be discussed in more detail in a later section of this chapter. Further, it has been reported that DBI is identical to acyl-*coenzyme A* (CoA) ester binding protein, and as such it has been argued that this protein plays no role as a ligand in signal transduction pathways (127). In addition, Snyder et al. (128) caution that the affinity of the PBR for some porphyrins is 1,000 times greater than its affinity for endozepine, that the endogenous ligands may, in fact, be porphyrins, and that the endozepine-like activity found in extracts may be due to the presence of small amounts of porphyrin. A further discrepancy concerning the role of the PBR in cholesterol transfer to the CSCC for steroid production will be discussed later in the section Lipoid Congenital Adrenal Hyperplasia. Lastly, while most investigations using ligands of the PBR have shown that such treatment is stimulatory, a number of investigations have demonstrated that treatment of steroidogenic tissues with PBR ligands can also be inhibitory to steroidogenesis (129–132).

Steroidogenic Acute Regulatory (StAR) Protein

Another group of proteins that has been thought to be involved in the acute regulation of steroid production in steroidogenic tissues is a family of mitochondrial proteins and phosphoproteins that have been described and characterized during the past decade. These proteins were perhaps first observed as being synthesized in response to ACTH stimulation of Y-1 adrenal tumor cells (35). However, the pioneering studies on this group of proteins were elegantly performed in Orme-Johnson's laboratory using radiolabeling and *two-dimensional polyacrylamide gel electrophoresis* (2-D PAGE). These studies demonstrated that these proteins consisted of a family of approximately 30-kd proteins that rapidly appeared in response to corticotropic hormone stimulation of rat adrenal cells and were cyclohex-imide sensitive (25). Later studies indicated that similar proteins were also synthesized in response to trophic hormone treatment in the corpus luteum (133), as well as in primary cultures of mouse testicular Leydig cells (26, 134). These proteins were then determined to be phosphoproteins in both adrenal and corpus luteum cells (27, 47). This group then used several amino acid analogues to demonstrate that steroidogenesis could be inhibited under conditions only partially inhibitory to protein synthesis, further indicating the necessity for the production of a labile protein in the acute regulation of steroidogenesis (39). Subcellular fractionation illustrated that these rapidly synthesized proteins were localized in the mitochondria of hormone-stimulated adrenal cells (48, 135). Recent observations have indicated that in ACTH stimulated rat adrenal cortex cells the 30-kd mitochondrial proteins arise as a result of the processing of two larger precursor forms having molecular weights of 37-kd and 32-kd (49). Much of the work on the acute regulation of steroidogenesis in adrenal cells was recently reviewed by Orme-Johnson (136). Lastly, it should be noted that in at least two additional laboratories, mitochondrial proteins similar or identical in molecular weights and isoelectric points have been described in hormone-stimulated small luteal cells and adrenal glomerulosa cells (137, 138).

In our laboratory the MA-10 mouse Leydig tumor cell line is employed as a model system with which to study the acute regulation of steroid production in response to hormone stimulation. These cells were derived from the M5480P tumor and have been shown to have functional LH/*chorionic gonadotropin* (CG) receptors and to produce large amounts of progesterone in response to stimulation (139). Observations made in our laboratory during the past 7–8 years indicate that MA-10 cells also synthesize a family of 37-kd, 32-kd, and 30-kd mitochondrial proteins in response to trophic hormone and cAMP analogue treatment and that the appearance and quantity of these proteins are highly correlative with the temporal appearance and quantitative levels of steroids produced (28, 29, 46, 50, 140–143).

However, while many of these earlier observations were most compelling, they remained correlative in nature; an unequivocal link between the synthesis and appearance of these mitochondrial proteins and increased steroidogenesis could not be made until recently. From a historical point of view, these correlations were found to exist in adrenal fasciculata cells, adrenal glomerulosa cells, primary cultures of luteal cells and Leydig cells, and MA-10 tumor Leydig cells and to include (i) the presence of similar (probably identical) proteins in response to hormone stimulation in primary cultures of adrenal fasciculata (25, 33, 39, 47–49, 133, 138), adrenal glomerulosa (139), luteal (27, 137), primary Leydig cell cultures (26, 134, 140), and MA-10 Leydig tumor cells (28, 29, 46, 50, 140–143); (ii) the appearance of the proteins following hormone stimulation in a time- and dose-dependent manner in rat adrenal (25) and MA-10 mouse Leydig tumor cells (28); (iii) the finding that the synthesis of the 30-kd proteins is sensitive to cycloheximide in rat adrenal (25), mouse Leydig cells (26), corpus luteum cells (27), and MA-10 cells (29); (iv) the constitutive presence of the 30-kd mitochondrial proteins in the constitutively steroid-producing R$_2$C rat Leydig tumor cell line (29); (v) the finding that the metal chelator orthophenanthroline, which inhibits the mitochondrial matrix protease, thus blocking the processing of the 37-kd protein to the 30-kd proteins, results in the disappearance of the 30-kd proteins and the total inhibition of steroidogenesis in MA-10 cells (142), whereas in R$_2$C cells steroidogenesis is not completely inhibited by this compound and significant amounts of the 30-kd proteins can be found in the mitochondria (142); (vi) inhibition of both steroidogenesis and the appearance of these proteins in the mitochondria in MA-10 cells in response to *carbonyl cyanide m-chlorophenyl-hydrazone* (*m*CCCP), a compound that disrupts the electrochemical potential across the inner mitochondrial membrane and prevents translocation of mitochondrial proteins (142); (vii) the loss of both constitutive steroid-producing capacity and the mitochondrial proteins in a "revertant" of the R$_2$C cell line (142); (viii) the correlation between steroid production and the mitochondrial 30-kd proteins in two stable constructs of the MA-10 cell line, one of which produces a mutant regulatory subunit of protein kinase A and the other of which constitutively overproduces a cAMP phosphodiesterase (143); (ix) the correlation between steroid production and the mitochondrial 30-kd proteins in MA-10 cells in response to treatment of stimulated MA-10 cells with threonine and serine analogues (46), hydrogen peroxide (144), and dimethyl sulfoxide (145).

As a result of these correlations, it became increasingly necessary that we attempt to establish a direct cause-and-effect relationship between the synthesis of these proteins and the production of steroids. With this goal in mind, we embarked on the purification, cloning, and expression of the 30-kd mitochondrial proteins. Within the past 2 years we have purified the protein to homogeneity, obtained amino acid sequence for several tryptic peptides, and used this sequence information to design degenerative oligonucleotides for cloning the cDNA. A cDNA library was generated using mRNA isolated from hormone stimulated MA-10 cells, and a 400-bp PCR product was amplified from the cDNA library using the degenerative oligonucleotides. The PCR product was then used to probe the library, and a 1,500-bp full-length cDNA clone was isolated. Comparison of the nucleic acid and deduced amino acid sequences to the GenEMBL and SWISS-PROT data bases revealed that the cDNA encoded a novel protein. Most important, however, was our observation that transient transfection and expression of this protein in MA-10 cells resulted in a significant increase in steroid production in the absence of hormone stimulation of any kind (146). We have since extended these studies to include observations that the transient transfection of the 30-kd protein can account for a rate and capacity of steroid production equal to that produced by hormone stimulation. We have also generated stable transfected MA-10 cell lines that constitutively synthesize the 30-kD protein and produce steroid constitutively at a level several times higher than basal parental MA-10 cells. Lastly, we have transiently transfected nonsteroidogenic monkey COS-1 kidney cells for expression of the 30-kd protein (in conjunction with P-450scc and adrenodoxin) and shown that these cells become highly steroidogenic only in the presence of the 30-kd protein. Therefore, for the first time ever in studies dealing with the acute regulation of steroid hormone production in response to the synthesis of a putative protein factor, we have demonstrated a direct cause and effect relationship between the expression of a specific protein and increased steroid production. As such, we have named this protein the *St*eroidogenic *A*cute *R*egulatory (StAR) protein (144).

In addition to the studies on StAR in MA-10 cells, we have also (i) isolated a cDNA for StAR from a human adrenal library; (ii) demonstrated that this cDNA is 86% identical to the mouse cDNA; (iii) shown that the tissue distribution of its mRNA is restricted to adrenal, gonadal, and possibly kidney in the human; (iv) shown that the coexpression of the human StAR cDNA with P-450scc and adrenodoxin in COS cells results in an increase in steroid production (147). We have also used fluorescence in situ hybridization to demonstrate that StAR resides on chromosome 8, region p11.2 in the human (147). Lastly, in vitro transcription, translation, and processing (using control mitochondria) have confirmed that the cDNA encodes all forms of the StAR protein previously reported (146, 148). We have also determined that while mRNA for StAR is undetectable by Northern analysis in unstimulated control cells, which make very little steroid, low levels of mRNA can be detected by *reverse transcriptase–polymerase chain reaction* (RT-PCR) (unpublished data). In addition, no difference was observed in the production of steroids in response to hormone stimulation in the presence and absence of the transcription inhibitor actinomycin D for the first 60–90 min. Following this time period steroid production in the inhibitor-treated cells plateaued, while control cells continued to make large amounts of steroid. Western analysis indicated no difference in the production of StAR protein in the first hour following actinomycin D treatment, but thereafter StAR was increased only in the noninhibitor treated cells, a pattern totally consistent with steroid production. Although the effect on mRNA levels has yet to be determined, Northern analysis indicates that no new mRNA for StAR is detected until approximately 2 h following stimulation. Therefore, it appears that the initial synthesis of StAR (and thus steroids) can occur from preexisting mRNA, which is present in control cells but that the continuing production of steroids following this initial period is dependent on new transcription. These observations confirm earlier studies that indicated that the initiation of steroidogenesis, while requiring de novo translation, does not require de novo transcription.

Lipoid Congenital Adrenal Hyperplasia

Perhaps the most striking evidence for the importance of StAR in the acute regulation of steroidogenesis is the results recently obtained from studies on the disease *lipoid congenital adrenal hyperplasia* (LCAH). LCAH is a lethal condition that results from a complete inability of the newborn infant to synthesize steroids. The lack of mineralocorticoids and glucocorticoids results in death within days to weeks of birth if not detected and treated with adequate replacement therapy. This condition is manifested by the presence of large adrenals containing very high levels of cholesterol and cholesterol esters and also by an increased amount of lipid accumulation in testicular Leydig cells, although this level is somewhat lower than that seen in adrenals. As isolated mitochondria from adrenals and gonads of affected patients cannot convert cholesterol to pregnenolone (149–152), this disease was understandably thought to be due to an abnormality of P-450scc enzyme activity, which converts cholesterol to pregnenolone (153). Recently, however, this enzyme has been shown to be normal in patients who suffered from this disease (154). Additionally, and most importantly, the mRNA encoding other proteins that either play a role or have been purported to play a role in the regulation of steroidogenesis such as adrenodoxin, adrenodoxin reductase, SAP, SCP$_2$, HSP-78, and PBR have also been shown to be present at apparently normal levels of abundance in these patients (154, 155). Recent clinical studies surprisingly showed that placental steroidogenesis persists in LCAH (156).

When we then observed that StAR was expressed normally in adrenals and gonads, but not in placenta (147), we postulated that LCAH was due to a disordered StAR protein. Testicular tissue of two patients and genomic DNA of a third patient with LCAH have mutations in the gene for StAR (157). These mutations result from C to T transitions in the gene sequences, which resulted in the premature insertion of stop codons. This resulted in the truncation of StAR protein by 28 amino acids in two of the patients and 93 amino acids in another. These truncations were confirmed by Western analysis following expression of the mutated cDNAs in COS-1 cells (157). In addition, virtually none of the precursor form of StAR expressed from the cDNAs of these patients was converted to the mature mitochondrial form. Expression of the StAR cDNA from these patients in COS-1 cells indicated that the protein produced was completely inactive in its ability to promote steroidogenesis, while the normal human protein resulted in an 8-fold increase in steroid production when expressed. Finally, the need for StAR activity could be circumvented by using freely diffusable 20α-hydroxycholesterol as a substrate for steroidogenesis (157). Therefore, in a most dramatic manner, the indispensable role of StAR in the production of steroids has been demonstrated.

Model of StAR Action

Because of our observations on the expression of StAR precursor followed by its processing to the mature mitochondrial forms (146), and because of the observations made during the studies on LCAH (157), we have formulated a model whereby StAR may act in the acute regulation of cholesterol transfer to the CSCC. We propose that in response to hormone stimulation, the 37-kd precursor protein is rapidly synthesized in the cystosol, probably using a preexisting mRNA. The 37-kd protein is targeted to the mitochondria via its signal sequence and interacts with a specific receptor on the mitochondrial outer membrane. As the transfer of this protein to the inner mitochondrial compartment begins, "contact sites" between the inner and outer membranes are formed and the signal sequence is removed by a matrix-processing protease forming the 32-kd form of the protein. Further processing of the protein removes the targeting sequence, and the mature 30-kd protein remains associated with either the inner mitochondrial or inter-membrane compartment. We propose that it is during the processing of the protein with the accompanying formation of "contact sites" that

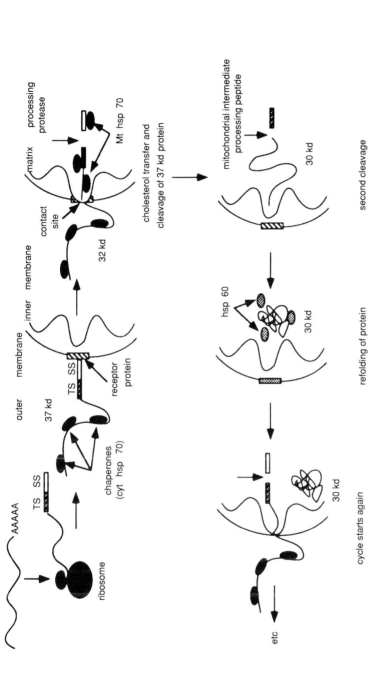

FIGURE 21.2. Proposed mechanism for the acute regulation of steroidogenesis. Upon stimulation of the Leydig cell with trophic hormone, a 37-kd protein is rapidly synthesized in the cytoplasm. This protein is accompanied by chaperon proteins, which prohibit folding of the 37-kd protein, a condition that would make transfer of the protein into the mitochondrion impossible. The 37-kd protein is then transported to the mitochondria, where it interacts with a specific receptor protein on the outer mitochondrial membrane. At this time the insertion process begins and contact sites between the outer and inner mitochondrial membranes are formed concomitant with the first cleavage event. The cleavage of the first signal precursor by the matrix protease results in the formation of a 32-kd intermediate form of this protein. It is during this time that cholesterol is able to transfer from the outer to the inner mitochondrial membrane. Lastly, the inner and outer membrane separate and the 32-kd protein is cleaved a second time to give the 30-kd product, which is no longer able to function in the further transfer of cholesterol.

cholesterol is able to transfer from the outer to the inner mitochondrial membrane (158) and hence be available to the CSCC.

Following processing of the 37-kd protein to the 30-kd proteins, the membranes once again separate and no further cholesterol transfer can occur. Thus, it is the continued synthesis and processing of additional precursor proteins that allows for the continued transport of cholesterol to the inner membrane. Since the half-life of the 37-kd and 32-kd precursors of the 30-kd mitochondrial proteins has been shown to be very short (49), this would explain the observation that steroidogenesis decays very quickly in the absence of new protein synthesis. In support of this model, we and others have demonstrated the presence of such precursor proteins (28, 49) and have shown that the 30-kd proteins are found associated with the inner mitochondrial compartment (28, 146). These observations, coupled with those indicating that the transport of mitochondrial proteins across the membranes occurs at contact sites (159–164), make this a viable model at this point in time. We should point out, however, that we have no information as to whether this transfer of cholesterol occurs in a passive manner when contact sites are formed or whether StAR has the capacity to act as a cholesterol-binding protein and hence carry cholesterol to the inner mitochondrial membrane. A summary of this model is shown in Figure 21.2.

In summary, we report at this time that the long-sought protein factor responsible for the transfer of cholesterol from cellular stores to the inner mitochondrial membrane and thus necessary for regulating the acute production of steroids has been unequivocally identified. The key future studies concerning StAR will be to determine the elements responsible for the regulation of this most important gene, and to determine the mechanism whereby StAR is able to effect the transfer of cholesterol to the inner mitochondrial membrane and the CSCC.

Acknowledgments. The authors would like to acknowledge the support of NIH grants HD 17481 (D.M.S.), HD 07688 (B.J.C.), HD 06274 (J.F.S.), DK 37922 and DK 42154 (W.L.M.), HD 28825 and Department of Pediatrics, University of California–San Francisco (D.L.).

References

1. Simpson ER, Waterman MR. Regulation by ACTH of steroid hormone biosynthesis in the adrenal cortex. Can J Biochem Cell Biol 1983;61:692–707.
2. Miller WL. Molecular biology of steroid hormone synthesis. Endocr Rev 1988;9:295–318.
3. Hanukoglu I. Steroidogenic enzymes: structure, function, and role in the regulation of steroid hormone biosynthesis. J Steroid Biochem Mol Biol 1992; 43:779–804.

4. Payne AH, Youngblood GI. Regulation of expression of steroidogenic enzymes in Leydig cells. Biol Reprod 1995;52:217–25.

5. Liscum L, Dahl NK. Intracellular cholesterol transport. J Lipid Res 1992;33:1239–54.

6. Freeman DA. Plasma membrane cholesterol: removal and insertion into the membrane and utilization as substrate for steroidogenesis. Endocrinology 1989;124:2527–34.

7. Stone D, Hechter O. Studies on ACTH action in perfused bovine adrenals: site of action of ACTH in corticosteroidogenesis. Arch Biochem Biophys 1954;51:457–69.

8. Karaboyas GC, Koritz SB. Identity of the site of action of cAMP and ACTH in corticosteroidogenesis in rat adrenal and beef adrenal cortex slices. Biochemistry 1965;4:462–8.

9. Garren LD, Gill GN, Masui H, Walton GM. On the mechanism of action of ACTH. Recent Prog Horm Res 1971;27:433–78.

10. Crivello JF, Jefcoate CR. Intracellular movement of cholesterol in rat adrenal cells. Kinetics and effects of inhibitors. J Biol Chem 1980;255:8144–51.

11. Jefcoate CR, DiBartolomeos MJ, Williams CA, McNamara BC. ACTH regulation of cholesterol movement in isolated adrenal cells. J Steroid Biochem 1987;27:721–9.

12. Privalle CT, Crivello JF, Jefcoate CR. Regulation of intramitochondrial cholesterol transfer to side-chain cleavage cytochrome P450scc in rat adrenal gland. Proc Natl Acad Sci USA 1983;80:702–6.

13. Privalle CT, McNamara BC, Dhariwal MS, Jefcoate CR. ACTH control of cholesterol side-chain cleavage at adrenal mitochondrial cytochrome P450scc. Regulation of intramitochondrial cholesterol transfer. Mol Cell Endocrinol 1983;53:87–101.

14. Lambeth JD, Xu XX, Glover M. Cholesterol sulfate inhibits adrenal mitochondrial cholesterol side-chain cleavage at a site distinct from cytochrome P450scc. Evidence for an intramitochondrial cholesterol translocator. J Biol Chem 1987;262:9181–8.

15. Lambeth JD, Seybert DW, Kamin H. Ionic effects on adrenal steroidogenic electron transport. The role of adrenodoxin as an electron shuttle. J Biol Chem 1979;254:7255–64.

16. Tuls J, Geren L, Lambeth JD, Millet F. The use of a specific fluorescence probe to study the interaction of adrenodoxin reductase and cytochrome P450scc. J Biol Chem 1987;262:10020–5.

17. Hanukoglu I, Hanukoglu Z. Stoichiometry of mitochondrials, cytochromes P450, adrenodoxin and adrenodoxin reductase in adrenal cortex and corpus luteum. Eur J Biochem 1986;157:27–31.

18. Rennert H, Chang YJ, Strauss JF. Intracellular cholesterol dynamics in steroidogenic cells: a contemporary view. In: Adashi EY, Leung PK, eds. The ovary. New York: Raven Press, 1993:147–64.

19. Schroeder F, Jefferson JR, Kier AB, Knittel J, Scallen TJ, Wood WG, Hapala I. Membrane cholesterol dynamics: cholesterol domains and kinetic pools. Proc Soc Exptl Biol Med 1991;196:235–52.

20. Phillips MC, Johnson WJ, Rothblat GH. Mechanisms and consequences of cellular cholesterol exchange and transfer. Biochim Biophys Acta 1987;906:223–76.

21. Ferguson JJ. Protein synthesis and adrenocorticotropin responsiveness. J Biol Chem 1963;238:2754–9.
22. Garren LD, Ney RL, Davis WW. Studies on the role of protein synthesis in the regulation of corticosterone production by ACTH in vivo. Proc Natl Acad Sci USA 1965;53:1443–50.
23. Simpson ER, McCarthy JL, Peterson JA. Evidence that the cycloheximidesensitive site of ACTH action is in the mitochondrion. J Biol Chem 1979;253:3135–9.
24. Arthur JR, Boyd GS. The effect of inhibitors of protein synthesis on cholesterol side-chain cleavage in the mitochondria of luteinized rat ovaries. Eur J Biochem 1976;49:117–27.
25. Krueger RJ, Orme-Johnson NR. Acute adrenocorticotropic hormone stimulation of adrenal corticosteroidogenesis. J Biol Chem 1983;258:10159–67.
26. Epstein LF, Orme-Johnson NR. Acute action of luteinizing hormone on mouse Leydig cells: accumulation of mitochondrial phosphoproteins and stimulation of testosterone biosynthesis. Mol Cell Endocrinol 1991;81:113–26.
27. Pon LA, Orme-Johnson NR. Acute stimulation of corpus luteum cells by gonadotropin or adenosine 3'5'-monophosphate causes accumulation of a phosphroprotein concurrent with acceleration of steroid synthesis. Endocrinology 1988;123:1942–8.
28. Stocco DM, Sodeman TC. The 30-kDa mitochondrial proteins induced by hormone stimulation in MA-10 mouse Leydig tumor cells are processed from larger precursors. J Biol Chem 1991;266:19731–8.
29. Stocco DM, Chen W. Presence of identical mitochondrial proteins in unstimulated constitutive steroid-producing R2C rat Leydig tumor and stimulated nonconstitutive steroid-producing MA-10 mouse Leydig tumor cells. Endocrinology 1991;128:1918–26.
30. Stevens VL, Xu T, Lambeth JD. Cholesterol trafficking in steroidogenic cells: reversible cycloheximide-dependent accumulation of cholesterol in a pre-steroidogenic pool. Eur J Biochem 1993;216:557–63.
31. Mendelson C, Dufau ML, Catt KJ. Dependence of gonadotropin-induced steroidogenesis on RNA and protein synthesis in the interstitial cells of the rat testis. Biochim Biophys Acta 1975;411:222–30.
32. Ferguson JJ, Morita Y. RNA synthesis and adrenocorticotropin responsiveness. Biochim Biophys Acta 1964;87:348–50.
33. Ney RL, Davis WW, Garren LD. Heterogeneity of template RNA in adrenal glands. Science 1966;153:896–7.
34. Schulster D. Corticosteroid and ribonucleic acid synthesis in isolated adrenal cells: inhibition by actinomycin D. Mol Cell Endocrinol 1974;1:55–64.
35. Nakamura M, Watanuki M, Hall PF. On the role of protein synthesis in the response of adrenal tumor cells to ACTH. Mol Cell Endocrinol 1978;12:209–19.
36. Cooke BA, Janszen FHA, van Driel MJA, van der Molen HJ. Evidence for the involvement of lutropin-independent RNA synthesis in Leydig cell steroidogenesis. Mol Cell Endocrinol 1979;14:181–9.
37. Schulster D, Richardson MC, Palfreyman JW. The role of protein synthesis in adrenocorticotrophin action: effects of cycloheximide and puromycin on the steroidogenic response of isolated adrenocortical cells. Mol Cell Endocrinol 1974;2:17–29.

38. Crivello JF, Jefcoate CR. Mechanism of corticotropin action in rat adrenal cells. 1. Effect of inhibitors of protein synthesis and of microfilament formation on corticosterone synthesis. Biochim Biophys Acta 1978;542:315–29.

39. Krueger RJ, Orme-Johnson NR. Evidence for the involvement of a labile protein in stimulation of adrenal steroidogenesis under conditions not inhibitory to protein synthesis. Endocrinology 1988;122:1869–75.

40. Rommerts FFG, Cooke BA, van der Molen HJ. The role of cAMP in the regulation of steroid biosynthesis in testis tissue. J Steroid Biochem 1974; 5:279–85.

41. Hsueh AJW, Adashi EY, Jones PBC, Welsh TH. Hormonal regulation of the differentiation of cultured ovarian granulosa cells. Endocr Rev 1984;5:76–127.

42. Marsh JM. The role of cyclic AMP in gonadal function. Adv Cyclic Nucl Res 1975;6:137–99.

43. Sala GB, Hayashi K, Catt KJ, Dufau ML. Adrenocorticotropin action in isolated adrenal cells. J Biol Chem 1979;254:3861–75.

44. Edelman AM, Blumenthal DK, Krebs EG. Protein serine/threonine kinases. Annu Rev Biochem 1987;56:567–613.

45. Griffin Green E, Orme-Johnson NR. Inhibition of steroidogenesis in rat adrenal cortex cells by a threonine analog. J Steroid Biochem Mol Biol 1991;40:421–9.

46. Stocco DM, Clark BJ. The requirement of phosphorylation on a threonine residue in the acute regulation of steroidogenesis in MA-10 mouse Leydig tumor cells. J Steroid Biochem Mol Biol 1991;46:337–47.

47. Pon LA, Hartigan JA, Orme-Johnson NR. Acute ACTH regulation of adrenal corticosteroid biosynthesis: rapid accumulation of a phosphoprotein. J Biol Chem 1986;261:13309–16.

48. Alberta JA, Epstein LF, Pon LA, Orme-Johnson NR. Mitochondrial localization of a phosphoprotein that rapidly accumulates in adrenal cortex cells exposed to adrenocorticotropic hormone or to cAMP. J Biol Chem 1989;264:2368–72.

49. Epstein LF, Orme-Johnson NR. Regulation of steroid hormone biosynthesis: identification of precursors of a phosphoprotein targeted to the mitochondrion in stimulated rat adrenal cortex cells. J Biol Chem 1991;266:19739–45.

50. Chaudhary LR, Stocco DM. Effect of different steroidogenic stimuli on protein phosphorylation in MA-10 mouse Leydig tumor cells. Biochim Biophys Acta 1991;1094:175–84.

51. Mrotek J, Hall PF. Response of adrenal tumor cells to ACTH: site of inhibition by cytochalasin B. Biochemistry 1977;16:3177–81.

52. Hall PF, Charponnier C, Nakamura M, Gabbiani G. The role of microfilaments in the response of adrenal tumor cells to ACTH. J Biol Chem 1979;254:9080–4.

53. Hall PF. The role of the cytoskeleton in hormone action. Can J Biochem Cell Biol 1984;62:653–65.

54. Hall PF. Cellular organization for steroidogenesis. Int Rev Cytol 1984;86:53–95.

55. Nagy L, Freeman DA. Cholesterol movement between the plasma membrane and the cholesteryl ester droplets of cultured Leydig tumor cells. Biochem J 1990;271:809–14.

56. Nagy L, Freeman DA. Effect of cholesterol transport inhibitors on steroido-genesis and plasma membrane cholesterol transport in cultured MA-10 Leydig tumor cells. Endocrinology 1990;126:2267–76.

57. Hall PF. The role of the cytoskeleton in the supply of cholesterol for steroido-genesis. In: Strauss JF, Menon KMJ, eds. Lipoprotein and cholesterol metabo-lism in steroidogenic tissues. Philadelphia: Strickley, 1985:207–17.

58. Hall PF. Testicular steroid synthesis: organization and regulation. In: Knobil E, Neill J, eds. The physiology of reproduction. New York: Raven Press, 1988:975–98.

59. Hall PF, Almahbobi G. The role of the cytoskeleton in the regulation of steroidogenesis. J Steroid Biochem Mol Biol 1992;43:769–77.

60. Soto EA, Kliman HJ, Strauss JF, Paavola LG. Gonadotropins and cyclic adenosine 3′,5′-monophosphate (cAMP) alter the morphology of cultured human granulosa cells. Biol Reprod 1986;34:559–69.

61. Almahbobi G, Hall PF. The role of intermediate filaments in adrenal steroido-genesis. J Cell Sci 1990;97:679–87.

62. Almahbobi G, Williams LJ, Hall PF. Attachment of steroidogenic lipid droplets to intermediate filaments in adrenal cells. J Cell Sci 1992;101:383–93.

63. Almahbobi G, Williams LJ, Hall PF. Attachment of mitochondria to interme-diate filaments in adrenal cells: relevance to the regulation of steroid synthesis. Exp Cell Res 1992;200:361–9.

64. Almahbobi G, Williams LJ, Han X-G, Hall PF. Binding of lipid droplets and mitochondria to intermediate filaments in rat Leydig cells. J Reprod Fertil 1993;98:209–17.

65. Vahouny GV, Chanderbhan R, Noland BJ, Scallen TJ. Cholesterol ester hy-drolase and sterol carrier proteins. Endocr Res 1985;10:473–505.

66. Vahouny GV, Chanderbhan R, Kharroubi A, Noland BJ, Pastuszyn A, Scallen TJ. Sterol carrier and lipid transfer proteins. Adv Lipid Res 1987;22:83–113.

67. Chanderbhan R, Noland BJ, Scallen TJ, Vahouny GV. Sterol carrier protein$_2$: delivery of cholesterol from adrenal lipid droplets to mitochondria for pregnenolone synthesis. J Biol Chem 1982;257:8928–34.

68. Vahouny GV, Chanderbhan R, Noland BJ, Irwin D, Dennis P, Lambeth JD, Scallen TJ. Sterol carrier protein$_2$: identification of adrenal sterol carrier pro-tein$_2$ and site of action for mitochondrial cholesterol utilization. J Biol Chem 1983;258:11731–7.

69. Vahouny GV, Dennis P, Chanderbhan R, Fiskum G, Noland BJ, Scallen TJ. Sterol carrier protein$_2$ (SCP$_2$)-mediated transfer of cholesterol to mito-chondrial inner membranes. Biochem Biophys Res Commun 1984;122:509–15.

70. McNamara BC, Jefcoate CR. The role of sterol carrier protein 2 in stimulation of steroidogenesis in rat adrenal mitochondria by adrenal cytosol. Arch Biochem Biophys 1989;275:53–62.

71. Yamamoto R, Kallen CB, Babalola GO, Rennert H, Billheimer JT, Strauss JF. Cloning and expression of a cDNA encoding human sterol carrier protein 2. Proc Natl Acad Sci USA 1991;88:463–7.

72. Chanderbhan RF, Kharroubi AT, Noland BJ, Scallen TJ, Vahouny GV. SCP$_2$: further evidence for its role in adrenal steroidogenesis. Endocr Res 1986;12:351–60.

73. Keller GA, Scallen TJ, Clarke D, Maher PA, Krisans SK, Singer SJ. Subcellular localization of sterol carrier protein-2 in rat hepatocytes: its primary localization to peroxisomes. J Cell Biol 1989;108:1353–61.

74. van Amerongen A, van Noort M, van Beckhoven JRCM, Rommerts FFG, Orly J, Wirtz KWA. The subcellular distribution of the nonspecific lipid transfer protein (sterol carrier protein 2) in rat liver and adrenal gland. Biochim Biophys Acta 1989;1001:243–8.

75. Fujiki Y, Tsuneoka M, Tashiro Y. Biosynthesis of nonspecific lipid transfer protein (sterol carrier protein 2) on free polyribosomes as a larger precursor in rat liver. J Biochem 1989;106:1126–31.

76. Mendis-Handagama SMLC, Zirkin BR, Scallen TJ, Ewing LL. Studies on peroxisomes of the adult rat Leydig cell. J Androl 1990;11:270–8.

77. Ohba T, Rennert H, Pfeifer SM, He Z, Yamamoto R, Holt JA, Billheimer JT, Strauss JF III. The structure of the human sterol carrier protein x/sterol carrier protein2 gene (SCP_2). Genomics 1994;24:370–4.

78. Trzeciak WH, Simpson ER, Scallen TJ, Vahouny GV, Waterman MR. Studies on the synthesis of SCP-2 in rat adrenal cortical cells in monolayer culture. J Biol Chem 1987;262:3713–20.

79. van Amerongen A, Demel RA, Westerman J, Wirtz KWA. Transfer of cholesterol and oxysterol derivatives by the non-specific lipid transfer protein (sterol carrier protein 2): a study on its mode of action. Biochim Biophys Acta 1989;1004:36–43.

80. Van Noort M, Rommerts FFG, van Amerongen A, Wirtz KWA. Regulation of SCP_2 in the soluble fraction of rat Leydig cells. Kinetics and possible role of calcium influx. Mol Cell Endocrinol 1988;56:133–8.

81. Rennert H, Amsterdam A, Billheimer JT, Strauss JF III. Regulated expression of sterol carrier protein 2 in the ovary: a key role for cyclic AMP. Biochemistry 1991;47:11280–5.

82. Pfeifer SM, Furth EE, Ohba T, Chang YJ, Rennert H, Sakuragi N, Billheimer JT, Strauss JF III. Sterol carrier protein 2: a role in steroid hormone synthesis? J Steroid Biochem Mol Biol 1993;47:167–72.

83. Pedersen RC, Brownie AC. Cholesterol side-chain cleavage in the rat adrenal cortex: isolation of a cycloheximide-sensitive activator peptide. Proc Natl Acad Sci USA 1983;80:1882–6.

84. Pedersen RC. Polypeptide activators of cholesterol side-chain cleavage. Endocr Res 1984;10:533–61.

85. Pedersen RC, Brownie AC. Steroidogenesis activator polypeptide isolated from a rat Leydig cell tumor. Science 1987;236:188–90.

86. Pedersen RC. Steroidogenesis activator polypeptide (SAP) in the rat ovary and testis. J Steroid Biochem 1987;27:731–5.

87. Mertz LM, Pedersen RC. Steroidogenesis activator polypeptide may be a product of glucose regulated protein 78 (GRP78). Endocr Res 1989;15:101–15.

88. Frustaci J, Mertz LM, Pedersen RC. Steroidogenesis activator polypeptide (SAP) in the guinea pig adrenal cortex. Mol Cell Endocrinol 1989;64:137–43.

89. Mertz LM, Pedersen RC. The kinetics of steroidogenesis activator polypeptide in the rat adrenal cortex. J Biol Chem 1989;264:15274–9.

90. Li X, Warren DW, Gregoire J, Pedersen RC, Lee AS. The rat 78,000 dalton glucose-regulated protein (GRP78) as a precursor of the rat steroidogenesis-

activator polypeptide (SAP): the SAP coding sequence is homologous with the terminal end of GRP78. Mol Endocrinol 1989;3:1944–52.

91. Anholt RRH, Pedersen PO, Souza EB, Snyder SH. The peripheral-type benzodiazepine receptor. J Biol Chem 1986;261:576–83.

92. Calvo DJ, Ritta MN, Calandra RX, Medina JH. Peripheral-type benzodiazepine receptors are highly concentrated in mitochondrial membranes of rat testicular interstitial cells. Neuroendocrinology 1990;52:350–3.

93. Verma A, Snyder SH. Peripheral type benzodiazepine receptors. Annu Rev Pharmacol Toxicol 1989;29:307–22.

94. Krueger KE, Whalin ME, Papadopoulos V. Regulation of steroid synthesis in the adrenals by mitochondrial benzodiazepine receptors. In: Costa E, Paul SM, editors. Neurosteroids and brain function. New York: Thieme Medical, 1991;8:155–60.

95. Krueger KE, Papadopoulos V. Mitochondrial benzodiazepine receptors and the regulation of steroid biosynthesis. Annu Rev Pharmacol Toxicol 1992; 32:211–37.

96. Papadopoulos V. Peripheral-type benzodiazepine/diazepam binding inhibitor receptor: biological role in steroidogenic cell function. Endocr Rev 1993; 14:222–40.

97. Amsterdam A, Suh BS. An inducible functional peripheral benzodiazepine receptor in mitochondria of steroidogenic granulosa cells. Endocrinology 1991;129:503–10.

98. Mukhin AG, Papadopoulos V, Costa E, Krueger KE. Mitochondrial benzodiazepine receptors regulate steroid biosynthesis. Proc Natl Acad Sci USA 1989;86:9813–6.

99. Papadopoulos V, Mukhin AG, Costa E, Krueger KE. The peripheral-type benzodiazepine receptor is functionally-linked to Leydig cell steroidogenesis. J Biol Chem 1990;265:3772–9.

100. Krueger KE, Papadopoulos V. Peripheral-type benzodiazepine receptors mediate translocation of cholesterol from outer to inner mitochondrial membranes in adrenocortical cells. J Biol Chem 1990;265:15015–22.

101. Papadopoulos V, Nowzari FB, Krueger KE. Hormone-stimulated steroidogenesis is coupled to mitochondrial benzodiazepine receptors. Trophic hormone action on steroid biosynthesis is inhibited by flunitrazepam. J Biol Chem 1991;266:3682–7.

102. Guarneri P, Papadopoulos V, Costa E. Regulation of pregnenolone synthesis in C6 glioma cells by 4′-chlorodiazepam. Proc Natl Acad Sci USA 1992;89:5118–22.

103. Yanagibashi K, Ohno Y, Nakamichi N, Matsui T, Hyashida K, Takamura M, Yamada K, Tou S, Kawamura M. Peripheral-type benzodiazepine receptors are involved in the regulation of cholesterol side chain cleavage in adrenocortical mitochondria. J Biochem 1989;106:1026–9.

104. Barnea ER, Fares F, Gavish M. Modulatory action of benzodiazepines on human term placental steroidogenesis in vitro. Mol Cell Endocrinol 1989;64:155–9.

105. Costa E, Guidotti A. Diazepam binding inhibitor (DBI): a peptide with multiple biological actions. Life Sci 1991;49:325–44.

106. Cavallaro S, Korneyev A, Guidotti A, Costa E. Diazepam-binding inhibitor (DBI)-processing products, acting at the mitochondrial DBI receptor, mediate

adrenocorticotropic hormone-induced steroidogenesis in rat adrenal gland. Proc Natl Acad Sci USA 1992;89:10598–602.

107. Papadopoulos V, Berkovich A, Krueger KE, Costa E, Guidotti A. Diazepam binding inhibitor and its processing products stimulate mitochondrial steroid biosynthesis via an interaction with mitochondrial benzodiazepine receptors. Endocrinology 1991;129:1481–8.

108. Papadopoulos V, Berkovich A, Krueger KE. The role of diazepam binding inhibitor and its processing products at mitochondrial benzodiazepine receptors: regulation of steroid biosynthesis. Neuropharmacology 1991;30:1417–23.

109. Brown AS, Hall PF. Stimulation by endozepine of the side-chain cleavage of cholesterol in a reconstituted enzyme system. Biochem Biophys Res Commun 1991;180:609–14.

110. Papadopoulos V, Guarneri P, Krueger KE, Guidotti A, Costa E. Pregnenolone biosynthesis in C6–2B glioma cell mitochondria: regulation by a mitochondrial diazepam binding inhibitor receptor. Proc Natl Acad Sci USA 1992;89:5113–7.

111. Boujrad N, Hudson JR, Papadopoulos V. Inhibition of hormone-stimulated steroidogenesis in cultured Leydig tumor cells by a cholesterol-linked phosphorothioate oligodeoxynucleotide antisense to diazepam-binding inhibitor. Proc Natl Acad Sci USA 1993;90:5728–31.

112. Yanagibashi K, Ohno Y, Kawamura M, Hall PF. The regulation of intracellular transport of cholesterol in bovine adrenal cells: purification of a novel protein. Endocrinology 1988;123:2075–82.

113. Besman MJ, Yanagibashi K, Lee TD, Kawamura M, Hall PF, Shively JE. Identification of des-(Gly-Ile)-endozepine as an effector of corticotropin-dependent adrenal steroidogenesis: stimulation of cholesterol delivery is mediated by the peripheral benzodiazepine receptor. Proc Natl Acad Sci USA 1989;86:4897–901.

114. Boujrad N, Gaillard JL, Garnier M, Papadopoulos V. Acute action of choriogonadotropin on Leydig tumor cells: induction of a higher affinity benzodiazepine-binding site related to steroid biosynthesis. Endocrinology 1994;135:1576–83.

115. Garnier M, Boujrad N, Ogwuegbu SO, Hudson JR, Papadopoulos V. The polypeptide diazepam-binding inhibitor and a higher affinity mitochondrial peripheral-type benzodiazepine receptor sustain constitutive steroidogenesis in the R2C Leydig tumor cell line. J Biol Chem 1994;269:22105–12.

116. Papadopoulos V, Boujrad N, Ikonomovic MD, Ferrara P, Vidic B. Topography of the Leydig cell mitochondrial peripheral-type benzodiazepine receptor. Mol Cell Endocrinol 1994;104:R5–R9.

117. McEnery MW, Snowman AM, Trifiletti RR, Snyder SH. Isolation of the mitochondrial benzodiazepine receptor: association with the voltage-dependent anion channel and the adenine nucleotide carrier. Proc Natl Acad Sci USA 1992;89:3170–4.

118. Kinnally KW, Zorov DB, Antonenko YN, Snyder SH, McEnery MW, Tedesschi H. Mitochondrial benzodiazepine receptor linked to inner membrane ion channels by nanomolar actions of ligands. Proc Natl Acad Sci USA 1993;90:1374–8.

119. Ohlendieck K, Riesinger I, Adams V, Krause J, Dieter B. Enrichment and biochemical characterization of boundary membrane contact sites from rat liver mitochondria. Biochim Biophys Acta 1986;860:672–89.

120. Sandri G, Siagri M, Panfili E. Influence of Ca^{-2+} on the isolation from rat brain mitochondria of a fraction enriched of boundary membrane contact sites. Cell Calcium 1988;9:159–65.

121. Moran O, Sandri G, Panfili E, Stuhmer W, Sorgato MC. Electrophysiological characterization of contact sites in brain mitochondria. J Biol Chem 1990;265:908–13.

122. Jefcoate CR, McNamara BC, Artemenko I, Yamazaki T. Regulation of cholesterol movement to mitochondrial cytochrome P450scc in steroid hormone synthesis. J Steroid Biochem Mol Biol 1992;43:751–67.

123. Hall PF, Papadopoulos V, Yanagibashi K. On the mechanism of action of ACTH. In: Imura H, Shizume K, Yoshida S, eds. Progress in endocrinology. Amsterdam: Elsevier Science, 1988:253–8.

124. Brown AS, Hall PF, Shoyab M, Papadopoulos V. Endozepine/diazepam binding inhibitor in adrenocortical and Leydig cell lines: absence of hormonal regulation. Mol Cell Endocrinol 1992;83:1–9.

125. Cavallaro S, Pani L, Guidotti A, Costa E. ACTH-induced mitochondrial DBI receptor (MDR) and diazepam binding inhibitor (DBI) expression in adrenals of hypophysectomized rats is not cause-effect related to its immediate steroidogenic action. Life Sci 1993;53:1137–47.

126. Oke BO, Suarez-Quian CA, Riond J, Ferrara P, Papadopoulos V. Cell surface localization of the peripheral-type benzodiazepine receptor in adrenal cortex. Mol Cell Endocrinol 1992;87:R1–R6.

127. Knudsen J, Nielsen M. Diazepam-binding inhibitor: a neuropeptide and/or an acylcoA ester binding protein? Biochem J 1990;265:927–8.

128. Snyder SH, Verma A, Trifiletti RR. The "peripheral-type" benzodiazepine receptor: a protein of mitochondrial outer membrane utilizing porphyrins as endogenous ligands. FASEB J 1987;1:282–8.

129. Shibata H, Kojima I, Ogata E. Diazepam inhibits potassium-induced aldosterone secretion in adrenal glomerulosa cell. Biochem Biophys Res Commun 1986;135:994–9.

130. Holloway CD, Kenyon CJ, Dowie LJ, Corrie JET, Gray CE, Fraser R. Effect of the benzodiazepines diazepam, des-n-methyldiazepam and midazolam on corticosteroid biosynthesis in bovine adrenocortical cells in vitro; location of site of action. J Steroid Biochem 1989;33:219–25.

131. Thomson I, Fraser R, Kenyon CJ. Inhibition of bovine adrenocortical steroidogenesis by benzodiazepines: a direct effect on microsomal hydroxylation or an inhibition of calcium uptake. J Endocrinol 1992;135:361–2.

132. Python CP, Rossier MF, Vallotton MB, Capponi AM. Peripheral-type benzodiazepines inhibit calcium channels and aldosterone production in adrenal glomerulosa cells. Endocrinology 1993;132:1489–95.

133. Pon LA, Orme-Johnson NR. Acute stimulation of steroidogenesis in corpus luteum and adrenal cortex by peptide hormones. J Biol Chem 1986;261:6594–9.

134. Pon LA, Epstein LF, Orme-Johnson NR. Acute cAMP stimulation in Leydig cells: rapid accumulation of a protein similar to that detected in adrenal cortex and corpus luteum. Endocr Res 1986;12:429–46.

135. Epstein LA, Alberta JA, Pon LA, Orme-Johnson NR. Subcellular localization of a protein produced in adrenal cortex cells in response to ACTH. Endocr Res 1989;15:117–27.
136. Orme-Johnson NR. Distinctive properties of adrenal cortex mitochondria. Biochim Biophys Acta 1990;1020:213–31.
137. Mittre H, Aunai P, Benhaim A, Leymarie P. Acute stimulation of lutropin by mitochondrial protein synthesis in small luteal cells. Eur J Biochem 1990;187:721–6.
138. Elliott ME, Goodfriend TL, Jefcoate CR. Bovine adrenal glomerulosa and fasciculata cells exhibit 28.5-kilodalton proteins sensitive to angiotensin, other agonists, and atrial natriuretic peptide. Endocrinology 1993;133:1669–77.
139. Ascoli M. Characterization of several clonal lines of cultured Leydig tumor cells: gonadotropin receptors and steroidogenic responses. Endocrinology 1981;108:88–95.
140. Stocco DM, Kilgore MW. Induction of mitochondrial proteins in MA-10 Leydig tumor cells with human choriogonadotropin. Biochem J 1988;249: 95–103.
141. Stocco DM, Chaudhary LR. Evidence for the functional coupling of cAMP in MA-10 mouse Leydig tumor cells. Cell Signal 1990;2:161–70.
142. Stocco DM. Further evidence that the mitochondrial proteins induced by hormone stimulation in MA-10 mouse Leydig tumor cells are involved in the acute regulation of steroidogenesis. J Steroid Biochem Mol Biol 1992;43: 319–33.
143. Stocco DM, Ascoli M. The use of genetic manipulation of MA-10 Leydig tumor cells to demonstrate the role of mitochondrial proteins in the acute regulation of steroidogenesis. Endocrinology 1993;132:959–67.
144. Stocco DM, Wells J, Clark BJ. Effects of hydrogen peroxide on steroidogenesis in mouse Leydig tumor cells. Endocrinology 1993;133:2827–32.
145. Stocco DM, King S, Clark BJ. Differential effects of dimethylsulfoxide on steroidogenesis in mouse MA-10 and rat R2C leydig tumor cells. Endocrinology 1995;136:2993–9.
146. Clark BJ, Wells J, King SR, Stocco DM. The purification, cloning and expression of a novel LH-induced mitochondrial protein in MA-10 mouse leydig tumor cells: characterization of the *St*eroidogenic *A*cute *R*egulatory protein (StAR). J Biol Chem 1994;269:28314–22.
147. Sugawara T, Holt JA, Driscoll D, Strauss JF III, Lin D, Miller WL, Patterson D, Clancy KP, Hart IM, Clark BJ, Stocco DM. Human steroidogenic acute regulatory protein: Functional activity in COS-1 cells, tissue-specific expression, and mapping of the structural gene to 8p11.2 and a pseudogene to chromosome 13. Proc Natl Acad Sci 1995;92:4778–82.
148. King SR, Ronen-Fuhrmann T, Timberg R, Clark BJ, Orly J, Stocco DM. Steroid production after in vitro transcription, translation, and mitochondrial processing of protein products of complementary deoxyribonucleic acid for steroidogenic acute regulatory protein. Endocrinology 1995;136: 5165–76.
149. Camacho AM, Kowarski A, Migeon CJ, Brough AJ. Congenital adrenal hyperplasia due to a deficiency of one of the enzymes involved in the biosynthesis of pregnenolone. J Clin Endocrinol Metab 1968;28:153–61.

150. Degenhart HJ, Visser HKA, Boon H, O'Doherty NJ. Evidence for deficient 20α-cholesterol-hydroxylase activity in adrenal tissue of a patient with lipoid adrenal hyperplasia. Acta Endocrinol 1972;71:512–8.

151. Koizumi S, Kyoya S, Miyawaki T, Kidani H, Funabashi T, Nakashima Y, Ohta G, Itagaki E, Katagiri M. Cholesterol side-chain cleavage enzyme activity and cytochrome P450 content in adrenal mitochondria of a patient with congenital lipoid adrenal hyperplasia (Prader disease). Clin Chim Acta 1977;77:301–6.

152. Hauffa PT, Miller WL, Grumbach MM, Conte FA, Kaplan SL. Congenital adrenal hyperplasia due to deficient cholesterol side-chain cleavage activity (20,22-desmolase) in a patient treated for 18 years. Clin Endocrinol 1985;23:481–93.

153. Miller WL, Levine LS. Molecular and clinical advances in congenital adrenal hyperplasia. J Pediatr 1987;111:1–17.

154. Lin D, Gitelman SE, Saenger P, Miller WL. Normal genes for the cholesterol side chain cleavage enzyme, P450scc, in congenital lipoid adrenal hyperplasia. J Clin Invest 1991;88:1955–62.

155. Lin D, Chang YJ, Strauss JF III, Miller WL. The human peripheral benzodiazepine receptor gene: cloning and characterization of alternative splicing in normal tissues and in a patient with congenital lipoid adrenal hyperplasia. Genomics 1993;18:643–50.

156. Saenger P, Klonari Z, Black SM, Compagnone N, Mellon SH, Fleischer A, Abrams CAL, Shackelton CHL, Miller WL. Prenatal diagnosis of congenital lipoid adrenal hyperplasia. J Clin Endocrinol Metab 1995;80:200–5.

157. Lin D, Sugawara T, Strauss JF, Clark BJ, Stocco DM, Saenger P, Rogol A, Miller WL. Role of steroidogenic acute regulatory protein in adrenal and gonadal steroidogenesis. Science 1995;267:1828–31.

158. Reinhart MP. Intracellular sterol trafficking. Experientia 1990;46:599–610.

159. Schwaiger M, Herzog V, Neupert W. Characterization of translocation contact sites involved in the import of mitochondrial proteins. J Cell Biol 1987;105:235–46.

160. Vestweber D, Schatz G. A chimeric mitochondrial precursor protein with internal disulphide bridges blocks import of authentic precursors into mitochondria. A means to quantitate translocation contact sites. J Cell Biol 1988;107:2037–43.

161. Rassow J, Guiard B, Weinhues U, Herzog V, Hartl FU, Neupert W. Translocation arrest by reversible folding of a precursor protein imported into mitochondria. A means to quantitate translocation contact sites. J Cell Biol 1989;109:1421–8.

162. Pon L, Moll T, Vestweber D, Marshallsay B, Schatz G. Protein import into mitochondria: ATP-dependent protein translocation activity in a submitochondrial fraction enriched in membrane contact sites and specific proteins. J Cell Biol 1989;109:2603–16.

163. Pfanner N, Rassow J, Wienhues U, Hergersberg C, Sollner T, Becker K, Neupert W. Contact sites between inner and outer membranes: structure and role in protein translocation into the mitochondria. Biochim Biophys Acta 1990;1018:239–42.

164. Hwang ST, Wachter C, Schatz G. Protein import into the yeast mitochondrial matrix: a new translocation intermediate between the two mitochondrial membranes. J Biol Chem 1991;266:21083–9.

22

Diazepam-Binding Inhibitor and Peripheral Benzodiazepine Receptors: Role in Steroid Biosynthesis

VASSILIOS PAPADOPOULOS, A. SHANE BROWN, BRANISLAV VIDIC, MARTINE GARNIER, STEPHEN O. OGWUEGBU, HAKIMA AMRI, AND NOUREDDINE BOUJRAD

Trophic hormone regulation of steroid synthesis can be thought of as being either acute, occurring within minutes and resulting in the rapid synthesis of steroids, or chronic, occurring over a long period of time and resulting in continued steroid production. The primary point of control in the acute stimulation of steroidogenesis by hormones involves the first step in this biosynthetic pathway, where cholesterol is converted to pregnenolone by the cholesterol *side-chain cleavage cytochrome P-450* (P-450scc) enzyme and auxiliary electron transferring proteins, localized on the inner mitochondrial membranes (1–4). More detailed studies have shown that the reaction catalyzed by P-450scc is not the rate-limiting step in the synthesis of steroid hormones, but rather the transport of the precursor, cholesterol, from intracellular sources to the inner mitochondrial membrane and the subsequent loading of cholesterol in the P-450scc active site (1–4). This hormone-dependent transport mechanism was shown to be mediated by *adenosine 3′:5′-cyclic monophosphate* (cAMP), to be regulated by a cytoplasmic protein, and to be localized in the mitochondrion where it regulates the intramitochondrial transport of cholesterol (1–4). This intramitochondrial cholesterol transport can be dissected in three steps: (i) transfer of cholesterol from the outer leaflet of the outer mitochondrial membrane to the inner leaflet of the membrane; (ii) translocation from the inner leaflet of the outer membrane to the outer leaflet of the inner membrane through the aqueous intramitochondrial space; and (iii) transfer and loading of cholesterol to the P-450scc present in the inner leaflet (matrix side) of the inner mitochondrial membrane. Figure 22.1 shows a graphic

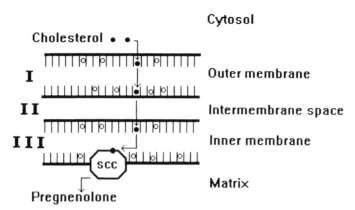

FIGURE 22.1. Steps that cholesterol follows from the cytoplasm to the inner mitochondrial membrane P-450scc. For details see text.

representation of the steps that cholesterol follows from the cytoplasm to the P-450scc inner mitochondrial membrane.

Definition of the Peripheral-Type Benzodiazepine Receptors (PBR)

Benzodiazepines have long been prescribed for their anxiolytic, anticonvulsant, and hypnotic actions. It has been well established that the major pharmacological effects of benzodiazepines are mediated by the γ-*aminobutyric acid* (GABA)$_A$ receptors in the *central nervous system* (CNS; 5, 6). In the search for specific binding sites for benzodiazepines outside the CNS another class of binding sites was first observed in the kidney (7), and later determined to be present in apparently all tissues, including the CNS (8–11). This class of binding sites is commonly referred to as the peripheral-type benzodiazepine recognition sites or receptors (PBR) due to their initial discovery in peripheral tissues.

PBRs were distinguished from GABA$_A$/benzodiazepine receptors by several criteria. Although both receptors bind diazepam with relatively high affinity, they exhibited very different binding specificities. In rodent species PBRs bind 4′-chlorodiazepam with high affinity, whereas GABA$_A$ receptors show low affinity for this benzodiazepine (10, 11). Conversely, clonazepam and flumazenil, which bind with high affinity to GABA$_A$ receptors, exhibit very low affinities for PBRs. PBRs also bind the imidazopyridine alpidem with high affinity and they have a low affinity for the imidazopyridine zolpidem (12). Conversely, GABA$_A$ receptors bind zolpidem with high affinity and have low affinity for alpidem. In addition, PBRs have high affinity for two classes of compounds, isoquinolines and indoleacetamides, which do not bind to the GABA$_A$ receptors (10, 11).

Isoquinolines were the major tool used for the identification and characterization of PBR (13).

In addition to these differences in drug specificity, it has been well established that $GABA_A$/benzodiazepine receptors, composed of 50- to 55-kd protein subunits, are coupled to synaptosomal chloride channels, whereas PBRs, an 18kd protein associated with other mitochondrial proteins, are not coupled to GABA recognition sites; their function will be addressed in this chapter. Subcellular fractionation studies demonstrated that PBRs were primarily localized on mitochondria (14, 15), and more specifically on the outer mitochondrial membrane (16), although it is likely that they are not exclusive to this organelle, and a plasma membrane location for this receptor was recently identified (17, 18).

The first identification of a molecular component associated with PBR was made possible by the development of a photoaffinity probe, the isoquinoline propanamide PK 14105 (19). This probe specifically labeled an 18-kd protein, which was subsequently purified (20, 21), and the corresponding cDNA was cloned from rat (22), human (23, 24), bovine (25), and murine (26) species. Expression studies with the *complementary DNA* (cDNA) probes demonstrated that the 18-kd protein contains the binding domains for PBR ligands, although, due to the constitutive expression of PBR in all cells used for transfections, the presence of other proteins important for PBR-binding expression cannot be excluded. The primary amino acid sequence deduced from the cDNA nucleotide sequence revealed that PBRs contain a predominance of hydrophobic amino acids predicting five transmembrane domains (22–26). In addition to the 18-kd protein, a number of laboratories have identified a 30- to 35-kd protein (8–11). The identification, characterization, and role of this protein will be discussed later in this chapter. In conclusion, PBR refers to a distinct and defined drug recognition site that, unlike the connotation of its name, is also found in the CNS.

Role of PBR in Steroidogenesis

Two important observations indicated that PBRs were likely to play a role in steroidogenesis: first, PBRs are found primarily on outer mitochondrial membranes, and second, we and others showed that PBRs are extremely abundant in steroidogenic cells (8–11). We then reported that a spectrum of ligands that bind to PBRs with affinities ranging from nanomolar to millimolar stimulate steroid biosynthesis in various cell systems (27, 28). The relationship between the affinities of these compounds for PBR and the concentrations of each compound required to stimulate steroidogenesis was examined and showed an excellent correlation, with a coefficient of $r = 0.9$, suggesting that these drugs, via binding to PBR, stimulate steroidogenesis. However, the stimulatory effect of PBR ligands was not additive to the stimulation by hormones and cAMP (29). Considering the mitochondrial localization of PBR, we then examined the direct effect of PBR ligands on mitochondrial steroid formation. PBR ligands were found to stimulate pregnenolone production by isolated mitochondria (28). This effect was greater with "cholesterol-loaded" mitochondria prepared from cells treated with hormone and the protein synthesis inhibitor cycloheximide (29). This treatment increases the amount of cholesterol present in the outer mitochondrial membrane (2, 4). The stimulatory effect of PBR ligands on intact mitochondria was not observed with mitoplasts (mitochondria devoid of the outer membrane), in agreement with the outer mitochondrial membrane localization of the receptor (28). In these studies we concluded that PBRs are implicated in the acute stimulation of adrenocortical and Leydig cell steroidogenesis possibly by mediating the entry, distribution, and/or availability of cholesterol within mitochondria.

To identify the exact step in mitochondrial pregnenolone formation activated by PBR ligands, we quantified the amount of cholesterol present in the outer and inner mitochondrial membranes before and after treatment with PBR ligands. The results obtained clearly demonstrated that the PBR ligand-induced stimulation of pregnenolone formation was due to PBR-mediated translocation of cholesterol from the outer to the inner mitochondrial membrane (29). PBR ligands, however, induced a massive translocation of cholesterol (10μg/mg of protein). Considering that only a portion, 10–20%, of this cholesterol will be used for steroidogenesis and that PBR is present in most tissues examined, these data indicate that PBR-mediated lipid translocation may also be involved in a more general mechanism such as membrane biogenesis. Thus, the abundance of PBR in steroidogenic tissues, together with the tissue-specific cholesterol transport, make PBR a regulator of this rate-determining process. Studies by different laboratories corroborated these observations (30, 31) and extended them to placental (32) and ovarian granulosa cells (33). Moreover, we showed that a similar mechanism regulates brain glial cell "neurosteroid" synthesis (34).

Role of PBR in Hormone-Stimulated Steroidogenesis

Despite the data presented on the effect of PBR ligands on basal steroid synthesis, it was still unclear whether PBRs participate in hormone-stimulated steroidogenesis. In search of a PBR ligand that may affect hormone-stimulated steroid production we found that flunitrazepam, a benzodiazepine that binds to PBR with high nanomolar affinity, inhibited hormone and cAMP-stimulated steroidogenesis (35). Radioligand binding studies revealed a single class of binding sites for flunitrazepam that was verified as being a PBR by displacement studies using a series of PBR ligands. Furthermore, this drug caused an inhibition in mitochondrial pregnenolone formation that was determined to result from a reduction of cholesterol transport to the inner mitochondrial membrane P-450scc. These observations demonstrated that the antagonistic action of flunitrazepam on hormone-stimulated steroidogenesis is mediated through the interaction of this compound with PBR. It should be noted, however, that flunitrazepam is also a weak stimulator of basal steroid production, suggesting that it acts as a partial agonist of the receptor-mediated steroid synthesis process. In conclusion, these studies suggested that hormone-induced steroidogenesis involves, at least in part, the participation of PBR.

Hormonal Regulation of PBR

We examined whether *human chorionic gonadotropin* (hCG) or cAMP regulates PBR expression in Leydig cells measured by ligand binding and RNA (Northern) blot analysis. Treatment of MA-10 cells from 10 min to 24 h with hCG was without any effect on PBR binding or message levels (36). However, the addition of hCG to MA-10 cells resulted in a very rapid increase in PBR-binding capacity (3-fold increase within 15 sec). This rapid increase gradually returned to basal levels within 60 sec. This stimulatory effect of hCG was dose dependent and the concentrations required were similar to those needed to stimulate steroidogenesis. As we and others reported, Scatchard analysis revealed, in addition to the known high-affinity (5.0 nM) benzodiazepine-binding site, a second higher-affinity (0.2 nM), hormone-induced, benzodiazepine-binding site. We then examined whether steroid synthesis could be detected in a similar time frame. MA-10 cells were incubated for 15 sec with aminoglutethimide, an inhibitor of P-450scc, together with hCG. Mitochondria were isolated from these cells, and after incubation in aminoglutethimide-free buffer an increase in the rate of pregnenolone formation was observed. Addition of a selective inhibitor of cAMP-dependent protein kinase blocked not only the hormone-induced PBR binding, but also steroid formation. Furthermore, addition of flunitrazepam abolished the hCG-induced rapid stimulation of steroid synthesis. These results demonstrate that, in Leydig cells, the most rapid effect of hCG and cAMP is the transient induction of a higher-affinity benzodiazepine binding site that occurs concomitantly with an increase in the rate of steroid formation (36). This, in turn, suggests that these hormones alter PBR to activate cholesterol delivery to the inner mitochondrial membrane and subsequent steroid formation.

PBR, a Substrate of the cAMP-Dependent Protein Kinase

Analysis of the amino acid sequence of the cloned rat (22), bovine (25), and murine (26) PBR, revealed the presence of putative phosphorylation motifs at the C-terminal domain of the protein. Interestingly, protein phosphorylation has been shown to be involved in the regulation of steroidogenesis. In mitochondrial preparations the cAMP-dependent protein kinase, but not other purified protein kinases, was found to phosphorylate the 18-kd PBR protein (37). In addition, the 18-kd PBR protein was found to be phosphorylated in digitonin-permeabilized Leydig cells and its phosporylation was stimulated by cAMP (37), suggesting that PBR is an in vitro and in situ substrate of *protein kinase A* (PKA). However, cloning of the human 18-kd PBR protein (23, 24) predicted an amino acid sequence missing the phosphorylation motif identified in the rat, mouse, and bovine sequences, suggesting that phosphorylation of the 18-kd PBR protein may not be an ubiquitous mechanism of regulation of PBR function.

PBR in a Constitutive Steroid-Producing Cell Model

In Leydig cell–derived tumors, steroid synthesis occurs independently of hormonal control since pituitary *luteinizing hormone* (LH) secretion is supressed by the excessive amount of steroids produced (38). R2C cells are derived from rat Leydig tumors and maintain their in vitro capacity to synthesize steroids constitutively in a hormone-independent manner (39). Thus, one can expect that constitutive steroidogenesis is driven by the unregulated expression of the hormonal mechanism that controls steroid synthesis or by an unknown separate mechanism. Radioligand binding assays on intact R2C cells revealed the presence of a single class of PBR binding sites with an affinity 10 times higher (K_d = 0.5 nM) than that displayed by the MA-10 PBR (K_d = 5 nM; 40). Photolabeling of R2C and MA-10 cell mitochondria with a photoactivatable PBR ligand showed that the 18-kd PBR protein was specifically labeled. This indicates that the R2C cells express a PBR protein that has properties similar to the MA-10 PBR. Moreover, a PBR synthetic ligand was able to increase steroid production in isolated mitochondria from R2C cells that express the 5-nM affinity receptor. Interestingly, mitochondrial PBR binding was increased by 6-fold upon addition of the postmitochondrial fraction, suggesting that a cytosolic factor modulates the binding properties of PBR in R2C cells and is responsible for the 0.5-nM affinity receptor seen in intact cells (40). In conclusion, these data demonstrate that ligand binding to the mitochondrial, higher-affinity PBR is involved in maintaining R2C constitutive steroidogenesis.

Structure of the PBR Complex

In parallel with the previously described studies we continued our efforts to better characterize the structure of the mitochondrial Leydig cell PBR. As noted above PBR was identified and characterized originally by its high affinity for two distinct classes of compounds, the benzodiazepines and the isoquinolines (8–11). High-affinity isoquinoline binding is diagnostic of the PBR, but the affinity of benzodiazepines for PBR is species specific, varying from high affinity (rodents) to low affinity (bovine) (10, 11). These species differences in benzodiazepine binding may be due to either structural differences in the 18-kd protein or differences in the components composing the PBR complex in the mitochondrial membranes. The 18-kd isoquinoline binding protein was identified as a PBR (10, 11). We isolated and sequenced a 626-base pair *complementary DNA* (cDNA), specifying an open reading frame of 169 amino acid residues from MA-10 Leydig cells (26). Expression of PBR cDNA in mammalian cells resulted in an increase in the density of both benzodiazepine and isoquinoline binding sites. To examine whether the increased drug binding was due to the 18-kd PBR protein alone or to other constitutively expressed components of the receptor, an in vitro system was developed using recombinant PBR protein (26). Isolated *maltose-binding protein* (MBP)-PBR recombinant fusion protein incorporated into liposomes, formed using lipids found in steroidogenic outer mitochondrial membranes but not MPB alone, maintained its ability to bind isoquinolines but not benzodiazepines. Addition of mitochondrial extracts in the liposomes resulted in the restoration of benzodiazepine binding. The protein responsible for this effect was then purified and identified as the 34-kd *voltage-dependent anion channel* (VDAC) protein, which by itself does not express any drug binding.

These findings provided the functional evidence for previous observations on 30- to 35-kd proteins nonspecifically labeled using irreversible isoquinolines and benzodiazepines (8–11). Among the ligands used to identify these proteins was flunitrazepam (8, 10, 11). Based on the observation that the 35-kd protein photolabeled with flunitrazepam could also bind radiolabeled dicyclohexylcarbodiimide, a reagent that covalently binds to VDAC, and specific reagents that inhibit VDAC function were able to abolish PBR ligand binding, the hypothesis that VDAC was part of PBR was advanced (8). Moreover, we observed that among the PBR ligands tested, only flunitrazepam could specifically antagonize, acting via PBR, hormone-stimulated cholesterol transport and steroidogenesis (35). Furthermore, the observation that the 18-kd PBR was isolated as a complex with the 34-kd VDAC and the inner mitochondrial membrane *adenine nucleotide carrier* (ADC) (41) suggested that PBR is not a single protein receptor but a multimeric complex.

These studies demonstrated that VDAC is functionally associated with the 18-kd PBR and is part of the benzodiazepine-binding site in the PBR. Benzodiazepine binding, however, will be expressed only in the presence of the 18-kd PBR protein that confers the other part of the recognition site. This model is also in agreement with the finding that the species difference in benzodiazepine binding may be due to five nonconserved amino acids in the C-terminal end of the 18-kd PBR protein (42). Although the 18-kd PBR and VDAC are required for drug binding, we cannot, however, exclude the possibility that, in vivo, other proteins may be transiently or permanently associated with the PBR complex and modulate drug binding in an "allosteric" manner.

VDAC is a large-conductance, large-diameter (about 3 nm) ion channel with thin walls formed by a β-sheet structure and located in the outer mitochondrial membrane, especially in the junctions between outer and inner membranes (contact sites) where it may complex with the adenine nucleotide carrier, hexokinase, and creatine kinase (43). VDAC forms a slightly anion-selective channel with complex voltage dependence and has been referred to as "mitochondrial porin" by analogy to bacterial porins. VDAC is believed to allow the transport of metabolites and small molecules between the cytoplasm and the inner mitochondrial membrane (43, 44).

Because of the interaction of 18-kd PBR with VDAC at the contact site level we will have to consider a potential role of other proteins shown to participate in contact site formation. First, the inner mitochondrial membrane ADC was shown to be structurally associated with PBR components (41). Second, the *inner mitochondrial megachannel* (IMC) (45) may coincide with the permeability transition pore or the multiple conductance channel activity (46), which are channels identified using the patch clamp technology, located in the inner membrane of the contact sites and representing activities regulated by voltage and ion (i.e., calcium) changes that result in pore opening and permeability increases. IMC is inhibited by PBR ligands (47) and is sensitive to the immunosupressant cyclosporin A (45). Interestingly, we observed that cyclosporin A is a noncompetitive inhibitor of PBR, suggesting that IMC may regulate PBR in an "allosteric" manner (Papadopoulos, unpublished data). On the basis of these observations we propose a model of the PBR complex, present at the contact sites of mitochondrial membranes, composed of the 18-kd PBR protein, VDAC, and two inner membrane proteins, ADC and IMC (Fig. 22.2).

PBR Topography in Mitochondrial Membranes

Native MA-10 Leydig cell mitochondrial preparations were examined by transmission electron and atomic force microscopic procedures in order to investigate the topography and organization of PBR. Mitochondria were immunolabeled with an anti-PBR antiserum coupled to gold-labeled secondary antibodies. Results obtained indicate that the 18-kd PBR protein is organized in clusters of four to six molecules (48). On many occasions, the interrelationship among the PBR molecules was found to favor the formation of a single pore. Since the 18-kd PBR protein is functionally associated with the pore forming 34-kd VDAC, which is preferentially located in the contact sites of the two mitochondrial membranes, these results suggest that

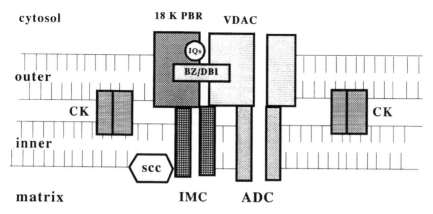

FIGURE 22.2. Components of the mitochondrial contact sites. The 18-kd PBR bears the isoquinoline (IQ) binding site and part of the benzodiazepine (BZ)/DBI binding site. VDAC bears the other part of the BZ/DBI binding site. The inner mitochondrial membrane ADC, shown to be structurally associated with PBR components and IMC, is located in the inner membrane of the contact sites. Creatine kinase (CK) is a structural component of the contact sites. P-450scc (scc) is present in the matrix side of the inner mitochondrial membrane.

the mitochondrial PBR complex may function as a pore. We then examined whether hormone-induced biochemical changes, such as increased PBR binding, correlated with appropriate morphological changes. Treatment with hCG for 15 sec induced the appearance of large clusters varying from 15 to 25 gold particles, or more, in contrast to the four to six particle clusters present in mitochondria from control cells. AFM analysis of these areas further demonstrated the reorganization of the membrane at the mitochondrial membrane sites (49).

The specificity of the effect of hCG was determined by treating cells with hCG and the selective inhibitor of cAMP-dependent protein kinase H-89, shown to block the hormone-induced PBR binding and steroid formation. H-89 also blocked the effect of hCG on PBR topography. In addition, flunitrazepam also blocked the effect of hCG on PBR distribution on mitochondrial membranes (Boujrad, et al., unpublished observations). Thus, it seems that hormones induce the rapid reorganization of mitochondrial membranes favoring the formation of contact sites that may facilitate cholesterol transfer from the outer to the inner mitochondrial membrane. An increase in the formation of contact sites between the mitochondrial membranes has been reported (50). Thus, free cholesterol from the outer mitochondrial membrane would transfer via the contact sites to the inner membrane where the P-450scc is located. It should also be noted that intramitochondrial translocation of phospholipids was recently shown to occur in a similar manner through mitochondrial contact sites (51).

PBR Modeling

Based on the known amino acid sequence of the human 18-kd PBR protein (23) a three-dimensional model of this receptor protein was recently developed using molecular dynamics simulations (52). According to this model the five transmembrane domains of PBR were modeled as five α helices that span one phospholipid bilayer of the outer mitochondrial membrane. This receptor model was then tested as a cholesterol carrier and it was shown that PBR can indeed accommodate a cholesterol molecule and function as a channel. These authors suggested that the receptor's function is to carry cholesterol molecules from the outer lipid monolayer to the inner lipid monolayer of the outer membrane thus acting as a "shield," hiding the cholesterol from the hydrophobic membrane inner medium. Considering the PBR complex formation at the level of the contact sites, this cholesterol movement could end in the inner mitochondrial membrane. This theoretical model further supports our experimental data about the role of PBR in the intramitochondrial cholesterol transport.

Targeted Disruption of the PBR Gene in Steroidogenic Cells

To further investigate the role of PBR in steroidogenesis, we developed a molecular approach based on the disruption of the PBR gene in the constitutive steroid-producing R2C rat Leydig cell line by homologous recombination (Garnier et al., unpublished observations). On the basis of the known rat PBR gene sequence (53), we designed two sets of primers that allowed us to amplify two fragments of the PBR gene from R2C cells genomic DNA by *polymerase chain reaction* (PCR). These PBR genomic DNA fragments were cloned and used to design the targeting construct. The targeting vector was constructed by positioning the *neo* gene, confering the neomycin resistance that allows for a positive selection of cells that have undergone homologous recombination, in between the two PBR genomic DNA fragments and the herpes simplex virus-tyrosine kinase gene, for negative selection against cells that have randomly integrated the targeting construct, at the 3'-end of the second PBR genomic DNA fragment. The targeting vector was then transfected in R2C cells and selection was performed with G418 and ganciclovir (54). Four G418/Ganc-resistant cell lines were generated. PBR expression, examined by ligand binding, was absent in all four cell lines. In addition, the PBR-negative R2C cells produced minimal amounts (10%) of steroids compared to normal R2C cells. However, addition of the hydrosoluble analogue of cholesterol 22R-hydroxycholesterol increased the steroid production by the PBR-negative R2C cells, indicating that the cholesterol transport mechanism was impaired.

The genomic DNA characterization of the PBR-negative R2C cells is under investigation.

Definition of Diazepam-Binding Inhibitor (DBI)

DBI is a 10-kd protein originally purified from the brain by monitoring its ability to displace diazepam from the allosteric modulatory sites for GABA action on $GABA_A$ receptors (55, 56). DBI was also independently purified and characterized for its ability to bind long-chain acyl-*coenzyme A* (CoA)-esters (57) and modulate insulin secretion (58). DBI is found in a variety of tissues and is highly expressed in steroidogenic cells (17, 18, 50–61).

Role of DBI in Steroidogenesis

In search of the cytoplasmic steroidogenesis-stimulating factor(s), a protein of 8.2-kd molecular size was isolated from bovine adrenals shown to stimulate transport of cholesterol into mitochondria and from the outer to the inner membrane (62). This 8.2-kd protein was shown to be identical to DBI, except for the loss of two amino acids (Gly-Ile) from the carboxy terminus (63). We examined the effect of isolated 10-kd DBI on mitochondria from adrenocortical and Leydig cells (60). Dose-response curves indicated that a 3-fold stimulation is obtained with low concentrations (0.1–1 µM) of DBI, whereas higher concentrations have a lower stimulatory effect on pregnenolone formation. The stimulation obtained was similar to those reported for the 8.2-kd des-(Gly-Ile)-DBI on bovine adrenocortical mitochondria (62, 64). Moreover, similar results were obtained using purified rat and bovine testes DBI (18). To exclude the possibility that the stimulatory effect of DBI was due to the α-helical structure of the protein, we used β-endorphin as a control since it also possesses α-helical structures. β-endorphin did not affect mitochondrial steroid synthesis (60).

We then showed that the 17 to 50 amino acid sequence of DBI bears the biological activity since the triacontatetraneuropeptide (TTN) (DBI_{17-50}) specifically stimulated mitochondrial steroidogenesis with a potency and efficacy similar to that of DBI (60). TTN together with other DBI peptide fragments were also found in adrenal and testis extracts and we noted that DBI could be processed in vitro by mitochondria. Binding studies of mitochondria also indicated that TTN binds specifically to PBR (65).

DBI Acts Via PBR

Binding of DBI to PBR was initially determined by examining the ability of DBI to displace high-affinity radiolabeled PBR drug ligands (18, 59, 65). Competition studies for specific binding indicated that DBI displaced radiolabeled benzodiazepines with an inhibitory constant of $1-2\,\mu M$. In subsequent studies we analyzed the binding of DBI to PBR under conditions identical to those used to examine the effects of DBI on mitochondrial steroid synthesis (34). We found that the inhibitory constant of DBI for PBR binding inhibition was 100 nM, a value that correlates well with the *median effective concentration* (EC_{50}) of DBI for mitochondrial steroid synthesis induction. In addition, the stimulatory effect of DBI was specifically blocked by flunitrazepam, the PBR ligand shown to inhibit hormone-stimulated steroidogenesis (60). This finding suggested that DBI stimulates mitochondrial pregnenolone synthesis acting via PBR.

To further demonstrate that DBI specifically binds to PBR, we performed cross-linking studies on Leydig cell mitochondria using metabolically labeled bioactive [^{35}S]DBI (40). Two protein complexes were specifically labeled within R2C Leydig cell mitochondria. The first was a protein complex with an apparent molecular size of 27 kd, recognized by an antiserum against PBR, suggesting that the 10-kd DBI formed a specific complex with the 18-kd PBR protein. A second complex, migrating at 65 kd, with an unidentified 55-kd protein cross-linked to radiolabeled 10-kd DBI was also formed. The characterization and role of this 55-kd protein in the DBI/PBR-mediated activation of mitochondrial steroid synthesis is under investigation.

DBI Levels Are Not Regulated by Hormones

In one of the original reports, it was suggested that the 8.2-kd des-(Gly-Ile)-DBI has a short half-life and its levels are acutely increased by hormones (62). However, the authors did not provide either quantitative data or metabolic labeling studies, which would be required to conclude that hormones have an effect on the rate of synthesis and turnover of DBI. We carefully investigated the effect of *adrenocorticotropic hormone* (ACTH) and LH on the synthesis and turnover of DBI using the hormone-responsive Y-1 and MA-10 steroidogenic cell lines (61). The time course of incorporation of ^{35}S-translabeled into DBI and its turnover rate when the isotope was removed were examined. Data obtained suggested that (i) DBI levels are not regulated by trophic hormones in these steroidogenic cell lines, and (ii) that DBI has a relatively long half-life ($>3\,h$), a finding incompatible with suggestions of a rapid turnover.

In Situ Role of DBI in Steroidogenesis

The findings that (i) hCG increases PBR ligand binding (36), (ii) DBI stimulates mitochondrial steroid formation acting via PBR (40, 60), and (iii) DBI is preferentially localized in the periphery of mitochondria (66) raise the possibility that trophic hormones, by altering PBR, increase PBR inter-action with DBI and that PBR-DBI interaction triggers steroidogenesis. To determine the in situ role of DBI in steroidogenesis, we suppressed cell DBI levels using antisense oligodeoxynucleoties. To overcome the uptake prob-lems usually encountered with oligodeoxynucleotide, we took advantage of the ability of steroidogenic cells to utilize exogenous cholesterol via the lipoprotein endocytotic pathway (67). Thus, we constructed *cholesterol-linked phosphorothioate oligodeoxynucleotides* (CHOL-ODNs) comple-mentary to either the sense or the antisense strand of the 24 nucleotides encoding mouse DBI, 9 bases immediately 5′ to the initiation codon ATG and 12 downstream of the ATG codon (68).

Treating MA-10 cells with CHOL-ODN antisense to DBI resulted in a dose-dependent reduction of DBI levels [*median effective dose* (ED_{50}) = $1\,\mu M$]. In contrast, CHOL-ODN sense to DBI did not affect its expression. Saturating amounts of hCG increased MA-10 progesterone production 150 times. Addition of increasing concentrations of CHOL-ODN sense to DBI or a nonrelated sequence did not reduce the MA-10 response to hCG. In contrast, a 2-fold increase in the amount of steroids produced was observed due to the cholesterol linked to the ODN, liberated in the cells and used as a substrate for steroid synthesis. However, in the presence of CHOL-ODN antisense to DBI and in amounts shown to reduce DBI levels, MA-10 cells lost their ability to respond to hCG ($ED_{50} = 1\,\mu M$). In these studies the hCG-stimulated cAMP levels and P-450scc activity were not affected by the CHOL-ODNs used (68).

Using similar technology we also decreased DBI levels in the R2C Leydig cells (40). DBI-depleted R2C cells did not produce steroids, suggesting that DBI plays a vital role both in the acute stimulation of steroidogenesis by trophic hormones and in constitutive steroid synthesis. Since we showed that DBI is not the long-sought labile factor, and that the site of hormone action is in the mitochondrion, we propose that hormones, by altering PBR, increase its interaction with DBI, which in turn triggers steroidogenesis.

Direct Effects of DBI on P-450scc

As noted above, PBR drug ligands did not have any direct effect on P-450scc activity when examined in mitoplasts (28). However, when prepara-tions of inner mitochondrial membranes were incubated with DBI, a 2-fold stimulation of the production of pregnenolone was observed. Evidence has been already discussed that indicates that the outer mitochondrial mem-brane PBR mediates the effects of PBR ligands and DBI on intact mito-chondria. However, the observation that DBI stimulates pregnenolone production by inner mitochondrial membranes implies that this protein can also act via an additional PBR-independent mechanism. Further evidence indicating that DBI acts directly on P-450scc was provided by observations in an in vitro reconstituted enzyme system (69, 70) where DBI stimulated the production of pregnenolone, suggesting that the non-PBR mechanism involved in steroidogenesis may involve direct activation of P-450scc, or an indirect mechanism that may act via increasing the availability of cholesterol or by altering the rate of reduction of P-450scc.

To identify a mechanism by which DBI may be active in the regulation of P-450scc activity, we examined the distribution of DBI within the mitochondria. Using anti-DBI antibodies we identified the 10-kd DBI in the outer mitochondrial membranes but not in the inner membranes of steroidogenic cells (Brown and Papadopoulos, unpublished observations). However, in inner mitochondrial membrane preparations, we did observe a 30-kd DBI-immunoreactive protein of 6.8 isoelectric point (71). Attempts to solubilize this protein indicated that it is deeply embedded within the inner mitochondrial membrane. Moreover, when cells were treated with hormones for 30 min prior to the preparation of mitochondria, the levels of this 30K-iDBI protein were reduced by 70% (71). In preliminary experiments isolated 30K-iDBI was found to increase the loading of the substrate (cholesterol) into the P-450scc active site (Brown and Papadopoulos, unpublished observations), suggesting that this hormone-induced decrease of the 30K-iDBI may trigger the cholesterol loading mechanism on the P-450scc.

Proposed Model

Considering the data presented in this chapter, we propose that, in response to hormones, the steroidogenic pool of cholesterol moves across the mitochondrial membranes in three steps. First, cholesterol enters the channel formed by the 18-kd PBR protein and transfers from the outer leaflet of the outer mitochondrial membrane to the inner leaflet of the outer membrane. This activity may be directly stimulated by hormones via modulation of the PBR affinity for the endogenous ligand DBI, which is continuously present around the mitochondria (72). Second, hormone-induced changes in PBR affinity will lead to changes in PBR topography and the rapid formation of contact sites between the outer and inner mitochondrial membranes. Thus, cholesterol will be "passively" transported from the outer to the inner membrane. We should also consider the role of DBI, as an acyl-CoA binding protein, on mitochondrial membrane contact site formation (57). DBI was shown to mediate intermembrane transport of long-chain acyl-CoA esters (72) and fatty acylation has been proposed as a mechanism employed in transport processes that require fusion of lipid bilayers (73). Thus, DBI may induce the formation of additional contact sites. In addition, DBI binding to the 18 kd/VDAC complex may also open the VDAC channel, allowing the transport of ions and low molecular weight molecules that may modulate P-450scc activity. Third, fragments from the hormone-sensitive 30K-iDBI protein will be released, within or near the inner mitochondrial membrane, and they will "prime" the P-450scc enzyme to take advantage of the increased availability of steroidogenic substrate and catalyze its conversion to pregnenolone at a greater rate. Thus, the stimulation will be amplified to generate the high amounts of steroids produced. A schematic representation of this model is shown in Figure 22.3.

It should be noted that the model proposed above does not exclude the presence of additional mechanisms involved in the process of acute regulation of steroidogenesis by hormones (74–78). It is possible that the hormone-induced increase in PBR binding and contact site formation triggers and/or represents the first in a series of events that will induce and sustain steroid synthesis for many hours: translocation from the cytoplasm to the mitochondrion, via the contact sites, of the 28-kd protein, shown to parallel steroid synthesis (75, 76), or the steroidogenesis activator polypeptide, *guanosine triphosphate* (GTP), and calcium shown to stimulate mitochondrial pregnenolone formation (74, 77, 78). Identifying and understanding the role of each component of the mitochondrial cholesterol transport apparatus and their interaction should allow us to piece together the puzzle of the steroidogenic pathway responsible for the hormonal acute stimulation of steroidogenesis.

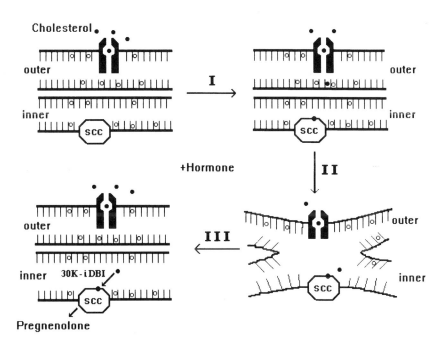

FIGURE 22.3. Hormone-induced movement of the steroidogenic pool of cholesterol across the mitochondrial membranes. For details see text.

Acknowledgment. The preparation of this manuscript was supported by grants from the National Institutes of Health (1RO1-ES07447 and 1KO4-HD01031) to V.P.

References

1. Simpson ER, Waterman MR. Regulation by ACTH of steroid hormone biosynthesis in the adrenal cortex. Can J Biochem Cell Biol 1983;61:692–707.
2. Hall PF. Trophic stimulation of steroidogenesis: in search of the elusive trigger. Recent Prog Horm Res 1985;41:1–39.
3. Kimura T. Transduction of ACTH signal from plasma membrane to mitochondria in adrenocortical steroidogenesis. Effects of peptide, phospholipid, and calcium. J Steroid Biochem 1986;25:711–6.
4. Jefcoate CR, McNamara BC, Artemenko I, Yamazaki T. Regulation of cholesterol movement to mitochondrial cytochrome P450scc in steroid hormone synthesis. J Steroid Biochem Mol Biol 1992;43:751–67.
5. Haefely W, Kulcsar A, Mohler H, Pieri L, Polc P, Schaffner R. Possible involvement of GABA in the central actions of benzodiazepine derivatives. In: Costa E, Greengard P, eds. Advances in biochemical psychopharmacology. New York: Raven Press, 1975;14:131–51.
6. Costa E, Guidotti A. Molecular mechanism in the recptor actions of benzodiazepines. Annu Rev Pharmacol Toxicol 1979;19:531–45.
7. Braestrup C, Squires RF. Specific benzodiazepine receptors in rat brain characterized by high-affinity [³H]diazepam binding. Proc Natl Acad Sci USA 1977;74:3805–9.
8. Verma A, Snyder SH. Peripheral type benzodiazepine receptors. Annu Rev Pharmacol Toxicol 1989;29:307–22.
9. Gavish M, Katz Y, Bar-Ami S, Weizman R. Biochemical, physiological, and pathological aspects of the peripheral benzodiazepine receptor. J Neurochem 1992;58: 1589–601.
10. Papadopoulos V. Peripheral-type benzodiazepine/diazepam binding inhibitor receptor: biological role in steroidogenic cell function. Endocr Rev 1993;14: 222–40.
11. Parola AL, Yamamura HI, Laird HE. Peripheral-type benzodiazepine receptors. Life Sci 1993;52:1329–42.
12. Krueger KE, Papadopoulos V. Cellular role and pharmacological implications of mitochondrial p-sites recognizing diazepam binding inhibitor as a putative endogenous ligand. In: Bartholini G, Garreau M, Morselli PL, Zivkovic B, eds. Imidazopyridines in anxiety disorders: a novel experimental and therapeutic approach. New York: Raven Press, 1993:39–48.
13. Le Fur G, Perrier ML, Vaucher N, Imbault F, Flamier A, Uzan A, et al. Peripheral benzodiazepine binding sites: effects of PK 11195, 1-(2-chlorophenyl)-N-(1-methyl-propyl)-3-isoquinolinecarboxamide. I. In vitro studies. Life Sci 1983;32:1839–47.
14. Anholt RRH, DeSouza EB, Oster-Granite ML, Snyder SH. Peripheral-type benzodiazepine receptors: autoradiograpic localization in whole-body sections of neonatal rats. J Pharmacol Exp Ther 1985;233:517–26.

15. Basile AS, Skolnick P. Subcellular localization of "peripheral-type" binding sites for benzodiazepines in rat brain. J Neurochem 1986;46:305–8.

16. Anholt RRH, Pedersen PL, DeSouza EB, Snyder SH. The peripheral-type benzodiazepine receptor: localization to the mitochondrial outer membrane. J Biol Chem 1986;261:576–83.

17. Oke BO, Suarez-Quian CA, Riond J, Ferrara P, Papadopoulos V. Cell surface localization of the peripheral-type benzodiazepine receptor in adrenal cortex. Mol Cell Endocr 1992;87:R1–R6.

18. Garnier M, Boujrad N, Oke BO, Brown AS, Riond J, Ferrara P, et al. Diazepam binding inhibitor is a paracrine/autocrine regulator of Leydig cell proliferation and steroidogenesis. Action via peripheral-type benzodiazepine receptor and independent mechanisms. Endocrinology 1993;132:444–58.

19. Doble A, Ferris O, Burgevin MC, Menager J, Uzan A, Dubroeucq MC, et al. Photoaffinity labeling of peripheral-type benzodiazepine binding sites. Mol Pharmacol 1987;31:42–9.

20. Antkiewicz-Michaluk L, Mukhin AG, Guidotti A, Krueger KE. Purification and characterization of a protein associated with peripheral-type benzodiazepine binding sites. J Biol Chem 1988;263:17317–21.

21. Riond J, Vita N, Le Fur G, Ferrara P. Characterization of a peripheral-type benzodiazepine binding site in the mitochondria of Chinese hamster ovary cells. FEBS Lett 1989;245:238–44.

22. Sprengel R, Werner P, Seeburg PH, Mukhin AG, Santi MR, Grayson DR, et al. Molecular cloning and expression of cDNA encoding a peripheral-type benzodiazepine receptor. J Biol Chem 1989;264:20415–21.

23. Riond J, Mattei MG, Kaghad M, Dumont X, Guillemot JC, Le Fur G, et al. Molecular cloning and chromosomal localization of a human peripheral-type benzodiazepine receptor. Eur J Biochem 1991;195:305–11.

24. Chang YJ, McCabe RT, Rennert H, Budarf ML, Sayegh R, Emanuel BS, et al. The human "peripheral-type" benzodiazepine receptor: regional mapping of the gene and characterization of the receptor expressed from cDNA. DNA Cell Biol 1992;11:471–80.

25. Parola AL, Stump DG, Pepperl DJ, Krueger KE, Regan JW, Laird HE II. Cloning and expression of a pharmacologically unique bovine peripheral-type benzodiazepine receptor isoquinoline binding protein. J Biol Chem 1991; 266:14082–7.

26. Garnier M, Dimchev AB, Boujrad N, Price MJ, Musto NA, Papadopoulos V. In vitro reconstitution of a functional peripheral-type benzodiazepine receptor from mouse Leydig tumor cells. Mol Pharmacol 1994;45:201–11.

27. Mukhin AG, Papadopoulos V, Costa E, Krueger KE. Mitochondrial benzodiazepine receptors regulate steroid biosynthesis. Proc Natl Acad Sci USA 1989;86:9813–6.

28. Papadopoulos V, Mukhin AG, Costa E, Krueger KE. The peripheral-type benzodiazepine receptor is functionally linked to Leydig cell steroidogenesis. J Biol Chem 1990;265:3772–9.

29. Krueger KE, Papadopoulos V. Peripheral-type benzodiazepine receptors mediate translocation of cholesterol from outer to inner mitochondrial membranes in adrenocortical cells. J Biol Chem 1990;265:15015–22.

30. Thompson I, Fraser R, Kenyon CJ. Regulation of steroidogenesis by benzodiazepines. J Steroid Biochem Molec Biol 1995;53:75–79.

31. Ritta MN, Calandra RS. Testicular interstitial cells as targets for peripheral benzodiazepines. Neuroendocrinology 1989;49:262–6.

32. Barnea ER, Fares F, Gavish M. Modulatory action of benzodiazepines on human term placental steroidogenesis in vitro. Mol Cell Endocrinol 1989;64:155–9.

33. Amsterdam A, Suh BS. An inducible functional peripheral benzodiazepine receptor in mitochondria of steroidogenic granulosa cells. Endocrinology 1991;128:503–10.

34. Papadopoulos V, Guarneri P, Krueger KE, Guidotti A, Costa E. Pregnenolone biosynthesis in C6 glioma cell mitochondria: regulation by a diazepam binding inhibitor mitochondrial receptor. Proc Natl Acad Sci USA 1992;89:5113–7.

35. Papadopoulos V, Nowzari FB, Krueger KE. Hormone-stimulated steroidogenesis is coupled to mitochondrial benzodiazepine receptors. J Biol Chem 1991;266:3682–7.

36. Boujrad N, Gaillard J-L, Garnier M, Papadopoulos V. Acute action of choriogonadotropin in Leydig tumor cells. Induction of a higher affinity benzodiazepine receptor related to steroid biosynthesis. Endocrinology 1994;135:1576–83.

37. Whalin ME, Boujrad N, Papadopoulos V, Krueger KE. Studies on the phosphorylation of the 18 KDa mitochondrial benzodiazepine receptor protein. J Recept Res 1994;14:217–28.

38. Ward JA, Krantz S, Mendeloff J, Haltiwanger E. Interstital cell tumor of the testes: report of two cases. J Clin Endocrinol Metab 1960;22:1622–9.

39. Freeman, DA. Constitutive steroidogenesis in the R2C leydig tumor cell line is maintained by the adenosine 3′:5′-cyclic monophosphate-independent production of a cycloheximide-sensitive factor that enhances mitochondrial pregnenolone biosynthesis. Endocrinology 1987;120:124–32.

40. Garnier M, Boujrad N, Ogwuegbu SO, Hudson JR, Papadopoulos V. The polypeptide diazepam binding inhibitor and a higher affinity peripheral-type benzodiazepine receptor sutain constitutive steroidogenesis in the R2C Leydig tumor cell line. J Biol Chem 1994;269:22105–12.

41. McEnery MW, Snowman AM, Trifiletti RR, Snyder SH. Isolation of the mitochondrial benzodiazepine receptor: association with the voltage-dependent anion channel and the adenine nucleotide carrier. Proc Natl Acad Sci USA 1992;89:3170–4.

42. Farges R, Joseph-Liausun E, Shire D, Caput D, Le Fur G, Loison G, et al. Molecular basis for the different binding poperties of benzodiazepines to human and bovine peripheral-type benzodiazepine receptors. FEBS Lett 1993;335:305–8.

43. Levitt D. Gramicidin, VDAC, porin and perforin channels. Curr Opin Cell Biol 1990;2:689–94.

44. Mannella CA, Forte M, Colombini M. Toward the molecular structure of the mitochondrial channel, VDAC. J Bioenerg Biomembr 1992;24:7–19.

45. Szabo I, Zoratti M. The giant channel of the inner mitochondrial membrane is inhibited by cyclosporin A. J Biol Chem 1991;266:3376–79.

46. Petronilli V, Constantini P, Scorrano L, Colonna R, Passamonti S, Bernardi P. The voltage sensor of the mitochondrial permeability transition pore is tuned by the oxidation-reduction state of vicinal thiols. J Biol Chem 1994;269:16638–42.

47. Kinnally KW, Zorov DB, Antonenko YN, Snyder SH, McEnenery MW,

Tedeshi H. Mitochondrial benzodiazepine receptor linked to inner membrane ion channel by nanomolar actions of ligands. Proc Natl Acad Sci USA 1993;90:1374–78.

48. Papadopoulos V, Boujrad N, Ikonomovic MD, Ferrara P, Vidic B. Topography of the Leydig cell mitochondrial peripheral-type benzodiazepine receptor. Mol Cell Endocrinol 1994;104:R5–R9.

49. Vidic B, Boujrad N, Papadopoulos V. Hormone-induced changes in the topography of the mitochondrial peripheral-type benzodiazepine receptor. Scanning 1995;17:V34–5.

50. Stevens VL, Tribble DL, Lambeth JD. Regulation of mitochondrial compartment volumes in rat adrenal cortex by ether stress. Arch Biochem Biophys 1985;242:324–7.

51. Simbeni R, Pon L, Zinser E, Paltauf F, Daum G. Mitochondrial membrane contact sites of yeast. Characterization of lipid components and possible involvement in intramitochondrial translocation of phospholipids. J Biol Chem 1991;266:10047–9.

52. Bernassau JM, Reversat JL, Ferrara P, Caput D, Lefur G. A 3D model of the peripheral benzodiazepine receptor and its implication in intra mitochondrial cholesterol transport. J Mol Graphics 1993;11:236–45.

53. Casalotti SO, Pelaia G, Yakovlev AG, Csikos T, Grayson DR, Krueger KE. Structure of the rat gene encoding the mitochondrial benzodiazepine receptor. Gene 1992;121:377–82.

54. Sedivy JM, Joyner AL. Gene targeting. New York: WH Freeman, 1992.

55. Guidotti A, Forchetti CM, Corda MG, Konkel D, Bennet CD, Costa E. Isolation, characterization, and purification to homogeneity of an endogenous polypeptide with agonistic action on benzodiazepine receptors. Proc Natl Acad Sci USA 1983;80:3531–3.

56. Shoyab M, Gentry LE, Marquardt H, Todaro G. Isolation and characterization of a putative endogenous benzodiazepinoid (Endozepine) from bovine and human brain. J Biol Chem 1986;261:11968–73.

57. Knudsen J, Hojrup P, Hansen HO, Hansen HF, Roepstorff P. Acyl-CoA-binding protein in the rat. Biochem J 1989;262:513–9.

58. Chen Z, Agerbeth B, Gell K, Andersson M, Mutt V, Ostenson C-G, et al. Isolation and characterization of porcine diazepam binding inhibitor, a polypeptide not only of cerebral occurrence but also common in intestinal tissues and with effects on regulation of insulin release. Eur J Biochem 1988;174:239–45.

59. Bovolin P, Schlichting J, Miyata J, Ferrarese C, Guidotti A, Alho H. Distribution and characterization of diazepam binding inhibitor (DBI) in peripheral tissues of rat. Regul Pept 1990;29:267–81.

60. Papadopoulos V, Berkovich A, Krueger KE, Costa E, Guidotti A. Diazepam binding inhibitor (DBI) and its processing products stimulate mitochondrial steroid biosynthesis via an interaction with mitochondrial benzodiazepine receptors. Endocrinology 1991;129:1481–8.

61. Brown AS, Hall PF, Shoyab M, Papadopoulos V. Endozepine/diazepam binding inhibitor in adrenocortical and Leydig cell lines: absence of hormonal regulation. Mol Cell Endocrinol 1992;83:1–9.

62. Yanagibashi K, Ohno Y, Kawamura M, Hall PF. The regulation of intracellular transport of cholesterol in bovine adrenal cells: purification of a novel protein. Endocrinology 1988;123:2075–82.

63. Besman MJ, Yanagibashi K, Lee TD, Kawamura M, Hall PF, Shively JE. Identification of des-(Gly-Ile)-endozepine as an effector of corticotropin-dependent adrenal steroidogenesis: stimulation of cholesterol delivery is mediated by the peripheral benzodiazepine receptor. Proc Natl Acad Sci USA 1989;86:4897–901.

64. Yanagibashi K, Ohno Y, Nakamichi N, Matsui T, Hayashida K, Takamura M, et al. Peripheral-type benzodiazepine receptors are involved in the regulation of cholesterol side chain cleavage in adrenocortical mitochondria. J Biochem 1989;106:1026–9.

65. Guidotti A, Berkovich A, Mukhin A, Costa E. Diazepam binding inhibitor: response to Knudsen and Nielsen. Biochem J 1990;265:928–9.

66. Rasmussen JT, Faergeman NJ, Kristiansen K, Knudsen J. Acyl-CoA-binding protein can mediate intermembrane acyl-CoA transport and donate acyl-CoA for β-oxidation and glycerolipid synthesis. Biochem J 1994;299:165–70.

67. Brown MS, Kovanen PT, Goldstein JL. Receptor-mediated uptake of lipoprotein-cholesterol and its utilization for steroid biosynthesis in the adrenal cortex. Recent Prog Horm Res 1979;35:215–57.

68. Boujrad N, Hudson JR, Papadopoulos V. Inhibition of hormone-stimulated steroidogenesis in cultured Leydig tumor cells by a cholesterol-linked phosphorothioate oligodeoxynucleotide antisense to diazepam binding inhibitor. Proc Natl Acad Sci USA 1993;90:5728–31.

69. Brown AS, Hall PF. Stimulation by endozepine of the side-shain cleavage of cholesterol in a reconstituted enzyme system. Biochem Biophys Res Commun 1991; 180:609–14.

70. Boujrad N, Hudson JR, Papadopoulos V. Mediation of the hormonal stimulation of steroidogenesis by the polypeptide diazepam binding inhibitor. In: Bartke A, ed. Function of somatic cells of the testis. New York: Springer-Verlag, 1994;186–94.

71. Brown AS, Leydman M, Papadopoulos V. Identification of an ACTH-dependent, diazepam binding inhibitor related, 30 Kd protein in bovine adrenocortical inner mitochondrial membranes. Abstracts of IX International Congress on Hormonal Steroids 1994:A176.

72. Schultz R, Pelto-Huikko M, Alho H. Expression of diazepam binding inhibitor-like immunoreactivity in rat testis is dependent on pituitary hormones. Endocrinology 1992;130:3200–6.

73. Pfanner N, Glick BS, Arden SR, Rothman JE. Fatty acylation promotes fusion of transport vesicles with Golgi cisternae. J Cell Biol 1990;110:955–61.

74. Pedersen RC, Brownie AC. Steroidogenesis activator polypeptide isolated from a rat Leydig cell tumor. Science 1987;236:188–90.

75. Pon LA, Orme-Johnson NR. Acute stimulation of steroidogenesis in corpus luteum and adrenal cortex by peptide hormones. J Biol Chem 1986;261:6594–9.

76. Clark BJ, Wells J, King SR, Stocco DM. The purification, cloning, and expression of a novel luteinizing hormone-induced mitochondrial protein in MA-10 mouse Leydig tumor cells. J Biol Chem 1994;269:28314–22.

77. Xu X, Xu T, Robertson DG, Lambeth DJ. GTP stimulates pregnenolone generation in isolated rat adrenal mitcohcondria. J Biol Chem 1989;264:17674–80.

78. Kowluru R, Yamazaki T, McNamara BC, Jefcoate CR. Metabolism of exogenous cholesterol by rat adrenal mitochondria is stimulated by physiological levels of free calcium and by GTP. Mol Cell Endocrinol 1995;107:181–8.

Author Index

357

Subject Index

ISBN 0-387-94648-9

EAN

9 780387 946481 >